Sociology

AS APPLIED TO

MEDICINE

Edited by Graham Scambler BSc PhD

Director,
Unit of Sociology,
Department of Psychiatry and Behavioural Sciences,
University College London,
London, UK

4th Edition

W. B. SAUNDERS COMPANY LTD

Edinburgh   London   New York   Philadelphia   St Louis   Sydney   Toronto

W. B. SAUNDERS
An imprint of Harcourt Publishers Limited

© W. B. Saunders Company Limited 1997
© Harcourt Publishers 1999

 is a registered trademark of Harcourt Publishers Limited

First edition published 1982
This edition published 1997
  Reprinted 1999

ISBN 0 7020 2275 6

British Library Cataloguing in Publication Data
A catalogue record for this book is available from the British Library.

Library of Congress Cataloging in Publication Data
A catalog record for this book is available from the Library of Congress.

Printed in China
GCC/02

CONTENTS

David Blane, MB, BS, MSc Senior Lecturer in Medical Sociology, Department of Psychiatry, Charing Cross and Westminster Medical School, 22–24 St Dunstan's Road, London, W6 8RP, UK

Ray M. Fitzpatrick, BA, MSc, PhD Fellow, Nuffield College, and Professor of Public Health and Primary Care, University of Oxford, Nuffield College, Oxford OX1 1NF, UK

Paul Higgs, BSc, PhD Lecturer in Medical Sociology, Unit of Medical Sociology, Department of Psychiatry and Behavioural Sciences, University College London Medical School, University College London, Wolfson Building, Riding House Street, London W1N 8AA, UK

Sheila Hillier, BSc, MSc (Econ), PhD Professor of Medical Sociology, St Bartholomews and Royal London School of Medicine and Dentistry, Department of Human Sciences & Medical Ethics, Turner Street, London E1 2AD, UK

David Locker, BDS, PhD Professor, Department of Community Dentistry, Faculty of Dentistry, University of Toronto, 124 Edward Street, Toronto, Ontario, M5G 1G6, Canada

Nicholas Mays, MA Director of Health Services Research, King's Fund Policy Institute, London W1M 0AN. Honorary Senior Lecturer, Department of Public Health and Policy, London School of Hygiene and Tropical Medicine, University of London, UK

Myfanwy Morgan, BA, MA, PhD Reader in Sociology of Health, United Medical and Dental Schools of Guy's and St Thomas' Hospitals, St Thomas' Campus, London, SE1 7EH, UK

Graham Scambler, BSc, PhD Senior Lecturer in Sociology and Director, Unit of Medical Sociology, Department of Psychiatry and Behavioural Sciences, University College London Medical School, University College London, Wolfson Building, Riding House Street, London, W1N 8AA, UK

Students of medicine and of other related disciplines may be forgiven for feeling that their schools and colleges insist that they learn more and more about an increasing number of aspects of the human condition in health and illness. There was a halcyon time, not so long ago, when the pre-clinical curriculum consisted of one course in human anatomy and another in physiology; the clinical phase involved merely learning the skills needed to recognize the signs and symptoms of a wide but ultimately limited range of diseases. Moreover, there was little institutional pressure on students to study since they were free to repeat examinations until they passed them.

The picture is very different today. Knowledge of the molecular structure of living beings and the factors which determine natural and pathological growth and decay has expanded exponentially in the last fifty years and continues to do so. Students are expected to know a good deal about the theories and research methods of the scientific disciplines, the 'ologies', which have led to this increased knowledge, as well as about the implications of their findings for medical practice. More and more disciplines claiming relevance to medical knowledge and practice jostle each other for a place in the pre-clinical curriculum; new clinical specialities want medical students to be exposed at some time during their clinical studies to what they have to offer. All make claims to the indispensable nature of their own contribution to the curriculum. Meanwhile, medical students are no longer free to work at their own pace. Examinations weed out those who cannot satisfy their teachers after a maximum of two failures. The pressures are those of the institution. Students of other health professions, such as nursing, dentistry, pharmacy and optometry, are exposed to broadly comparable pressures in the process of qualifying as practitioners.

Sociology is one of the disciplines which has recently claimed the attention of the medical and other related health professions and their students. Its formal introduction into the curriculum as a basic medical science, which by the 1980s had taken place in most of the medical schools of the United Kingdom, was a radical innovation. Compared with most of the other new subjects it involves a break away from the traditional preparation for medicine based exclusively on the detailed study of parts of the biological organism which we call the human body. Its focus is not on the human individual *per se*: it is on the two-way relationships between the individual and society. Sociology as applied to medicine is concerned specifically with those aspects of the relationship which influence the experiences of health and illness in individuals and the response to them of others − relatives, doctors, nurses, administrators and governments.

Not surprisingly, not all those already involved in medical education welcomed the advent of sociological teaching. Some of the staff involved in teaching the traditional laboratory based or clinical subjects saw in it an intrusion of a largely unknown and untested quantity competing for the students' limited span of attention time. They were unfamiliar with its methods or potential and sceptical about its contribution to the making of a good practitioner. Some students, expecting the medical curriculum to resemble in essence the pre-medical natural science courses they had taken prior to entry, also needed to be persuaded that sociology was relevant to their preparation as future doctors, especially when they felt themselves to be under pressure to absorb all that the teachers of subjects which were more thoroughly examined put before them.

Such early doubts have not entirely disappeared, but they have substantially diminished. Indeed, the General Medical Council's recommendations for medical education in the 1980s are even more insistent than earlier recommendations on the necessity for broadening the students' basic understanding of the social context of health and illness and of the social determinants of medical practice and health service provision. This then is the major task and challenge for those responsible for the teaching of sociology as applied to medicine, and the contributors to this book are to be congratulated for providing a concise introduction to the subject.

In this book, which will form an admirable basic text upon which teachers and students can build, the contributors have shown how some of the theories, concepts and methods developed by sociologists can illuminate aspects of human experience in health and illness. They look at how such socially determined factors as marital status, social class and family composition influence the pattern of morbidity and mortality. They show that medical perceptions of what constitutes mental or physical illness are not necessarily shared by the populations served and that the absence of shared perceptions may frustrate much medical effort. They look at the variety of ways in which old age, death and ethnicity are regarded and treated and the dilemmas which such variety can pose for practitioners. They explore the social origins of contemporary systems of health care in order to obtain greater understanding of their present problems. They examine too the various interpretations which can be placed upon the collective and individual behaviour of members of the medical profession, and on the expansion of medical concern and metaphors into many aspects of social life. This list does not exhaust their concerns and there are many other developments in the sociology of health and illness which cannot be covered in a volume of this size.

It seems to me impossible to argue that acquaintance with such findings and with the methods and conceptual frames of the discipline on which they are based is not an essential ingredient in the preparation of the doctor for medical practice whether it be in general practice, an age-band or body-system speciality, or community medicine. He or she needs it at the very least for protection against the very real hazard of frustration and unhappiness when it proves difficult to implement medical measures; but above all it is needed if the medical and other health-related professions are to make their greatest potential contribution to the welfare of the populations they are privileged to serve.

Margot Jefferys

August 1981

When the first edition of this textbook was published in 1982, sociology had only recently established itself on the curricula of medical, nursing and other schools and colleges preparing students for work in the health service. By the time the second edition was produced in 1986, not only had its contribution to education and training been consolidated, but it had also been associated with a rapidly expanding body of research in the health field, some of which was incorporated into the revised text. The pace of acquisition of new knowledge continued, and the third edition in 1991 was reorganized to allow for this, with new chapters on chronic conditions, community care and the organization and funding of health care.

For this fourth edition we have retained the format of the third, but have substantially updated and revised each chapter. In addition, we have been joined by Paul Higgs, who brings a fresh perspective to the chapters on the health and circumstances of older people, and on the limitations of medical knowledge. Once again we are indebted to our students and colleagues for comments on previous editions and for their continuing feedback.

We are conscious too of our debts to Donald Patrick who, as senior co-editor of the first and second editions, was instrumental in getting the venture off the ground, and to Margot Jefferys for her support both then and since and for her considerable contribution to the establishment of our discipline in the education programmes of medical and other students of the health professions.

Graham Scambler

SOCIAL ASPECTS OF DISEASE

Society and Changing Patterns of Disease

RAY M. FITZPATRICK

One of the most important recent developments in ideas about health care and illness has been the widespread recognition that social and economic conditions have a major effect on patterns of disease and death rates. A wide range of sources – historical, medical and sociological – have provided the evidence for such influences. This chapter considers how lines of influence from society and the economy can be traced to patterns of disease.

The starting point of this analysis is the dramatic variation to be found in death rates both in the past and at present. For example, the death rate per annum has virtually halved in England and Wales over the last 150 years: in 1851 it was 22.7 per 1000 population and by 1990 it had fallen to 11.9. Another way to express the difference over this period is in terms of the average number of years an individual could expect to live at birth, i.e. life expectancy. In 1840 a man and woman could, on average, expect to live to 40 and 43 years, respectively, whereas by 1990 life expectancy had risen to 72 and 77 years, respectively. Such differences in overall mortality rates, however, disguise a more complex picture if we look at particular age groups. The higher death rates of the mid-nineteenth century were much more severe in particular age groups, especially in infancy and childhood. Thus, future life expectancy for those who have reached the age of 45 years has improved slightly over the last 100 years, but not nearly as dramatically as has the life expectancy of a child at birth.

The higher death rates and lower life expectancies are not of course simply an historical phenomenon. At present, many third world countries have crude death rates much higher than those of England; for example, Ethiopia 23.6 per 1000 and Sierra Leone 23.4 per 1000. Third world countries with higher death rates resemble nineteenth-century England and Wales in that infant and child mortality are one of the main reasons for lower life expectancy.

VARIATION IN DISEASE PATTERNS IN HUMAN SOCIETY

The diseases encountered by humans have not remained the same over time. The history of humans might be viewed as a progressive victory over disease, but this is an over-simplification. Although some diseases are less important than in the past, others have become more important. Complex social and biological processes have altered the balance between humans and disease. A number of authorities (Powles 1973; McKeown 1979) now agree on three characteristic disease patterns in historical sequence.

Preagricultural disease patterns

Before about 10 000 BC, indeed for most of the evolution of humans as a distinct species, humans lived as hunter–gatherers, that is without any form of settled agriculture for subsistence. Although conclusions based on such early evidence are somewhat speculative, anthropologists and epidemiologists have argued that the infectious diseases which were later to become major causes of illness and death were relatively uncommon at this stage of social evolution. Furthermore, diseases which are sometimes described as diseases of civilization, such as heart disease and cancer, were less common than at the present time (Powles 1973). It is likely that mortality in adults arose from environmental and safety hazards, for example hunting accidents and exposure.

Diseases in agricultural society

Knowledge of the diseases which plagued agricultural societies is more certain. These were predominantly the infectious diseases, which for purposes of discussion can be divided into the following:

1. air-borne diseases, such as tuberculosis;
2. water-borne diseases, such as cholera;
3. food-borne diseases, such as dysentry;
4. vector-borne (i.e. carried by rats or mosquitoes) diseases, such as plague and malaria.

In England and Wales, and in Europe generally, the plague was a particularly important cause of death and at its most virulent, in the Black Death of 1348, it killed one-quarter of the English population. It last occurred on any large scale in England and Wales in 1665 and disappeared from Europe shortly after. The plague was spread by the fleas carried by black rats. Its disappearance was due to the replacement of the black rat by the brown rat which was much less prone to infest human habitations.

Malaria was never as great a health problem in England and Wales as it has been in the tropics where conditions are ideal for the natural life cycle of both vector and parasite. By the mid-nineteenth century, when reliable vital statistics were available in England and Wales and the country's economy was changing from agricultural to industrial, the major causes of death were tuberculosis, bronchitis, pneumonia, influenza and cholera.

The modern industrial era of disease

By the mid-twentieth century, infectious diseases had become relatively unimportant causes of death in England and Wales and in the western world in general, although some infectious diseases such as influenza remained common causes of death, particularly in the elderly. The infectious diseases have been replaced as major causes of death by the so-called degenerative diseases, cancer and cardiovascular disease.

Because of these changes in patterns of death the major medical problems of today are such chronic illnesses as atherosclerosis, diabetes and osteoarthritis. These are all problems involving multiple risk factors, rather than a single cause. Their onset is quite early in life; they tend to be progressive; and they appear in all modern societies. Fries (1983) argues that there appear to be quite definite limits to the extension of the human lifespan, so that life expectancy at age 100 years has barely changed in the last 80 years. However, if one looks at such indices as age at first heart attack or age-specific lung cancer rates in the USA, there have been quite definite improvements in recent years. Fries concludes that health policy should make the compression of morbidity a major objective. Combining medical and social approaches to reducing the risk factors for chronic illnesses such as atherosclerosis would result in a life in which serious illness and decline in functioning were increasingly confined to later ages and the years of vigorous life extended.

This dramatic increase in importance of the chronic degenerative diseases is characteristic of almost all countries that have undergone industrialization, although the exceptions and the variations in rates from one country to another provide important and intriguing problems for the medical and social scientist. Japan, for example, has a much lower incidence of heart disease than comparable industrialized societies. On the other hand, the level of stomach cancer is considerably higher in Japan compared with, for example, the USA.

Explaining changes in disease prevalence

It would be all too easy to regard changes in disease patterns as the inevitable consequences of medical and technical progress without further explanation. Close examination of the major influences on disease patterns, however, uncovers a complex picture which is increasingly recognized as important for the understanding of disease in the contemporary world. The study of how disease patterns have changed indicates the pervasive influence of social and economic factors on disease prevalence.

Three main factors seem important in the changes in disease patterns that followed the transition from nomadic hunting and gathering to agricultural life. First, the development of cereals such as wheat allowed agricultural societies to feed more mouths and hence support higher population densities. Evidence from epidemiological studies, however, shows that many infectious organisms thrive when human populations grow above certain densities. Second, agricultural work necessitated permanent settlement, whereas hunter–gatherers periodically moved settlement in search of fresh food sources. However, in the absence of sanitation and awareness of its importance, permanent settlement often led to the contamination of water supplies by waste products, which increased the risks of infection from a number of organisms. Third, the development of cereals as the major source of food, whilst supporting greater numbers of people, paradoxically narrowed the range and quality of diet, a factor which crucially reduced resistance to infection.

More careful examination is needed to explain the remarkable changes in death rates and the decline in significance of mortality from infectious disease that occurred with the transition from agricultural to industrial economies. The nineteenth and twentieth centuries' victory over death and diseases still represents the most dramatic improvement in health in the history of human kind. Death rates for the various infectious diseases did not decline simultaneously. Tuberculosis, the most common cause of death in the nineteenth century, began to decline in the first half of that century, as indicated in Fig. 1.1.

There are a limited number of possible explanations for such a marked decline in mortality from an infectious organism. Box 1.1 shows the competing explanations that have been offered, not only for the decline of tuberculosis but for the wide range of infectious diseases for which mortality rates dramatically declined in the course of the nineteenth century in Britain and other parts of western Europe. It is possible that a change occurred in the virulence of the organism itself or that the genetic immunity of the population improved. Both these possibilities are generally discounted. There is no theoretical reason why the organisms responsible for tuberculosis and a number of other infectious diseases should fortuitously change in their virulence at approximately the same period. It is very unlikely that genetic immunity could improve in such a short time since the selection processes implied would require dramatic increases in mortality rates across a range of diseases. For these reasons, the first and third explanations in Box 1.1 are normally rejected as unlikely. The most convincing explanation for the decline in mortality from tuberculosis and, later in the century, from air-borne diseases such as pneumonia, is that of greater acquired resistance. An increased resistance to infection resulted from improvement in nutritional intake as agricultural techniques improved and transportation of produce became

Fig. 1.1 *Pulmonary tuberculosis: annual death rates for England and Wales, 1838–1970. (Reproduced with permission from McKeown, 1979.)*

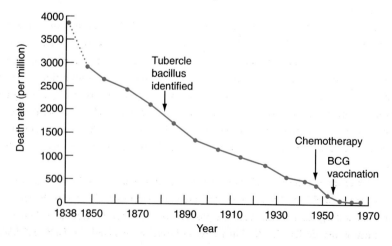

BOX 1.1

POSSIBLE EXPLANATIONS FOR THE DECLINE OF MORTALITY FROM
INFECTIOUS DISEASE IN BRITAIN IN THE NINETEENTH CENTURY

- Decline in virulence of organisms: organisms responsible for diseases, e.g. tuberculosis, bronchitis, became less lethal due to changes in biological properties.

- Reduction in exposure of humans to infectious organisms: for example, through changes in domestic housing and urban planning or through reduced contamination of food and water supplies.

- Genetically induced increase in resistance of humans to infection: human genes associated with resistance to infection may be favoured by Darwinian selection processes and thus individual and population resistance increased over time.

- Acquired resistance of humans to infection: general fitness brought about by improved nutrition resulted in greater resistance in terms of probability of (a) being infected and/or (b) recovering from infection.

- Specific medical interventions: rates of recovery from infectious diseases were improved by developments in medical treatment and therefore mortality rates were reduced.

---

faster and more efficient. Much of the nineteenth century also saw unprecedented increases in real wages and standard of living in Britain. It is also possible to argue for the significance of nutrition with contemporary evidence. In many third world countries today, diseases such as measles or tuberculosis have a much higher fatality, especially among the very young in populations whose resistance is reduced by malnutrition. McKeown cites the conclusion of the World Health Organization report that one-half to three-quarters of all statistically recorded deaths of infants and young children are attributed to a combination of malnutrition and infection (McKeown 1979).

However, the role of the second possible explanation in Box 1.1 – reduced exposure to infectious organisms – is also of importance. The incidence of illness and mortality from water-borne diseases such as cholera declined somewhat later in the nineteenth century, largely as the result of concerted efforts by the public health movement to prevent the contamination of drinking water supplies by sewage; gastroenteric infectious diseases came under control by the beginning of the twentieth century, resulting in a dramatic impact on infant mortality. The sterilization and more hygienic transportation of milk in particular, and improved food hygiene in general, constitute another form of environmental change that produced the decline in infectious disease mortality.

Thus, most of the decline in death rates achieved in this country and in the western world generally by the Second World War can be attributed to environmental factors such as improvements in food and hygiene, which were the products of economic development. Other social changes, such as the decline in the birth rate, reduced the demand for food and housing resources. Improved housing and better personal hygiene also played their role in reducing mortality rates.

Historians still dispute the precise nature of the changes that brought about the decline in mortality rates just described. The nature of that debate can, with some simplification, be termed one between the 'public health' form of explanation and the 'invisible hand' version of events (Box 1.2). The debate is of more than purely historical interest because it mirrors and has implications for current debates. Even now, some would argue that improvements in the economy and wealth are the most effective ways of producing improvements in the health of modern populations ('the invisible hand' (Guha, 1994)). Others would argue that more direct and political intervention is required by a modern public health movement to address the ills described later in this chapter (Szreter, 1988). Box 1.2 shows how difficult it is to disentangle claims even with historical hindsight!

BOX 1.2

THE DEBATE BETWEEN 'PUBLIC HEALTH' AND 'THE INVISIBLE HAND' TO EXPLAIN IMPROVED LIFE EXPECTANCY IN NINETEENTH CENTURY BRITAIN

The 'public health' explanation emphasizes deliberate government interventions

- The public health movement improved water supplies, housing standards, regulation of food sold to public

- Increased income of working classes sometimes coincided with deteriorating death rates because of migration into more unhygienic industrial towns

The 'invisible hand' explanation emphasizes benefits of rising incomes

- Some areas of London enjoyed improved death rates in the nineteenth century before reforms to water supplies

- Studies of claims to insurance societies show that while working class sickness rates due to infectious disease were stable, deaths from the same causes declined

- In some nineteenth century towns such as Mansfield, deaths from infectious disease remained high despite excellent water supplies

- The greatest benefit of improved diet is upon capacity of infants and children to survive infectious disease

---

THE HISTORICAL ROLE OF MEDICINE

To this point nothing has been said about the role that medical intervention (the last possible explanation listed in Box 1.1) has played in the relationship between man and disease. At first glance, this might seem an important omission, given that medical knowledge was accumulating throughout the period and that hospitals had grown in number since the latter part of the eighteenth century. The evidence that McKeown and others have gathered, however, suggests that very little of the decline in mortality rates can be attributed to improvements in medical care. They list a range of evidence against the role of specific medical interventions having a substantial effect on mortality.

- Hospitals and surgical procedures were actually harmful. When Florence Nightingale began to reform the hygienic conditions in hospitals, it was widely thought that hospitals constituted a risk to health; in other words, one stood a high risk of crossinfection, contracting a disease from other patients, since wards were unsegregated as well as unhygienic. Similarly, in spite of the advances in surgery made possible by the development of anaesthetics, there is little evidence that surgical procedures made any impact on life expectancy in the nineteenth century (McKeown and Brown 1969).

- Drugs were largely ineffective. Before the twentieth century a large armoury of medicines appears to have been available to the Victorian doctor. However, only a few, such as digitalis, mercury and cinchona, used in the treatment of heart disease, syphilis and malaria, respectively, would be recognized by modern standards as having specific efficacy and, in any case, dosages were unlikely to have been appropriate.

The first drugs which can be shown to have influenced mortality rates did not appear until the end of the 1930s. The antibiotics used in the treatment of a wide range of bacterial infections were developed in the 1930s and 1940s. Prophylactic immunization against such diseases as whooping cough and polio date from the 1950s. In the case of these medical breakthroughs, however, it is easy to overstate the contribution that they made to mortality rates. The decline in mortality for most infectious diseases took place before the introduction of antibiotics. For tuberculosis the period of decline can be seen in Fig. 1.1, and the mortality rates for bronchitis, pneumonia and influenza are shown in Fig. 1.2. Moreover, it is difficult to distinguish between

Fig. 1.2 Bronchitis, pneumonia and influenza: death rates for England and Wales, 1848–1971. (Reproduced with permission from McKeown, 1979.)

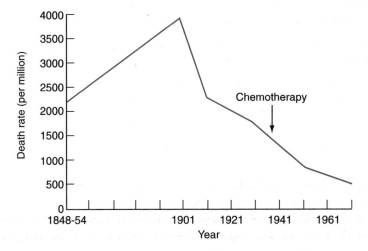

the improvements in disease mortality that can be attributed to the introduction of treatment or immunization and those due to the continuing influence of improving social and economic conditions. Most likely, the immunization programmes for diphtheria and polio brought about the greatest improvement which can be attributed to specific medical intervention.

DISEASE RATES AND SOCIAL FACTORS IN MODERN SOCIETY

The association between diseases and social and economic circumstances is not a purely historical phenomenon. In many parts of the third world life expectancy at birth is much lower than in Europe or North America. Many aspects of the environment in the third world provide much more favourable conditions for the spread of infectious diseases than those that prevailed in historical Europe. For example, tropical ecology is particularly favourable for such vectors of disease as the mosquito (malaria) and tsetse fly (sleeping sickness). Nevertheless it is the extremely low standard of living above all else that produces high mortality rates in countries such as Bangladesh and Ethiopia.

In countries like Britain, the social and environmental factors that are responsible for many kinds of commonly occurring disease are somewhat different and may require different explanation. The association between standard of living and the risk of disease, however, is still apparent in the social-class differences in illness and mortality rates discussed in Chapter 8. It is evident that environmental factors, whether in the home or at work, continue to play an important role in influencing the risks of illness and mortality.

The report of the Research Working Group on Inequalities in Health (DHSS 1981) makes clear in many of its recommendations which aspects of the social and economic environment it considers responsible for inequalities in health in Britain. Its proposed strategy largely targets poverty and low income.

- Benefits such as the maternity grant and child benefits need to be increased in order to reduce child poverty.
- Major programmes are needed in housing improvement, the prevention of accidents to children and the provision of school meals.
- More action is needed to prevent accidents in the work place, largely in manual occupations.

These recommendations are a clear reminder that, for large sections of society, health is harmed by material deprivation in terms of income, diet and housing, rather than because of the 'diseases of affluence'.

Although environmental conditions associated with poverty increase the risk of disease, many kinds of disease are now associated with behaviour which may have little or nothing to do with poverty. Increasingly, the mass media are focusing attention on the role that over-eating or inappropriate diet, smoking and excessive alcohol consumption have in a wide variety of disorders such as heart disease, diabetes, lung cancer and cirrhosis of the liver.

The association between smoking and lung cancer has been established beyond all reasonable doubt. It is important to recognize, however, that contemporary health risks associated with behaviour are just as certainly a function of current social conditions as were the infectious health risks associated with the social conditions of the nineteenth century. This is an essential point to grasp, since it is all too easy to view behaviour such as smoking simply as reflecting an individual's decisions and preferences. To focus on an individual smoker would not only lead to erroneous and oversimplified explanations of the causes of his or her behaviour, but more importantly it might lead to misguided or naive attempts to change that behaviour (Box 1.3).

The example of smoking illustrates that disease is as much a reflection of the economy today as it has been in the past. Diet is another example. It has been estimated (Lock and Smith 1976) that 56% of women and 52% of men in Britain over the age of 40 years are at least 15% overweight. The mortality risks of men who are 10% overweight are one-fifth higher than average, especially in mortality associated with diabetes and vascular disease. Clearly, over-eating may be a major health risk. Burkitt (1973) and others have argued that inappropriate diet is also a problem. He argues that diverticular disease, cancer of the bowel, diabetes and indeed various venous diseases such as varicose veins and deep vein thrombosis may all be linked to lack of fibre. Populations which have diets with high fibre content seem relatively free of many such diseases. In Britain the daily fibre intake from bread has been reduced to about one-tenth of its level in 1850, whereas we have almost doubled our consumption of sugar and other refined carbohydrates. Again the statistics of change do not reveal the causal links. Changes in diet have reflected

---

BOX 1.3

SMOKING: A PRODUCT OF THE ECONOMY AS MUCH AS OF INDIVIDUAL BEHAVIOUR?

Who smokes is socially patterned

- 17% of men and 15% of women in social class I are smokers (see Chapter 8 for the definition of the five social classes).

- 49% of men and 36% of women in social class V are smokers.

- Attitudes and behaviour are influenced by:
  Advertising and marketing strategies
  Governmental health warnings
  Taxation

- Effective health policies require evidence of social factors, e.g. there is no point in increasing spending on health education to alter the behaviour of groups who do not respond to such influences.

Economic significance of cigarettes

- An analysis of smoking should include political, economic and health issues.

- An increase in taxation would make cigarettes cost-prohibitive to some, but this would result in a decline in revenue.

- A reduction in smoking would lead to a decrease in National Health Service costs but an increase in pensions as greater numbers would live to old age.

- A reduction in the tobacco industry would reduce the amount of sickness absence but lead to unemployment in areas dependent on the industry.

changes in the food-producing industries which are now concentrated in a small number of multinational companies more concerned with producing standardized and well-accepted, easily transported commodities: nutritional values have taken second place to the expansion of profits.

Another essentially modern form of health hazard may be identified in the 6000 deaths and 80 000 serious injuries that occur annually as a result of road traffic accidents. Doll (1983) makes the point that the rate per million of deaths on the roads is actually lower now than it was in the 1930s and is in this sense a testament to the beneficial effects of legislation with regard to prevention. Nevertheless, some 2000 hospital beds are occupied each day by the victims of road traffic accidents (Butler and Vaile 1984) which represents a considerable demand on health-care resources. Risks of accidents are 18 times higher to motorcyclists than to car drivers, and much more still could be achieved to prevent accidents to this group by, for example, legislation on training and testing riding ability.

It may seem that an analysis of the relationship of social and economic factors to health is unhelpful because it points to features of our economic system that are central, firmly established and difficult to change. If this is the case, then another parallel is suggested with the nineteenth-century problems of environmental disease. The changes in sanitation, urban planning and building that were required to transform the pattern of infectious diseases in Victorian times were similarly regarded as unrealistic and resisted for long periods by politicians and business interests; but the reforms were slowly adopted and growing awareness of the relationship between commercially promoted behaviours such as smoking and unhealthy eating in our own time should help to speed the process of securing reforms.

A multidisciplinary committee has produced a major report to assess the effectiveness of existing public health policies and to stimulate new national strategies (Smith and Jacobson 1988). Six areas of current life-styles that influence health were identified, for which research evidence of harmful effects is strong and support for the feasibility of action is clear cut:

- tobacco
- diet
- physical activity
- alcohol
- sexuality
- road safety.

Similarly, five areas of preventive services were identified where evidence is very strong that public health interventions could now produce dramatic improvements:

- maternity services
- dental health
- immunization
- early cancer detection (breast and cervix)
- high-blood-pressure detection.

The approach in each of these 11 priority areas is to identify precise quantitative targets and make specific recommendations to public bodies and institutions. Thus one of a number of specific nutritional targets is to increase the total dietary fibre intake from 20 g per person per day to 30 g. The list of agencies to whom nutritional targets and specific actions are recommended includes the food industry, local authorities, health authorities and government. Their view is that agencies need specific targets to stimulate action and to provide a ready means of monitoring results.

THE ECONOMY AND HEALTH POLICY IN MODERN SOCIETY

Some of the most recent research on the relationship between the economy and health suggests that, even in modern societies, economic factors play the predominant role in determining patterns of illness, and that the role of health services is negligible by comparison. Four different views of how the economy generally, and patterns of employment and income in particular, may affect health are evaluated here (Box 1.4).

BOX 1.4

ALTERNATIVE MODELS OF THE ECONOMY AND HEALTH

- Unemployment is major cause of ill-health

- Rapid economic growth is a major cause of ill-health

- Particular forms of employment are causes of ill-health
  'job-strain' model
  'effort–reward imbalance' model

- Income distribution is a major cause of ill-health

Unemployment and health

Brenner (1977) has argued that most of the variation in annual overall mortality rates for the USA can be statistically explained in terms of changes in the annual level of employment, provided that a time lag of 5 years is allowed for unemployment to have its effect on health. This impact is produced in two ways: first, unemployment reduces family income and, therefore, material standard of living; second, the individual loses a sense of meaning and purpose found at work and experiences increased fears about the future and tension at home. This results in greater vulnerability to ill health. From USA data, Brenner concluded that a 1% increase in unemployment, if sustained for 5 years, was statistically responsible for nearly 37 000 extra deaths. Similar results have been found from analyses of data collected in England and Wales and Sweden (Brenner 1979).

Rapid economic growth and health

This work has been challenged by Eyer (1977), who argues that the influence on health of experience such as unemployment generally occurs within a much shorter time than the 5-year lag that Brenner allows. If this is the case, the association between unemployment and mortality is considerably reduced. Instead, Eyer argues that death rates increase at the time of business booms when employment rates are high. The association between employment and mortality he explains in terms of four connected social factors that attend business cycles.

1. Economic booms increase workers' migration, which weakens social networks that normally protect individuals against disease.
2. 'Stress' through overwork in times of business peaks increases ill health.
3. The unhealthy consumption of alcohol and tobacco increases.
4. Conversely, during low periods of the economy, social networks are strong and act to protect individuals.

Forms of employment and health

Increasingly it is argued that it is the nature of work processes that need to be examined for possible health effects. One very influential theory is associated with the work of Karasek and Theorell (1990). According to the 'job-strain' model, individuals who have very demanding jobs but who see themselves as having very little control over their work, experience not only higher levels of stress than others but also elevated cardiovascular disease. A number of studies have been carried out in Sweden and the United States to support this approach. A related model – the effort–reward imbalance model – argues rather similarly that those whose work is demanding and stressful but who perceive themselves as insufficiently rewarded for their efforts are also more prone to distress as well as cardiovascular disease (Siegrist et al. 1990). Rewards are not primarily monetary but prospects of status enhancement or promotion. Both models, when tested on work forces, have been found to demonstrate the highest levels of risk in semi- and unskilled manual workers.

Income distribution and health

One final model of the effects of the economy on health argues that it is the relative degree of inequality in incomes within a country that influences health (Wilkinson 1994). The evidence to support this model comes from international comparisons of countries where it is claimed that countries with the smallest spread and least inequality of incomes from top to bottom (Japan, Sweden) have higher life expectancies than those with large income differentials such as the USA and the UK. The emphasis of the model is, therefore, not on how absolute income influences health but how people attach meaning to disadvantage in ways that actually harm them.

Of the four models outlined, only the role of unemployment has been researched to any great extent. The other three need further investigation. Bunn (1979) examined national statistics for the incidence of ischaemic heart disease in Australia. He found that economic recessions and their associated problems of high unemployment were associated not only with subsequently higher levels of heart disease mortality, but also with increased rates of drug prescribing. The latter he interpreted as a potential indicator of the stress of the recession, which resulted in increased general practice prescribing. One of the most convincing pieces of statistical evidence to support this research is the Office of Population Censuses and Surveys (OPCS) Longitudinal Study (OPCS 1984). This found that men who were unemployed in 1971, and their wives, experienced a 20% higher mortality rate than those men employed in the following 10 years (Moser et al. 1987).

Other studies, instead of looking at correlations in national statistics, have examined at close hand the experiences of unemployed families. Fagin (1981) examined in detail a small sample of families in which the male breadwinner had been without work for at least 16 weeks. In many families the breadwinners developed clinical depression, loss of self-esteem, insomnia and suicidal thoughts, much of which necessitated psychotropic drug treatment by their general practitioners. Physical symptoms included asthmatic attack, backache and skin lesions. The health of younger children in some families also seemed to be affected.

MODERN MEDICINE AND HEALTH

The issues raised by these contrasting approaches are far from resolution. All four models at least agree in placing the main responsibility for health and illness on economic policy rather than on the health services. This controversial position is partly shared by more radical writers who are more concerned with analysing directly the contribution of modern medicine to health. Perhaps the best known is Illich (1977), who argues that medicine has played a very small role in improving health and that its contribution has actually been negative, insofar as it has:

1. raised public expectations of 'wonder cures' which in reality are ineffective;
2. extended too far the kinds of problem that are thought to be medical;
3. been responsible for large amounts of iatrogenic (medically induced) illness;
4. decreased the ability of individuals to cope with their own illness by fostering a debilitating dependency on the expert (see Chapter 12).

Illich's own solution is first to break down the monopoly of medicine in health care, so that there is a 'free market' in which anyone can practise healing, and second to reverse the social trend towards dependency by restoring the value of personal responsibility.

This approach, which is attractive to many advocates of 'alternative medicine' and self-help groups, is rejected as mistaken and utopian by writers such as Navarro (1975) because it wrongly blames the medical profession and a 'gullible' public for aspects of ill health which are best understood as products of a capitalist economy. It is this which directly creates much illness, maintains an unequal distribution of illness and encourages a very inappropriate health-care system for treating illness once it has occurred. Hence Navarro advocates radical political changes in society as the only solution to the kinds of problems that have been identified in this chapter.

Other writers such as McKeown and Powles place more emphasis on the need to reform health care rather than concerning themselves with wider issues of social change. First, they argue that, since much disease is environmentally caused, preventive medicine in teaching, research and practice should concentrate on the prevention of disease rather than treatment after it has occurred. Not only has prevention had a significant impact in the past, it appears to be a simple, more humane and sound means of reducing disease for the present.

Second, these analysts also maintain that health-care resources and energy have become too concentrated on high technology and hospital-based acute medicine at the expense of preventive and community resources. In the light of the evidence reviewed above, it seems that there is an unwarranted faith in technological medicine. With the possible exception of antibiotics and immunization, few improvements in health can be attributed to breakthroughs in laboratory medicine. Cochrane (1972) argues that all too few medical procedures have been submitted to rigorous evaluation of their effectiveness (see Chapter 18).

Third, it is argued that another shift in the emphasis of medicine is needed, that from cure to care. Since medicine can claim few cures to be effective, it must confront the task of caring for the sick with greater zeal and effectiveness. Caring necessitates concern with the quality of life of the ill and reduction in any handicap or disadvantage consequent to disease. However, financial and other resources, reflecting medical values, are at present spent more in efforts in acute medicine than in the psychiatric or geriatric units. Medical education perpetuates such values because it is conducted predominantly in acute hospitals where consultants maintain traditional values in their teaching.

Clearly these arguments are controversial and have not gone unchallenged. Lever (1977) has argued that inferences about current health planning based on historical patterns are hazardous. To prove that environmental factors were the most important determinants of mortality in the past does not necessarily prove that environmental measures will produce such beneficial effects in the present. Given limited funds for health services, a major shift towards environmental and preventive health care would be a major gamble. Whatever the merits of such points, it has to be acknowledged that at present insufficient resources have been committed to such preventive services as health education and occupational medicine, compared with expenditure on hospital technology, to allow any serious examination of their potential role.

It might also be argued that analysts like McKeown are too pessimistic in their interpretation of the impact of medical treatments, which have been shown to have led to markedly improved survival rates for many forms of childhood cancers and Hodgkin's disease and cancer of the testis amongst adult cancers (Doll 1990). Moreover, the debate has tended to focus on death rates, thereby ignoring substantial benefits that may have been derived from medical treatments in improving individuals' quality of life, for example by mitigating symptoms of pain, discomfort or disability (see Chapter 18).

At present much work remains to be done regarding the influence that social and economic factors exert on health. At the same time controversial debates continue unresolved about the priorities in efforts and expenditure that are most appropriate to modern patterns of illness.

REFERENCES

Brenner, M.   (1977) Health costs and benefits of economic policy. *Int. J. Health Serv.*, **7,** 581–623.
Brenner, M.   (1979) Mortality and the national economy. *Lancet*, **ii,** 568–73.
Bunn, A.   (1979) Ischaemic heart disease mortality and the business cycle in Australia. *Am. J. Public Health*, **69,** 772–81.
Burkitt, D.   (1973) Some diseases characteristic of modern Western civilization. *Br. Med. J.*, **1,** 274–8.
Butler, J. & Vaile, M.   (1984) *Health and Health Services*. London: Routledge & Kegan Paul.
Cochrane, A.   (1972) *Effectiveness and Efficiency: Random Reflections on the Health Service*. London: Nuffield Provincial Hospitals Trust.
Department of Health and Social Security (DHSS)   (1981) *Inequalities in Health*. London: HMSO.
Doll, R.   (1983) Prospects for prevention. *Br. Med. J.*, **286,** 81–8.
Doll, R.   (1990) Are we winning the fight against cancer? An epidemiological assessment. *Eur. J. Cancer*, **26,** 500–8.
Eyer, J.   (1977) Does unemployment cause the death rate peak in each business cycle? *Int. J. Health Serv.*, **7,** 625–62.
Fagin, L.   (1981) *Unemployment and Health in Families*. London: Department of Health and Social Security.
Fries, J.   (1983) The compression of morbidity. *Milbank Q.*, **61,** 397–419.

Guha, S.   (1994) The importance of social intervention in England's mortality decline: the evidence reviewed. *Soc. Hist. Med.*, **7**, 89–114.

Illich, I.   (1977) Limits to Medicine. *Medical Nemesis: The Expropriation of Health*. Harmondsworth: Penguin.

Karasek, R. & Theorell, T.   (1990) *Healthy Work*. New York: Basic Books.

Lever, A.   (1977) Medicine under challenge. *Lancet*, **i**, 353–5.

Lock, S. & Smith, T.   (1976) *The Medical Risks of Life*. Harmondsworth: Penguin.

McKeown, T.   (1979) *The Role of Medicine: Dream, Mirage or Nemesis*, 2nd edn. Oxford: Blackwell Scientific.

McKeown, T. & Brown, R.   (1969) Medical evidence related to English population changes in the eighteenth century. In: *Population in Industrialisation*, ed. M. Drake. London: Methuen.

Moser, K., Goldblatt, P., Fox, A. & Jones, D.   (1987) Unemployment and mortality: comparison of the 1971 and 1981 longitudinal study census samples. *Br. Med. J.*, **294**, 86–90.

Navarro, V.   (1975) The industrialization of fetishism or the fetishism of industrialization: a critique of Ivan Illich. *Int. J. Health. Serv.*, **5**, 351–71.

Office of Population Censuses and Surveys   (1984) *Mortality Statistics*. London: HMSO.

Powles, J.   (1973) On the limitations of modern medicine. *Sci. Med. Man*, **1**, 1–30.

Siegrist, J., Peter, R., Junge, A. et al.   (1990) Low status control, high effort at work and ischaemic heart disease: prospective evidence from blue-collar men. *Soc. Sci. Med.*, **31**, 1127–39.

Smith, A. & Jacobson, B. (eds)   (1988) *The Nation's Health: A Strategy for The 1990s*. London: Kings Fund.

Szreter, S.   (1988) The importance of social intervention in Britain's mortality decline c. 1850–1914: a reinterpretation of the role of public health. *Soc. Hist. Med.*, **1**, 1–38.

Wilkinson, R.   (1994) The epidemiological transition: from material scarcity to social disadvantage? *Daedalus*, **123**, 61–78.

Social Causes of Disease

DAVID LOCKER

In Chapter 1 evidence was presented to indicate that the improvements in health observed during the eighteenth and nineteenth centuries were the product of rising standards of living and sanitary reform. This illustrates the general principle that the health of a population is closely tied to the physical, social and economic environment. This chapter expands on this point of view by examining some of the social factors which have been linked to health and disease. Over the past 40 years research in this field has grown significantly, with relatively new disciplines such as social epidemiology and psychophysiology devoted to the investigation of the links between the social environment, psychological and emotional states, physiological change and disease. The broad implication of this work, and the view of health it embodies, is that health and illness are social, as well as medical, issues.

THEORIES OF DISEASE CAUSATION

Before the rise of modern medicine, disease was attributed to a variety of spiritual or mechanical forces. It was interpreted as a punishment by God for sinful behaviour or the result of an imbalance in body elements or 'humours'. Cholera, which was epidemic during the early nineteenth century, was ascribed to a life of vice or a weak moral character or believed to be due to 'miasma', that is, bad air arising out of dirt and decaying organic matter.

Ideas about disease emerging during the nineteenth century were influenced by two developments which provided a philosophical and empirical basis for the biomechanical approach characteristic of modern medical practice. These developments were the 'Cartesian revolution', which gave rise to the idea that the mind and body were independent, and the doctrine of specific aetiology, which flowed from the discovery of the microbiological origins of infectious disease. These effectively denied the influence of social and psychological factors in disease onset. Rather, the body was viewed as a machine to be corrected when things go wrong by procedures designed to neutralize specific agents or modify the physical processes causing disease. These ideas have been progressively challenged as the monocausal view of disease has been modified by multicausal models of disease onset. The key features of these theories of disease are summarized in Box 2.1.

BOX 2.1

THEORIES OF DISEASE CAUSATION: KEY IDEAS

Germ theory
 Disease is caused by transmissable agents.
 A specific agent is responsible for one disease only.
 Medical practice consists of identifying and neutralizing these agents.

Epidemiological triangle
 Exposure to an agent does not necessarily lead to disease.
 Disease is the result of an interaction between agent, host and environment.
 Disease can be prevented by modifying factors which influence exposure and susceptibility.

Web of causation
 Disease results from the complex interaction of many risk factors.
 Any risk factor can be implicated in more than one disease.
 Disease can be prevented by modifying these risk factors.

General susceptibility
 Some social groups have higher mortality and morbidity rates from all causes.
 This reflects an imperfectly understood general susceptibility to health problems.
 This probably results from the complex interaction of the environment, behaviours and life-styles.

Socioenvironmental approach
 Health is powerfully influenced by the social and physical environments in which we live.
 Risk conditions integral to those environments damage health directly and through the physiological, behavioural and psychosocial risk factors they engender.
 Improving health requires political action to modify these environments.

The germ theory of disease

During the second half of the nineteenth century, the work of Ehrlich, Koch and Pasteur revealed that the prevailing health problems of the time were the product of living organisms which entered the body through food, water, air or the bites of insects or animals. In 1882, Koch identified and isolated the bacillus causing tuberculosis, and between 1897 and 1900 the organisms responsible for 22 infectious diseases were identified. This work gave rise to the idea that each disease has a single and specific cause. This is embodied in Koch's postulates, a set of rules for establishing causal relationships between a micro-organism and a disease. These state that, to be ascribed a causal role, the agent must always be found with the disease in question and not with any other disease. This doctrine with its monocausal approach came to dominate medical research and practice. As a result, research effort moved from the community to the laboratory and concentrated on the identification of the noxious agents responsible for a given disease, while medical practice became devoted to the destruction or eradication of that agent from individuals already affected (Najman 1980).

Multicausal models of disease

Although the infectious organism theory of disease made a significant contribution to explaining and solving the major health problems of its time, it has serious limitations in terms of our understanding of disease processes. The most important of these is that not all those exposed to pathogens become ill: an organism or other noxious agent is a necessary, but not a sufficient, cause of disease. The **epidemiological triangle** approach sees disease as the product of an interaction between an agent, a host and the environment. Host and environmental factors determine exposure and/or susceptibility to the noxious agent in question. In this respect, all diseases, including infections, are multifactorial and have multiple causes. One of the benefits of this broader view is that the health of a population may be promoted by procedures which modify susceptibility and exposure as well as by procedures which attack the agent involved in the disease. That is, disease can be prevented as well as cured.

The epidemiological triangle is useful in understanding infectious disorders, but is less useful with respect to chronic, degenerative disorders such as heart disease, stroke and arthritis, for here no specific agent can be identified against which individuals and populations may be protected. Many contemporary medical problems are better understood in terms of a **web of causation** (MacMahon and Pugh 1970). According to this concept, disorders such as heart disease develop through complex interactions of many factors which form interlocking chains. These factors may be biophysical, social or psychological and may promote or inhibit the disease at more than one point in the causal process. This is illustrated with respect to heart disease in Fig. 2.1. Since many of these factors can be modified, prevention offers better prospects for health than cure. It is also important to note that many of the factors implicated in heart disease have been identified as increasing the risk of other disorders, such as stroke and cancer.

The theory of general susceptibility

The theory of general susceptibility has emerged over the past 20 years and departs in important ways from monocausal and multicausal models of disease. It is not concerned with identifying single or multiple risk factors associated with specific disorders, but seeks to understand why some social groups seem to be more susceptible to disease and death in general. For example, numerous studies have shown that social class, measured by occupation, education, income or area of residence, is closely related to health, even in countries with nationalized and egalitarian health–care systems such as the National Health Service (NHS) in the UK (see Chapter 8).

Fig. 2.1 *The web of causation: risk factors for heart disease. LDL/HDL = Low density lipoproteins/high density lipoproteins. (Reproduced with permission from Mausner and Kramer, 1985.)*

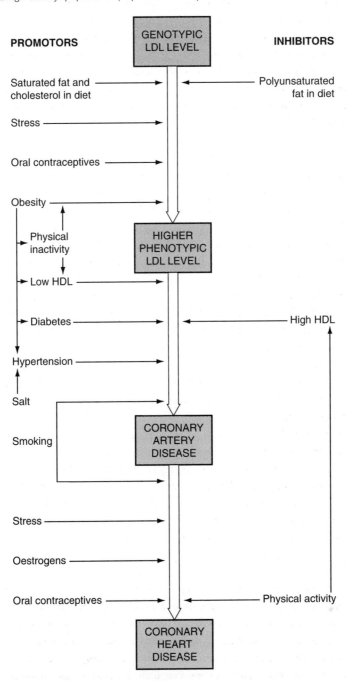

The socioenvironmental approach

During the late 1980s, the theory of general susceptibility became more explicitly formulated as the socioenvironmental approach. This forms the basis for the health promotion strategies described in Chapter 17. The socioenvironmental model has as its basis risk conditions which emanate from the social and physical environments in which we live. These have a direct effect on health and well-being and also affect health through the numerous psychosocial, behavioural and physiological risk factors which they engender (Fig. 2.2).

The main implication of this model is that material deprivation and a lack of control over important dimensions of one's life are the main issues that need to be addressed in promoting the health of the population. It is no accident that those countries where the income gap between the rich and the poor is narrowest have the lowest overall mortality rates. As a consequence, social and political change, including income redistribution, may be necessary to modify the health experience of lower socioeconomic groups.

These theories of the causes of disease have been presented in a more or less historical sequence. From the brief descriptions offered it is clear that the role ascribed to the physical, social and psychological environment increases as we have progressed from the germ theory to the theory of general susceptibility. The latter completely overturns the doctrine of specific aetiology central to the former, for broad non-specific social and psychological factors are seen to be associated with a variety of disease outcomes.

It would, however, be a mistake to assume that the role of social and psychological factors as causes of disease has been realized only in modern times. Many of the so-called 'pre-scientific' explanations of disease gave recognition to the part played by such factors. In many cultures, disease is still seen in social terms, as the outcome of a lack of harmony in social relationships. In the context of modern medical history the idea that disease can be brought about by psychological influences was integral to the work of Freud, who explained disorders such as asthma and gastric ulcers as the product of unresolved psychological conflict. Freud's work gave rise to the notion that some diseases were 'psychosomatic' whereas others were not. The contemporary view is that social and psychological factors are implicated in all diseases, although the mechanisms by which they influence health are complex and variable.

SOCIAL AND PSYCHOLOGICAL FACTORS AND HEALTH

The research effort invested in studies of social and psychological factors and health is enormous and the body of work that has been produced is difficult to summarize. One reason for this is that a wide variety of factors having a potential influence on health have been studied. As the discussion of theories of disease indicated, these factors fall into three broad types: socioenvironmental, behavioural and psychological.

Clearly, there are close links between many of these factors, and contemporary models of illness attempt to specify how and when they are involved in the mechanisms leading to disease. Even though behaviours such as smoking are individual acts, a number of social and cultural factors influence whether someone will become a smoker and continue to smoke. These factors include 'cultural themes associated with smoking such as relaxation, adulthood, sexual attractiveness and emancipation; the socioeconomic structure of tobacco production, processing,

Fig. 2.2 The socioenvironmental approach. *(Reproduced with permission from The University of Toronto from Labonte, 1993.)*

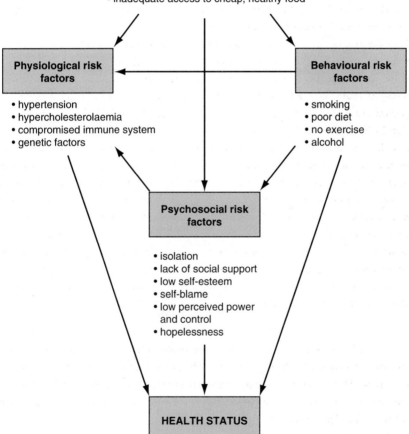

distribution and legislation; explicit and continual advertising by the tobacco companies and the influence of peers, siblings and significant others' (Syme 1986).

Some of the social factors having an influence on health and explanations of their role as causes of disease are reviewed below.

Social and cultural change

Most of the early studies of social factors and disease onset were concerned with the effects of social and cultural change. They included studies of industrialization and urbanization, migration and social, occupational and geographical mobility. The major disease outcome studied was coronary heart disease since this is predominantly a disease of industrialized, urbanized nations. Some populations isolated from western culture have low blood pressure which does not rise with age. However, blood-pressure levels and coronary heart disease rates increase when these populations move to urban settings (Prior 1974).

A number of studies conducted during the 1960s and early 1970s found higher rates of disease among people who changed jobs, place of residence or life circumstances. For example, one study found that men reared on farms who moved to urban centres to take middle-class jobs had higher rates of coronary heart disease than men who continued to work on the farm or who took up labouring jobs in cities (Syme et al. 1964). Similar observations have been made with respect to cancer. Men raised on farms who moved to cities had higher rates of lung cancer than those who did not, even at comparable levels of smoking (Haenszel et al. 1962). However, a study of the impact of oil development in the north of Scotland showed that rapid social change did not have negative consequences on the health of the population if the community was well integrated prior to the change, if the change was anticipated and planned, and if it had more advantages than disadvantages for the community.

A number of mechanisms might be responsible for the negative effects of social and cultural change on health. The adverse effects may be the direct result of change itself, a product of the circumstances to which individuals move or the product of personal characteristics which predispose individuals to both mobility and poor health. One study which attempted to evaluate these explanations compared rates of heart disease among Japanese immigrants to California and Hawaii with those of Japanese men still living in Japan (Marmot et al. 1975). Coronary heart disease and mortality rates were highest among those living in California and lowest in Japan. This difference was not explained by differences in risk factors such as cholesterol levels, diet, blood pressure or smoking. However, among those living in California, some had become 'acculturated' and had adopted western lifestyles, whereas others retained traditional Japanese ways. The former had disease rates up to five times as high as the latter. This suggests that being mobile is not, in itself, the important factor.

Social support

One of the earliest studies of the relationship between social environment and health was undertaken by the French sociologist Durkheim and published in 1897. In this work Durkheim pioneered the use of statistical methods for exploring and explaining differences in suicide rates across different social groups. Although suicide is an individual act, these differences in rates have persisted over time and across cultures. Durkheim explained suicide in terms of the social organization of these groups, particularly the extent to which individuals were integrated into the group, and the way in which this encouraged or deterred individuals from suicide. High rates of suicide were associated with groups which had very high and very low levels of integration.

More recent studies of social ties and health have focused on the relationship between social support and individual well-being. Some of this early work looked at differences in health according to marital status. The single, widowed and divorced have higher mortality rates than the married, the differences being much larger for men than for women (Table 2.1). These differences, which were first observed and reported in the mid-nineteenth century, have been remarkably consistent over time, and are consistent across cultures and health-care systems. Only a small part of the differences in mortality rates can be explained by the selective effects of marriage (Morgan 1980).

TABLE 2.1 *Mortality, all causes: ratio of mortality rate of the unmarried to the mortality rate of the married; whites aged 25–64 years, USA, 1960.*

Maritial status	Sex	Ratio
Single	Male	1.96
	Female	1.68
Widowed	Male	2.64
	Female	1.77
Divorced	Male	3.39
	Female	1.95

Reproduced with permission from The University of Chicago Press from Gove (1979).

One possible explanation of these differences is that marital status has an influence on psychological states and life-styles (Gove 1979). Studies have shown that the married tend to be happier and more satisfied with life than the unmarried, they are less likely to be socially isolated and have more social ties. In a society in which marriage and family life are a central value, being married gives meaning and significance to daily life, promotes a sense of well-being and is a source of social and emotional support. This explanation tends to be supported by data on marital status and specific causes of death. Variations in mortality rates are large where psychological states or aspects of life-style play a direct role in death, as in suicide or death from accidents, or are associated with acts such as smoking or alcohol consumption. Large differences are also observed with respect to diseases such as tuberculosis, where family factors may influence entry into medical care, willingness to undergo treatment or the availability of help and support (Table 2.2).

The high death rates of widowed men have also been confirmed in studies which have documented the mortality experience of recently bereaved men. Parkes et al. (1969) found that mortality rates of widowers aged 55 years and over were 40% higher than those of men the same age in the 6 months following the loss of a spouse.

TABLE 2.2 Mortality, specific causes: ratio of mortality rate of the unmarried to the mortality rate of the married; whites aged 25–64 years, USA, 1960.

			Cause		
Marital status	Suicide	Lung cancer	Cirrhosis	Tuberculosis	Diabetes
Single					
Male	2.00	1.45	3.29	5.37	2.69
Female	1.51	1.11	1.19	3.31	2.03
Widowed					
Male	5.01	2.24	4.61	7.70	2.46
Female	2.21	1.20	3.45	3.31	1.71
Divorced					
Male	4.75	3.07	8.84	9.27	4.32
Female	3.43	1.11	4.43	3.10	1.67

Reproduced with permission from The University of Chicago Press from Gove (1979).

An influential study which clearly demonstrated that integration into the community has a direct effect on health was undertaken by Berkman and Syme (1979). They followed a random sample of adults over a 9-year period. At the start of the study a social network score was calculated for each subject based on marital status, contacts with friends and relatives and membership of religious and other social groups. Over the 9-year period of the study those with low network scores were more likely to die than those with high network scores. After controlling for other factors such as weight, cigarette smoking, alcohol consumption, physical activity, health practices and health status at baseline, mortality rates for the socially isolated were two to three times higher than those with extensive social networks.

Other evidence suggests that social integration and social support have a broad influence on health. They have been linked to heart disease (Reed et al. 1983), complications of pregnancy (Nuckolls et al. 1972) and emotional illness (Henderson et al. 1978). A 2-year follow-up study of people with disabilities living in an urban community found that people with few social contacts were more likely to deteriorate in physical and psychosocial functioning than people with high levels of contact with others (Patrick et al. 1986). However, the greatest and most significant difference between those with and without social support occurred among those reporting an adverse life event during the period of the study.

Social support refers to a fairly broad category of events and includes practical assistance, financial help, the provision of information and advice and psychological support. The mechanisms by which it enhances or protects health are not known. One hypothesis concerning this mechanism has emerged in the context of studies of the negative health impact of stressful life circumstances. This research suggests that social support has no direct influence on health but acts as a buffer against adverse events that would otherwise have health-damaging effects. In their research on the social origins of depression, Brown and Harris (1978) found that social support was protective only in the context of a severe life event. Although this and other studies strongly suggest that social support enhances coping and the ability to tolerate stressful life circumstances, further research is needed to specify what types of support buffer which kinds of life problems and precisely how they promote health and well-being.

Life events

A more comprehensive attempt to assess the influence of life experiences such as bereavement and unemployment is to be found in studies of life events and health. This approach emerged at the end of the 1960s with the development of instruments such as the Social Readjustment Rating Scale (SRRS) (Holmes and Rahe 1967). This scale consists of a list of 42 events, each of which involves personal loss or some degree of change in roles or personal relationships. Each event is given a score depending on how much life change it involves. The top of the scale is the death of a wife or husband and is given a score of 100. Divorce has a score of 73 and losing a job a score of 45. Scores for an individual are totalled to give a numerical estimate of the amount of life change experienced in a defined period, usually the past year. A number of studies have shown that there is some relationship between scores on this scale and future changes in health.

There have been a number of criticisms of this method of measuring the frequency and severity of life events. Perhaps the most important is that scales such as the SRRS fail to take account of variations in the meaning and significance of life events. The birth of a child, for example, may be a positive event for some women but a negative event for others, depending on the social context in which it occurs. More sophisticated measures of life events have been developed which take account of variations in the meaning of life events based on contextual factors (Brown and Harris 1978).

A second criticism of the SRRS is that it focuses on major life events and ignores less severe but more common life difficulties. A measure which attempts to tap such difficulties is the Hassles Scale (Kanner et al. 1981). Its proponents claim that measures of life stress based on daily 'hassles' are better predictors of changes in physical and psychological health than measures based on major life events.

Clearly, the measurement of life stress is a complex issue and establishing a relationship between such stress and negative health outcomes is methodologically challenging. Many studies which have shown such a relationship have design weaknesses which make interpretation of their results difficult.

One particularly noteworthy study is that conducted by Brown and Harris (1978) which was mentioned above in connection with social support. This was an investigation of the social and economic circumstances causally implicated in the onset of depression in women. Using measures which were context sensitive, they were able to show a clear relationship between life events with long-term threatening implications and the onset of depression in women. Events with short-term implications, no matter how stressful, were not associated with depression. However, whether or not a woman became depressed after an event involving long-term threat depended on the presence of four 'vulnerability factors'. These were: the absence of a close, confiding relationship with a spouse or other person, loss of mother before age 11 years, lack of employment outside the home, and having three or more children under the age of 15 living at home. The greater the number of these factors present, the greater was the likelihood of depression following an event with long-term threatening implications. Brown and Harris (1978) believe that these vulnerability factors produce ongoing low self-esteem and an inability to cope with the world. These interact with life events to produce generalized feelings of hopelessness and, subsequently, depression.

This model also explains why working-class women have higher rates of depression than middle-class women. They are more likely to experience severe life events and, because their lives are more likely to be characterized by one or more of these vulnerability factors, they are more prone to become depressed as a result.

Life events have also been implicated in the mechanisms leading to physical disorders (Creed 1985). They have been linked to disturbances in the control of diabetes (Bradley 1979), to diseases such as duodenal ulcer (Murphy and Brown 1980) and to abdominal pain leading to appendicectomy (Creed 1981). Murphy and Brown (1980) suggested that the development of physical conditions was dependent on the prior development of a psychiatric disorder, whereas Creed (1985) suggested that life stress was an important component of functional disorders.

Occupational hierarchies and the organization of work

The physical environments in which people work are often hazardous and damaging to health. Air pollution at work, exposure to carcinogens, working with machinery and industrial accidents take a large toll on the health of manual workers. However, the social environments in which we work can also have a negative impact on health. Evidence in support of this point of view comes from a study of British civil servants which explored the links between the organization of work and health outcomes (Marmot and Theorell 1988). It confirmed work conducted in Sweden which showed that cardiovascular disease was more common among those who had a low level of control over their work (Johnson and Hall 1988). None of the subjects in the British study were living in poverty; nevertheless, there were differences in health status according to occupational grade. Those in the lowest grade had mortality rates three times that of those in the highest grade and higher rates of diseases such as lung cancer and bronchitis. Rates of smoking were twice as high in low compared to high grade workers. Another noteworthy finding was that although blood pressure levels were similar for low and high grade civil servants when at work, they declined much more for the latter than the former when they were at home. This study concluded that a lack of freedom to make decisions at work, particularly when jobs are stressful or psychologically demanding, is linked both to at-risk behaviours such as smoking, physiological risk factors such as high blood pressure and health outcomes such as heart disease.

Unemployment

Although the physical and social environments in which we work can have a negative effect on health, so can unemployment. There are two main reasons why unemployment could conceivably affect health (Marmot and Madge 1987). First, it is related to standards of living and the material conditions of life, and second it is a stressful event which may become chronic and deprive an individual of a social role, meaningful daily existence and contact with others.

Two approaches are evident in studies of unemployment and health and both are subject to problems in interpretation, largely because it is difficult to separate the effects of unemployment from the effects of other social and economic conditions (Marmot and Madge 1987). The first of these approaches attempts to demonstrate an association between unemployment rates and mortality rates and the way these co-vary with the ups and downs of the economic cycle. The most recent of this work was conducted by Brenner (1979) and is reviewed in Chapter 1. The second approach attempts to assess the health of people who are, or have recently become, unemployed. Since ill health can lead to unemployment as well as vice versa, such studies need to be conducted carefully before it can be concluded that unemployment is a cause of poor health. Nevertheless, evidence from well-designed research does suggest that the unemployed experience more illness, have higher blood pressure and increased mortality (Arber 1987; Moser et al. 1987; Jin et al. 1996; Turner 1995).

THE SOCIAL CAUSES OF DISEASE: BIOLOGICAL PATHWAYS

Psychoneuroimmunology, an emerging and controversial field of knowledge, is beginning to provide evidence of the biological pathways linking social factors and disease and filling in the gaps in the stress–illness model. Although there are a number of formulations of this model, most assume that stressors (threatening environmental circumstances) give rise to strains (psychological and physiological changes) which increase an individual's susceptibility to disease. There is evidence to suggest that stress, or its outcome in the form of depression, leads to a number of changes in the human body. It interferes with the normal functioning of hormonal and immune systems, leads to increased heart rate and respiration, dilatation of blood vessels to the muscles and alterations in gastrointestinal function. These changes are believed to cause disease directly or render an individual more prone to disease.

As some of the research reviewed above suggests, this essentially simple model is more complex than it seems. Clearly, the link between stressors and illness is mediated by a number of factors which may increase or decrease an individual's vulnerability when faced with a stressor. Social factors such as social support and psychological variables such as personality characteristics, perceptual processes and coping styles, interact in complex ways to affect health outcomes. Moreover, as the socioenvironmental approach suggests, behavioural responses to environmental stressors in the form of health-damaging activities such as smoking also play an important role (Najman 1980).

PEOPLE, PLACES AND HEALTH

Although a great deal has been made of the links between social and physical environments and health, it is rare for these environments themselves to be the focus of research. The overwhelming tendency has been to look at the characteristics of individuals rather than the characteristics of the places in which they live. However, as evidence begins to accumulate, it is clear that the immediate neighbourhood in which one lives can have an impact on health. Simply put, poor people living in wealthier neighbourhoods have better health than similarly poor people living in poor neighbourhoods (Blaxter 1990). MacIntyre et al. (1993) have argued that findings such as these indicate a need for research to discover precisely which features of local areas either damage or promote health. Although some research is available which tries to link aspects of the physical environment, such as air pollution or water hardness, to diseases such as bronchitis and cancer, there is very little work that tries to identify the social, cultural or economic characteristics of areas that affect health. The importance of such work is clear; we may be able to improve health by changing places rather than people.

As an example of this kind of research, MacIntyre et al. (1993) compared two areas of Glasgow to identify differences in the living environments they provided. One was in the north west of the city and had relatively low mortality rates; the other was in the south west of the city and had high mortality rates. They found differences between the areas such that living in the north west would be more conducive to good health than living in the south west. Healthy foodstuffs were more available and cheaper in the north west, there were more sporting and recreational facilities, better transport services, better health services, less crime and a less hostile environment. Even though two people might have the same personal characteristics (the same income, family size and composition, and housing tenure, for example) the one living in the north west would be advantaged compared to the one in the south west in ways likely to be related to physical and mental health.

The main conclusion to be drawn from the research summarized here is that patterns of health and disease are largely the product of social and environmental influences. Although health and illness may involve biological agents and processes, they are inseparable from the social settings in which people live. Ultimately, it is these which influence the challenges people encounter in daily life and their capacity to manage them. Changing these environments is one way in which the health of a community can be improved.

REFERENCES

Arber, S.   (1987) Social class, non-employment and chronic illness: continuing the inequalities in health debate. *Br. Med. J.*, **294**, 1069–73.

Berkman, L. & Syme, S.   (1979) Social networks, host resistance and mortality: a nine-year follow-up of Alameda County residents. *Am. J. Epidemiol.*, **109**, 186–204.

Blaxter M.   (1990) *Health and Lifestyles*. London: Tavistock-Routledge.

Bradley, C.   (1979) Life events and the control of diabetes mellitus. *J. Psychosom. Res.*, **23**, 159–62.

Brenner, M.   (1979) Mortality and the national economy. *Lancet*, **ii**, 568–73.

Brown, G. & Harris, T.   (1978) *The Social Origins of Depression*. London: Tavistock.

Creed, F.   (1981) Life events and appendicitis. *Lancet*, **i**, 1381–5.

Creed, F.   (1985) Life events and physical illness: a review. *J. Psychosom. Res.*, **29**, 113–24.

Gove, W.   (1979) Sex, marital status and mortality. *Am. J. Sociol.*, **79**, 45–67.

Haenszel, W., Loveland, D. & Sirken, M.   (1962) Lung cancer mortality as related to residence and smoking histories: I. White males. *J. Natl. Cancer Inst.*, **28**, 947–1001.

Henderson, S., Byrne, D., Duncan-Jones, P., Adcock, S., Scott, R. & Steale, G.   (1978) Social bonds in the epidemiology of neurosis. *Br. J. Psychiatry*, **132**, 463–6.

Holmes, T. & Rahe, R.   (1967) The social readjustment rating scale. *J. Psychosom. Res.*, **11**, 231–218.

Jin, R.L., Shah, C.P. & Sroboda, T.J.   (1996) The impact of unemployment on health: a review of the evidence. *Canadian Medical Association Journal*, **153**, 529–40.

Johnson, J. & Hall, E.   (1988) Job strain, work place social support and cardiovascular disease: a cross-sectional study of a random sample of the Swedish working population. *Am. J. Public Health*, **78**, 1336–42.

Kanner, A., Coyne, J., Schaefer, C. & Lazarus, R.   (1981) Comparison of two modes of stress measurement: daily hassles and uplifts versus major life events. *J. Behav. Med.*, **4**, 1–39.

Labonte, R.   (1993) *Health Promotion and Empowerment: Practice Frameworks*. Centre for Health Promotion, University of Toronto. Issues in Health Promotion no. 3.

MacIntyre S., MacIver, S & Soomans, A.   (1993) Area, class and health: should we be focusing on places or people? *J. Soc. Pol.*, **22**, 213–34.

MacMahon, B. & Pugh, T.   (1970) *Epidemiological Principles and Methods*. Boston, MA: Little, Brown.

Marmot, M. & Madge, N.   (1987) An epidemiological perspective on stress and health. In: *Stress and Health: Issues in Research Methodology*, ed. S. Kasl & C. Cooper. Winchester: Wiley.

Marmot, M. & Theorell, T.   (1988) Social class and cardiovascular disease: the contribution of work. *Int. J. Health Serv.*, **18**, 37–45.

Marmot, M., Syme, L. & Kagan, A.   (1975) Epidemiological studies of heart disease and stroke in Japanese men living in Japan, Hawaii and California. Prevalence of coronary and hypertensive disease and associated risk factors. *Am. J. Epidemiol.*, **102**, 514–25.

Mausner, J. & Kramer, S.   (1985) *Epidemiology: An Introductory Text*. Philadelphia: W.B. Saunders.

Morgan, M.   (1980) Marital status, health, illness and service use. *Soc. Sci. Med.*, **14A**, 633–43.

Moser, K., Goldblatt, P. & Fox, A.   (1987) Unemployment and mortality: a comparison of the 1971 and the 1981 longitudinal study census samples. *Lancet*, **ii**, 1324–8.

Murphy, E. & Brown, G.   (1980) Life events, psychiatric disturbance and physical illness. *Br. J. Psychiatry*, **136**, 326–38.

Najman, J.   (1980) Theories of disease causation and the concept of general susceptibility: a review. *Soc. Sci. Med.*, **14A**, 231–7.

Nuckolls, K., Cassel, J. & Kaplan, B.   (1972) Psychosocial assets, life crises and the prognosis of pregnancy. *Am. J. Epidemiol.*, **95**, 431–41.

Parkes, C., Benjamin, B. & Fitzgerald, R.   (1969) Broken heart: a statistical survey of increased mortality among widowers. *Br. Med. J.*, **1**, 740–4.

Patrick, D., Morgan, M. & Charlton, J.   (1986) Psychosocial support and change in the health status of physically disabled people. *Soc. Sci. Med.*, **22**, 1347–54.

Prior, I.   (1974) Cardiovascular epidemiology in New Zealand and the Pacific. *N Z Med. J.*, **80**, 245–52.

Reed, D., McGee, D., Yano, K. & Feinleib, M.   (1983) Social networks and coronary heart disease among Japanese men in Hawaii. *Am. J. Epidemiol.*, **117**, 384–96.

Syme, S.   (1986) Social determinants of health and disease. In: *Public Health and Preventative Medicine*, ed. J. Last. Norwalk, CT: Appleton-Century-Crofts.

Syme, S., Hyman, M. & Enterline, P.   (1964) Some social and cultural factors associated with the occurrence of coronary heart disease. *J. Chron. Dis.*, **17**, 277–89.

Turner, J.B.   (1995) Economic context and the impact of unemployment. *Journal of Health and Social Behaviour*, **35**, 213–19.

SOCIAL FACTORS IN MEDICAL PRACTICE

PART

2

Health and Illness Behaviour

3

GRAHAM SCAMBLER

Definitions of 'health' and 'illness' vary within cultures, subcultures and communities, and even within households, between generations for example. There may be gaps too between lay and medical concepts. The primary focus of this chapter is on lay beliefs about, and attitudes toward, health and illness, and on the various ways in which these, together with a host of other social factors, can influence people's behaviour when faced with what they perceive to be threats to their well-being.

Consideration is given first to differences in people's perspectives on health and illness. A brief review is then given of studies of the prevalence of illness and disease in the community. Special attention is paid to those factors known to influence help-seeking behaviour, and especially to those known to affect whether or not people who define themselves as ill consult a physician, usually a general practitioner. Finally, self-help and sources of help other than allopathic medicine are considered, ranging from informal lay networks to alternative therapies.

PERCEPTIONS OF HEALTH AND ILLNESS

The modern study of how lay people define health and illness was pioneered by Herzlich (1973) with her research with 80, largely middle-class, adults in France. Analysing their accounts of health and illness, she found that illness was generally perceived as external and as a product of a way of life, notably urban life. This covered not merely pathological agents such as germs, but also accidents and diseases like cancer and various mental disorders. Health, on the other hand, was perceived as internal to the individual, with three different and discernible dimensions: an absence of illness ('health in a vacuum'); a 'reserve of health', determined by constitution and temperament; and a positive state of well-being or 'equilibrium'.

Several studies in Britain have since led to similar distinctions. Pill and Scott (1982) interviewed mothers of families with young children from working-class backgrounds. They encountered definitions of health in terms of the absence of illness. A functional definition of health was also common, that is, in terms of the capacity to perform or cope with normal roles. As in Herzlich's study, a positive definition of health was apparent as well, although among Pill and Scott's sample it was associated with being cheerful and enthusiastic rather than with a state of equilibrium.

Such a positive dimension was missing, however, from the accounts of mothers and daughters in socially disadvantaged families questioned by Blaxter and Paterson (1982). References were made to health as the absence of illness, but the majority seemed to have a functional definition of health. They also had a functional definition of illness, many of them distinguishing between normal illness, which they accommodated, and serious illness, like cancer, heart disease and tuberculosis, which called for radical adjustment and change. These conceptions of health and illness, especially the lack of a positive definition of health, clearly reflected the high prevalence of health problems among the sample.

Reviewing these and other studies, Blaxter (1990) writes: 'Health can be defined negatively, as the absence of illness, functionally, as the ability to cope with everyday activities, or positively, as fitness and well-being'. She adds that health also has moral connotations, as salient in modern urban communities as among pre-modern or primitive societies. There is a sense in which people feel a duty to be healthy and experience illness as failure. Health can be seen in terms of will-power, self-discipline and self-control.

Increasingly relevant too, it might be added, is an emphasis on what has been called 'body maintenance'. This is linked to innovative forms of entrepreneurial activity and to 'consumerism'. The body becomes a site of pleasure and a representation of happiness and success. As Nettleton (1995) puts it, 'to look good is to *feel* good'. Health education echoes the commercialization of body maintenance. Thus Featherstone (1991) argues that common to the media treatment of body maintenance and to health education is the 'encouragement of self-surveillance of bodily health and appearance as well as the incentive of lifestyle benefits'. He goes on to refer to the 'transvaluation' of activities like jogging and slimming, which have been freshly evaluated in light of their putative health benefits. The most conspicuous example of the commercialization of healthy life-styles is probably the 'fitness industry', its products ranging from exercise machines and videos to special stylish clothing.

ILLNESS AND DISEASE IN THE COMMUNITY

The *National Health and Lifestyle* survey found that 71% of participants defined their health as at least 'good' (Blaxter 1990). This did not mean that none of these people had symptoms of illness or, indeed, medically defined disease. For example, many disabled and/or elderly people defined their health as 'excellent', clearly meaning 'my health is excellent despite my disability/considering my advanced years'. Comparisons were made between participants' own assessments of their health and a series of objective measures. Although there was a general correspondence between the two, most obviously at the extremes, 10% of men and 7% of women in the top category of health, objectively measured, described their health as only 'fair' or 'poor'; and as many as 40%

of those with undoubted health problems, objectively measured, described their health as 'good' or 'excellent'.

In the more recent *Health Survey for England, 1993* (OPCS 1993) all informants were asked to rate their health according to five categories: 'very good', 'good', 'fair', 'bad' or 'very bad'. Over three-quarters of men (77%) and women (76%) rated their health as 'good' or 'very good', only 1% of each rating it as 'very bad'. The likelihood of an informant reporting good general health decreased with age among both men and women (Fig. 3.1).

Fig. 3.1 *Self-reported general health by age and sex. (Reproduced with permission of the Controller of HMSO and the Office for National Standards from OPCS 1995.)*

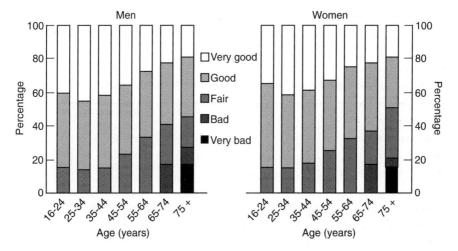

Members of the same sample were also asked about any long-standing illness or disability that had troubled them, or was likely to affect them, over a period of time; 40% of men and 41% of women reported such an illness or disability. Again, reporting increased with age. However, even among those aged 16–24, a relatively high proportion reported having a long-standing illness: 23% of men and 22% of women. For those aged 75 or more, the figures were 63% for men and 67% for women.

As far as acute sickness is concerned, participants in the Health Survey were asked if they had 'had to cut down on any of the things you usually do (about the house/at work or in your free time) because of illness or injury' during the two weeks prior to interview. This sometimes included recurrence or long-standing illness. Acute sickness, thus defined, was reported by 12% of men and a rather higher proportion, 16%, of women. For both men and women the likelihood of reporting acute sickness increased slightly with age. Whereas 11% of men and 12% of women aged 16–24 reported acute sickness, the figures for those over 75 were 16% for men and 21% for women.

The Health Survey also revealed that 16%, 13% of men and 19% of women, had consulted a general practitioner in the two weeks prior to interview. Women aged 16–34 were significantly more likely to have consulted a general practitioner in the last 14 days than men in the same age group; but many of these consultations were probably for purposes such as contraception and normal pregnancy and not related to illness.

The rate of reporting of individual symptoms of illness is, of course, considerably higher. The findings by Wadsworth et al. (1971) remain typical of retrospective studies in this area. Of their sample of 1000 adults 95% had experienced symptoms in the 14 days prior to interview and only one in five had consulted a doctor. In a prospective study (Scambler et al. 1981) a sample of women aged 16−44 years kept 6-week health diaries in which they recorded any disturbances in their health. Symptoms were recorded on an average of one day in three. Table 3.1 shows the 10 most frequently recorded symptoms and also how often these precipitated medical consultations and the ratio of medical consultations to symptom episodes. Overall, there was one medical consultation for every 18 symptom episodes.

TABLE 3.1 *Symptom episodes and medical consultations recorded in health diaries.*

Main types of symptoms recorded	No of symptom episodes	Percentage of total number of symptom episodes	Mean length of symptom episodes (days)	No of occasions on which symptom episode precipitated medical consultation	Ratio of medical consultations to symptom episodes
Headache	180	20.9	1.3	3	1:60
Changes in energy, tiredness	109	12.6	1.4	0	—
Nerves, depression or irritability	74	8.6	1.7	1	1:74
Aches or pains in joints, muscles, legs or arms	71	8.2	1.6	4	1:18
Women's complaints like period pain[a]	69	8.0	1.7	7	1:10
Stomach aches or pains	45	5.2	1.5	4	1:11
Backache	38	4.4	1.6	1	1:38
Cold, flu, or running nose	37	4.3	4.1	3	1:12
Sore throat	36	4.2	2.4	4	1:9
Sleeplessness	31	3.6	1.5	1	1:31
Others	173	20.0	1.9	21	1:8
Total	863	100.0	1.7	49	1:18

Reproduced with permission from Scambler et al. (1981).
[a] *Stomach aches and pains and backache were classified as period pains if so defined by the women themselves.*

It might be thought that most symptoms not precipitating consultations are mild and not indicative of disease requiring medical intervention. Ingham and Miller (1979) found that symptom severity for seven selected symptoms was indeed greater in consulters than in non-consulters. There is convincing evidence, however, that general practitioners are often not consulted for disease which would undoubtedly respond to treatment. Epsom (1978) carried out an investigation of the health status of a sample of adults using a mobile health clinic. Of the 3160 people investigated, 57% were referred to their general practitioners for further tests and possible treatment. Major diseases detected included seven instances of pre-invasive cervical cancer, one confirmed case of carcinoma of the breast and one active case of pulmonary tuberculosis. A follow-up study of those referred to their general practitioners indicated that 38% of the findings had not previously been known to the general practitioners, and that 22% of the findings made known to the general practitioners for the first time were judged serious enough to warrant hospital referrals. This and other studies confirm that a significant clinical iceberg exists: the professional health services treat only the tip of the sum total of ill health.

The existence of a clinical iceberg has important implications. Most obviously there is the problem of unmet need: many people of all ages are enduring avoidable pain, discomfort and handicap. There is a gap in other words between the need for and the demand for health care. It must be remembered, however, that any substantial increase in the existing level of demand would swamp the primary care services. Many general practitioners also argue that there is currently a widespread tendency for people to consult for trivial, unnecessary or inappropriate reasons: in one national study, one-quarter of the general practitioners questioned felt that half or more of their surgery consultations fell into this category (Cartwright and Anderson 1981). Basic to these issues, of course, is the question of how to define 'need'.

UNDERSTANDING ILLNESS BEHAVIOUR

A number of studies have documented the sociodemographic characteristics of users and non-users of medical services. It is known, for example, that women consult more than men, children and the elderly more than young adults and the middle-aged; social class, ethnic origin, marital status and family size are other factors which have been shown to be related to utilization. These studies tell us who does and does not make use of the services, rather than why. To begin to answer the more complex question of why people seek or decline to seek professional help is to begin to theorize about illness behaviour.

It is crucial to recognize that whether or not people consult their doctors does not depend only on the presence of disease, but also on how they, or others, respond to its symptoms. Mechanic (1978) has listed 10 variables known to influence consulting behaviour (see Box 3.1). Mechanic acknowledges that this list is far from exhaustive and that in reality different variables tend to interact together. He also introduces a basic underlying distinction between 'self-defined' and 'other-defined' illness: the major difference is that, in the latter, individuals tend to resist the definitions that others attempt to impose upon them, and it may be necessary to bring them into treatment under great pressure, even involuntarily. Since it is not possible to explore all the multifarious and interrelated influences on illness and consulting behaviour here, six broad categories have been selected for emphasis.

BOX 3.1

MECHANIC'S VARIABLES KNOWN TO INFLUENCE ILLNESS BEHAVIOUR

1. Visibility, recognizability, or perceptual salience of signs and symptoms.

2. The extent to which the symptoms are perceived as serious (that is, the person's estimate of the present and future probabilities of danger).

3. The extent to which symptoms disrupt family, work and other social activities.

4. The frequency of the appearance of the signs or symptoms, their persistence, or their frequency or recurrence.

5. The tolerance threshold of those who are exposed to and evaluate the signs and symptoms.

6. Available information, knowledge and cultural assumptions and understandings of the evaluator.

7. Basic needs that lead to denial.

8. Needs competing with illness responses.

9. Competing possible interpretations that can be assigned to the symptoms once they are recognized.

10. Availability of treatment resources, physical proximity, and psychological and monetary costs of taking action (not only physical distance and costs of time, money and effort, but also such costs as stigma, social distance and feelings of humiliation).

Reproduced with permission of The Free Press from Mechanic (1978).

Cultural variation

The significance of cultural factors in determining how symptoms are interpreted has been well documented, perhaps most convincingly in studies of ethnicity and the experience and reporting of pain. In a pioneering study conducted in New York, Zborowski (1952) found that patients of Old-American or Irish origin displayed a stoical, matter-of-fact attitude towards pain and, if it was intense, a tendency to withdraw from the company of others. In contrast, patients of Italian or Jewish background were more demanding and dependent and tended to seek, rather than shun, public sympathy. Subsequent research has both corroborated Zborowski's findings and afforded support for the more general view that there is a marked cultural difference in the interpretation of and response to symptoms between so-called Anglo-Saxon and Mediterranean groups. It is tempting to assume that such cultural variation is explicable in terms of socialization alone, namely that differences in illness behaviour merely reflect different culturally learned styles of coping with the world at large. The authors of a study of Anglo-Saxon, Anglo-Greek and Greek groups in Australia, however, have suggested that other factors may also be important. They found, for example, that immigrant status and, relatedly, the stress of adapting to a majority culture, played a significant part in accounting for the different patterns of illness behaviour among the Anglo-Saxon and Mediterranean groups (Pilowski and Spence 1977). In short, cultural patterns may vary depending on the social context.

Phenomenology of symptoms and knowledge of disease

Studies have indicated that symptoms which present in a 'striking' way, for example, a sharp abdominal pain or a high fever, are more likely to be interpreted as illness and to receive prompt medical attention than those which present less dramatically. Consultation in such circumstances may simply be a function of the pain or discomfort; alternatively, it may be a function of the degree of incapacitation or disruption engendered by the pain or discomfort (see 'Triggers' below). Many distressing symptoms are not indicative of serious disease; but, equally, some serious diseases, for example, some cancers, rarely appear in a striking fashion: their onset may be slow and insidious. The actions of potential patients are thus also dependent on their knowledge of disease, and on their capacity to differentiate between diseases which are threatening/non-threatening and which can/cannot be effectively treated.

'Triggers'

Although many of the symptoms people experience are recognized as indicating disease processes, it is not necessarily the case that treatment is sought. What, when and if action to resolve any problems is undertaken often depends on a number of other factors. Zola (1973) has looked at the timing of decisions to seek medical care. He found that most people tolerated their symptoms for quite a time before they went to a doctor, and that the symptoms themselves were often not sufficient to precipitate a consultation: something else had to happen to bring this about. He identified five types of 'trigger':

1. the occurrence of an interpersonal crisis (e.g. a death in the family);
2. perceived interference with social or personal relations;
3. 'sanctioning' (pressure from others to consult);
4. perceived interference with vocational or physical activity; and
5. a kind of 'temporalizing of symptomatology' (the setting of a deadline, e.g. 'If I feel the same way on Monday . . .', or 'If I have another turn . . .').

The decision to seek professional help is, then, very much bound up with an individual's personal and social circumstances. Zola also found that, when doctors paid insufficient attention to the specific trigger which prompted an individual or which an individual used as an excuse to seek help, there was a greater chance that the patient would eventually break off treatment.

Perceptions of costs and benefits

Doctors and other health-care personnel tend to assume that a rational individual will report any symptoms which are causing him or her distress or anxiety; in other words, they take it for granted that the restoration of 'good health' is a natural first priority. Good health, however, is one goal among others; it is not always supreme. At any given time a person may deem obtaining treatment, which may perhaps involve hospitalization, to be less important or urgent than, for example, looking after young children or a dependent mother at home, preparing for an examination, being at work or going on holiday. Thus the value an individual attaches to good health varies in accordance with his or her perception of the benefits versus the costs of its accomplishment. The 'health belief model' represents one sustained attempt to bring together all these factors – from the demographic to the psychological – which influence an individual's assessment of the costs and benefits involved in seeking help.

Lay referral and intervention

It is comparatively rare for someone to decide in favour of a visit to the surgery without first discussing his or her symptoms with others. Scambler et al. (1981) found that three-quarters of those participating in their study discussed their symptoms with some other person, usually a relative, before seeking professional aid. Freidson (1970) has claimed that, just as doctors have a professional referral system, so potential patients have lay referral systems: 'the whole process of seeking help involves a network of potential consultants from the intimate confines of the nuclear family through successively more select, distant and authoritative laymen until the "professional" is reached'. Freidson has himself produced a model in terms of: (a) the degree of congruence between the subculture of the potential patient and that of doctors; and (b) the relative number of lay consultants interposed between the initial perception of symptoms and the decision whether or not to go to the doctor. Thus, for example, a situation in which the potential patient participates in a subculture which differs from that of doctors and in which there is an extended lay referral system would lead to the 'lowest' rate of utilization of medical services. In line with this example, one Scottish study reported that a high degree of interaction with interlocking kinship and friendship networks might well have 'inhibited' women in social class V from using antenatal care services (McKinlay 1973).

Occasionally lay persons may take it upon themselves to intervene and to initiate medical consultations (see Mechanic's other-defined illness above). This is most common when symptoms are perceived to be serious or life-threatening or when the sufferer is temporarily incapable of self-help: parents may take action on behalf of a child, a wife on behalf of a husband who is psychotic or who has experienced a tonic–clonic seizure. Scambler (1989) found that four out of five first consultations for epilepsy were other-initiated, many of them involving the calling of an ambulance. It has been suggested, however, that lay persons who are not members of the sufferer's family may be less likely than those who are to tolerate delays in help-seeking resulting from the normalization or denial of symptoms. Finlayson and McEwen (1977), for example, have described how the wives of some men tried in vain to persuade their husbands to see a doctor in the hour preceding myocardial infarction.

Access to healthcare facilities

Ease of access to healthcare facilities has obvious implications for usage. Tudor-Hart (1971) has argued that what he terms an inverse care law applies in Britain; that is, the provision of health care is inversely related to the need for it (i.e. poor facilities in depressed areas characterized by high morbidity and good, or better, facilities in affluent areas characterized by low morbidity). He relates this to the market economy: the more prosperous areas attract the most resources, including skilled health workers, in both primary and secondary care. Empirical support for this 'law' has accumulated steadily. More specifically, it has often been shown that, as the distance between home and general practice increases, the likelihood of consultation diminishes; this is particularly true for elderly or disabled people, who are relatively immobile (Whitehead 1992).

SELF-CARE, SELF-HELP AND ALTERNATIVE THERAPY

Evidence cited earlier showed that only a small minority of all symptoms are presented to a doctor. This suggests that self-care, and especially self-medication, may be of considerable importance. Wadsworth et al. (1971) found that self-treatment with non-prescribed medicines and home remedies is indeed extremely common. Dunnell and Cartwright (1972) found lower consultation rates among people who reported self-medication. They also found that in a 2-week period the ratio of non-prescribed to prescribed medicines taken by adults was approximately two to one; 67% of their sample had taken one or more non-prescribed medicines during this period. Moreover, only one in ten of the non-prescribed medicines consumed had been first suggested by a doctor; most were recommended by members of lay referral systems. The data suggested that adults tended to use self-medication as an alternative to medical consultation. Anderson et al. (1977) provide support for this interpretation, but add that, whereas self-medication seems to be more popular among non-users than among users of the primary-care services, non-users are also less inclined than users to obtain medical help for potentially serious symptoms. Dunnell and Cartwright found that, for children, self- or parent-medication seemed to be used more as a supplement to medical consultation.

Of particular interest too is the rapid growth of self-help groups. Some, like Alcoholics Anonymous, have been established for a long time and are well known, but there are many newer and less well-known groups – for people with schizophrenia, skin diseases, depression, hypertension, cancer, the parents of handicapped children, victims of disasters, and so on. Some of these were the brainchildren of health workers who are still active within them, but many operate quite independently of the formal health services; in fact, the impetus for the formation of a number of groups has been the lack of adequate understanding, care, treatment or support from the various health professions. Some commentators regard self-help groups as a poor substitute for people who are starved of 'real' services. Others, like Robinson (1980), argue that 'it is the professional health services which should be seen as specific technical, organizational or expert assistance'; they contend that self-help should be regarded as one of the basic components of primary health care.

Kelleher (1994) notes that although many of the activities of self-help groups can be seen as complementary to the work of health professionals, some also reflect 'a subversive readiness to question the knowledge of doctors and to assert that experiential knowledge has value'. Developing this theme, he suggests that self-help groups may constitute a new social movement. His argument is that modern medicine, like other 'expert systems', has become increasingly limited in its capacity to comprehend human suffering and to engage with patients; it pays far too little attention, for example, to how people with chronic illnesses define their own situations experientially and 'cope' on an everyday basis. Self-help groups, whether or not they comprise a social movement, allow people to diverge from the medical perspective and, if necessary, to challenge and interrogate it.

Apart from simply ignoring symptoms, another alternative to consulting a doctor or pursuing some form of self-care or self-help is to rely on alternative or non-orthodox therapies. Thomas et al. (1991) estimated that in 1987 there were 1909 registered, non-medical practitioners of non-orthodox health care, that is, of acupuncture, chiropractic, homoeopathy, medical herbalism, naturopathy and osteopathy, working in Britain (Table 3.2). The same authors report that of the 70 600 patients seen by this group of practitioners in an average week, 78% were attending for musculoskeletal problems. Two-thirds of the patients were women. About 36% of the patients had not received previous medical care for their main problem; 18% were receiving concurrent non-orthodox and medical care. It has been estimated that alternative or non-orthodox medicine is growing five times as rapidly as orthodox allopathic medicine. Recent survey evidence indicates that one in seven of the population currently go to alternative practitioners for care (Saks 1994).

The increasing popularity of non-orthodox therapy may in part be a function of people's disillusionment with biomedicine. Practitioners themselves stress also their longer consultations and a holistic orientation which concerns itself 'with complete wellness, not just symptomatology' (Bakx 1991). Saks (1994) cautions, however, that although alternative therapists, like self-help groups, are now offering a real challenge to the mode of practice of orthodox medicine, there is little evidence as yet that the legitimacy of medical authority is being seriously undermined.

To summarize, it has been shown that very often the decision whether or not to consult a doctor is not simply a function of the degree of pain or disability associated with symptoms or of their perceived seriousness. What Hannay (1980) has termed 'incongruous referral

TABLE 3.2 *Main treatment offered and use of multiple treatments by the membership of the professional association for estimated numbers (%) of registered non-orthodox practitioners.*

Main treatment	Registered practitioners		Practitioners in each group offering multiple treatments and having membership of only one association	
	No.	%	No.	%
Acupuncture	507	27	100	20
Chiropractic	290	15	6	2
Homoeopathy	93	5	12	13
Medical herbalism	115	6	45	39
Naturopathy with osteopathy	128	7	41	32[a]
Osteopathy	680	36	34	5
Member of more than one association	96	5	—	
Total	1909	100	238	12

Reproduced with permission from Thomas et al. (1991).
[a] *Practitioners offering at least one treatment in addition to naturopathy and osteopathy.*

behaviour' is commonplace. The heterogeneous assembly of factors which are known to influence decisions about medical consultation has been indicated. It has been stressed too, however, that the study of illness behaviour is not concerned exclusively with whether or not people visit doctors. On the basis of anthropological work, Kleinman (1985) suggested that there are typically three major arenas of care in what he calls 'local health care systems': popular, folk and professional (Fig. 3.2).

Most health care takes place in the popular sector, which embraces self-care, including self-medication, and those self-help groups which function independently of professional health workers. The folk sector comprises non-professional 'specialists' who offer some form of alternative or non-orthodox therapy. Professionalization, Kleinman contends, has a tendency to distance practitioners from patients and to lead to a focus on (medically defined) disease as opposed to (patient defined) illness. Of the professional sector in western societies he writes: 'Western-oriented biomedicine seems to be the more extreme example of this trend, perhaps because biomedical ideology and norms are more remote from (one almost wants to say estranged from) the life world of most patients'. He considers that the major challenge is to 're-work medicine's paradigm of clinical practice to make it more responsive to indigenous patient values, beliefs and expectations'. Agree or disagree, there is no question that the study of illness behaviour must address itself to the popular and folk as well as to the professional sectors of local health-care system.

Fig. 3.2 *Local health care systems. (Reproduced with permission from Tavistock Publications from Kleinman 1985.)*

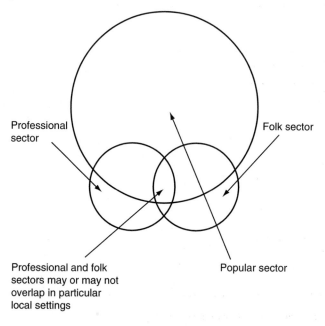

Professional sector

Folk sector

Professional and folk sectors may or may not overlap in particular local settings

Popular sector

Health care system

REFERENCES

Anderson, J., Buck, C., Danaher, K. & Fry, J. (1977) Users and non-users of doctors – implications for care. *J. R. Coll. Gen. Pract.*, **27**, 155–9.

Bakx, K. (1991) The 'eclipse' of folk medicine in Western society. *Sociol. Health Illness*, **13**, 20–57.

Blaxter, M. (1990) *Health and Lifestyles*. London: Tavistock/Routledge.

Blaxter, M. & Paterson, E. (1982) *Mothers and Daughters*. London: Heinemann Educational.

Cartwright, A. & Anderson, R. (1981) *General Practice Revisited: A Second Study of Patients and their Doctors*. London: Tavistock.

Central Statistical Office (1990) *Social Trends 20*. London: HMSO.

Dunnell, K. & Cartwright, A. (1972) *Medicine-Takers, Prescribers and Hoarders*. London: Routledge & Kegan Paul.

Epsom, J. (1978) The mobile health clinic: a report on the first year's work. In: *Basic Readings in Medical Sociology*, ed. D. Tuckett & J. Kauffert. London: Tavistock.

Featherstone, M. (1991) The body in consumer culture. In: *The Body: Social Processes and Cultural Theory*, ed. M. Featherstone, M. Hepworth & B. Turner. London; Sage.

Finlayson, A. & McEwen, J. (1977) *Coronary Heart Disease and Patterns of Living*. London: Croom Helm.

Freidson, E. (1970) *Profession of Medicine*. New York: Dodds, Mead.

Hannay, D. (1980) The iceberg of illness and trivial consultations. *J. R. Coll. Gen. Pract.*, **30**, 551–4.

Herzlich, C. (1973) *Health and Illness*. London: Academic Press.

Ingham, J. & Miller, P. (1979) Symptom prevalence and severity in a general practice. *Epidemiol. Commun. Health*, **33**, 191–8.

Kelleher, D. (1994) Self-help groups and their relationship to medicine. In: *Challenging Medicine,* ed. J. Gabe, D. Kelleher & G. Williams. London: Routledge.

Kleinman, A. (1985) Indigenous systems of healing: questions for professional, popular and folk care. In: *Alternative Medicines: Popular and Policy Perspectives*, ed. J. Salmon. London: Tavistock.

McKinlay, J. (1973) Social networks, lay consultation and help-seeking behaviour. *Soc. Forces*, **53**, 255–92.

Mechanic, D. (1978) *Medical Sociology*, 2nd edn. New York: Free Press.

OPCS (Office of Population Censuses and Surveys). *Health Survey for England, 1993*. London; HMSO.

Nettleton, S. (1995) *The Sociology of Health and Illness*. Cambridge: Polity Press.

Pill, R. & Scott, N. (1982) Concepts of illness causation and responsibility: some preliminary data from a sample of working-class mothers. *Soc. Sci. Med.*, **16**, 43–52.

Pilowski, I. & Spence, N. (1977) Ethnicity and illness behaviour. *Psychol. Med.*, **7**, 447–52.

Robinson, D. (1980) The self-help component of primary care. *Soc. Sci. Med.*, **14A**, 415–21.

Saks, M. (1994) The alternatives to medicine. In: *Challenging Medicine*, ed. J. Gabe, D. Kelleher & G. Williams. London: Routledge.

Scambler, A., Scambler, G. & Craig, D. (1981) Kinship and friendship networks and women's demand for primary care. *J. R. Coll. Gen. Pract.*, **26**, 746–50.

Scambler, G. (1989) *Epilepsy*. London: Routledge.

Thomas, K., Carr, J., Westlake, L. & Williams, B. (1991) Use of non-orthodox and conventional health care in Great Britain. *Br. Med. J.*, **302**, 207–10.

Tudor-Hart, J. (1971) The inverse care law. *Lancet*, **i**, 405–12.

Wadsworth, M., Butterfield, W. & Blaney, R. (1971) *Health and Sickness: The Choice of Treatment*. London: Tavistock.

Whitehead, M. (1992) *The Health Divide*, 2nd edn. London: Penguin.

Zborowski, M. (1952) Cultural components in response to pain. *J. Soc. Issues*, **8**, 16–30.

Zola, I. (1973) Pathways to the doctor: from person to patient. *Soc. Sci. Med.*, **7**, 677–89.

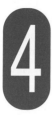

The Doctor–Patient Relationship

MYFANWY MORGAN

The essential unit of medical practice is viewed as the occasion when, in the intimacy of the consulting room, or sick room, a person who is ill, or believes himself to be ill, seeks the advice of a doctor whom he trusts. Such meetings are a frequent and regular occurrence, with over half a million consultations occurring between general practitioners and their patients in the UK every working day and a large number also taking place at a hospital level. Their success or otherwise depends not only on the doctors' clinical knowledge and technical skills, but also on the nature of the social relationship that exists between doctor and patient.

This chapter first examines the general societal expectations that influence the behaviours of doctors and patients in the medical consultation, and describes some of the conflicts that may be experienced by doctors in responding to both the demands and expectations of the wider community and the needs and interests of individual patients. It then considers the forms and determinants of the interaction between individual doctors and patients in the consultation, and the significance of these social processes for patients' satisfaction and the clinical and psychosocial outcomes of medical care.

SOCIAL ROLES OF DOCTORS AND PATIENTS

Parsons (1951) was one of the earliest sociologists to examine the relationship between doctors and patients. His interest arose from a concern with how society is able to function smoothly and respond to problems of deviance. Parsons regarded social functioning as partly achieved through the existence of institutionalized roles with socially prescribed patterns of behaviour. We are, therefore, all aware how people are likely to behave when they occupy the role of father, teacher, shop assistant, etc. and of their expectations of us when we occupy the complementary role of child, pupil or customer. Parsons regarded doctors and patients as similarly occupying social roles which facilitate interaction as they define the expectations and obligations of each participant. In addition, they form a mechanism for coping with the problem of illness by ensuring that patients return to health and normal role performance as quickly as possible.

Parsons' description of the roles of doctor and patient is presented as an 'ideal type' model. This abstracts and presents what are regarded as the fundamental features of a particular social organization or social role and is an important method of analysing and describing very complex social phenomena.

Parsons' model of the sick role and doctor's role

Parsons depicted the role of sick people as involving four general expectations. First, sick people are allowed, and may even be required, to give up some of their normal activities and responsibilities, such as going to work or playing football for the local team, and secondly they are regarded as being in need of care. These two expectations and privileges are, however, contingent on the sick person fulfilling the obligations of wanting to get well as quickly as possible, seeking professional medical advice and, most importantly for the doctor–patient relationship, co-operating with the doctor (Table 4.1).

TABLE 4.1 *Parsons' analysis of the roles of patients and doctors.*

Patient: sick role	Doctor: professional role
Obligations and privileges	*Expected to*
1. Must want to get well as quickly as possible	1. Apply a high degree of skill and knowledge to the problems of illness
2. Should seek professional medical advice and co-operate with the doctor	2. Act for welfare of patient and community rather than for own self-interest, desire for money, advancement, etc.
3. Allowed (and may be expected) to shed some normal activities and responsibilities (e.g. employment and household tasks)	3. Be objective and emotionally detached (i.e. should not judge patients' behaviour in terms of personal value system or become emotionally involved with them)
4. Regarded as being in need of care and unable to get better by his or her own decisions and will	4. Be guided by rules of professional practice
	Rights
	1. Granted right to examine patients physically and to enquire into intimate areas of physical and personal life
	2. Granted considerable autonomy in professional practice
	3. Occupies position of authority in relation to the patient

Reprinted with permission from The Free Press from Parsons (1951).

Parsons points out that the specific expectations of the sick person, such as the number and type of activities the ill person is expected to give up, will be influenced by the nature and severity of the condition. It is also recognized that not all illness requires people to relinquish their normal social roles and occupy the status 'sick'. For example, much minor illness is coped with without recourse to the doctor and does not require any changes to a person's everyday life (Chapter 3). Similarly, people with a chronic illness may need to consult the doctor regularly, but rather than occupying a permanent sick role they are generally expected to try to achieve their maximum level of functioning, and to occupy the status 'sick' only if they experience a change in their usual health. Parsons thus viewed the sick role as a *temporary* social role which has been instituted by society with the aim of returning sick people to a state of health and restoring them to fully functioning members of society as quickly as possible. The sick role is also regarded as a *universal* role, in that its obligations and expectations apply to all sick people whatever their age, gender, ethnicity, occupation or status in other spheres.

Parsons viewed the role of the doctor as complementary to the role of patient. Whereas the patient is expected to co-operate fully with the doctor, doctors are expected to apply their specialist knowledge and skills for the benefit of the patient, and to act for the welfare of the patient and community rather than in their own self-interest. Doctors are also expected to be objective and emotionally detached and to be guided by the rules of professional practice. Conformity with these general expectations is depicted as an essential requirement for carrying out the tasks of diagnosis and treatment, which often involve the need to know intimate details about the patient that are not usually known between strangers and may, for example, require the conduct of an intimate physical examination or information about the patient's personal affairs. Parsons also viewed doctors as enjoying considerable autonomy in executing their professional skills and occupying a position of authority in relation to the patient.

Parsons' analysis thus identifies the general expectations that guide the behaviour of doctors and patients, and shows how these roles facilitate interaction in the consultation as both parties are aware how each other is expected to behave, and also serve to reduce the potentially disruptive effects of illness in society. The latter is partly achieved through the role of the doctor in officially legitimating illness and acting as a gatekeeper to the sick role, thus preventing inappropriate occupancy and enjoyment of the privileges of the sick role, such as time off work or financial benefits. The expectations placed on both doctors and patients also ensure that people who are officially sanctioned as sick are returned to a state of health and normal role performance as quickly as possible, thus contributing to the smooth functioning of society (see Chapter 13).

Conflicts in the doctor's role

Whereas Parsons' analysis emphasizes the consensual nature of the roles and relationships between doctors and patients, in reality tensions and strains often exist. One set of tensions arises from the conflicting demands placed on doctors, who are required to act in the best interests of their patients and also have a duty to serve the interests of the state. As Parsons recognized, doctors serve the state as agents of social control in their role as gatekeepers to the sick role with authority to determine who is 'healthy' and who is 'sick', but also have an obligation to act in the best interests of individual patients. When patients request, or even demand, a sick note, problems can arise for the doctor in determining whether disease exists and the designation of 'sick' and privileges of the sick role can be justified. For example, back pain is the major reason for time off work, but it is often difficult to determine its cause or severity except by relying on patients' reports which may present problems in determining the legitimacy of patients' claims to the sick role. In such situations of uncertainty should doctors give priority to the interests of the patient, or to their societal function in ensuring that people do not malinger or occupy the sick role inappropriately? Similarly, should doctors inform the licensing authority if they are aware that a patient diagnosed with epilepsy is driving a car and thus contravening the state's regulations, and should they inform patients thinking of being tested for human immunodeficiency virus (HIV) of the potential problems of being diagnosed as a carrier for insurance premiums when this might discourage testing? In addition, doctors may experience conflicts between their own values and those of some of their patients in relation to abortion, homosexuality, AIDS and other conditions or behaviours invested with moral evaluations.

A further source of conflict for doctors arises from the competing interests of individual patients and the larger patient population. For example, doctors are often involved in rationing scarce resources of staff time, beds and medical equipment and may have to decide which patients should be given a transplant or undergo other medical procedures, as well as the priority to be assigned to treating different cases. In the absence of clear and explicit criteria, such choices rest on the judgement of individual clinicians. A recent illustration is the decision made by some consultants not to administer tests and carry out coronary artery by-pass surgery on people who continue to smoke. This is based on the argument that scarce resources should not be spent on people who smoke, as such people have longer hospital stays and less chance of recovery, and treating them deprives patients who have never smoked or who have stopped smoking (Underwood and Bailey 1993). However, such reasoning raises questions of how far the notion of culpability and self-inflicted ill health should extend. For example, what is the situation in the prescribing of nebulizers to asthmatic smokers and the treatment of drunken victims of road accidents?

Doctors may also experience conflicts between maintaining the confidentiality of the doctor–patient relationship and disclosing information to a patient's parent or spouse. This raises the question of whether medical confidentiality is absolute, or whether there are any situations when interests are best served by passing on information about a patient. For example, are there are any circumstances in which a clinic doctor should disclose that a patient has acquired immunodeficiency syndrome (AIDS), or is positive for HIV, when this is against the patient's wishes? Such situations frequently pose dilemmas for doctors and raise questions concerning their primary duties and responsibilities, as well as possibly presenting conflicts in relation to their own beliefs and values. However, there are powerful arguments to support the view that priority should be given to maintaining the confidentiality of the doctor–patient relationship. In particular this has the benefit of preserving patients' trust in doctors and their willingness to consult and discuss their problems freely in the future, for destroying this trust undermines the very foundation of the relationship between doctor and patient (Lockwood 1985).

CLINICAL AND PSYCHOSOCIAL OUTCOMES OF THE CONSULTATION

An important aspect of the consultation is the information communicated by patients, with a good history often being central to diagnosis and treatment decisions, and is itself sufficient for the doctor to make a correct diagnosis in more than half of all patients (Myerscough 1992). However, unless patients feel at ease and are encouraged to talk freely they may not disclose the problems that are troubling them or express their worries and concerns. This is illustrated by a study of general practice patients, which showed that 60% of the patients who reported symptoms in answer to a brief questionnaire had not mentioned some of these in the consultation. Major reasons given for this included feeling that it was not appropriate to ask (36%), feeling hurried (27%), being frightened that the doctor would think less well of them (14%) and being frightened of a bad reaction from the doctor (14%) (Tuckett et al. 1985). It is also well known that some patients, if they feel very embarrassed or worried about a problem, will present a condition which forms a 'ticket of entry' to the consultation. Whether such patients disclose their 'real' problem or this remains 'hidden' often depends on what they perceive as the general atmosphere of the consultation and opportunities for a sensitive discussion.

Barriers to communication and a failure to elicit patients' worries and interpretation of symptoms may sometimes lead doctors to believe that patients have consulted inappropriately. For example, mothers often consult about a childhood cough, with 30% of all consultations for children aged less than 11 years being for respiratory conditions. Many of these consultations are for a condition that is 'trivial' from a biomedical perspective. However, a study of mothers who had consulted their general practitioner for this reason revealed that this was often due to fears that their child would experience long-term chest damage, or even die from choking in phlegm or vomit or through an asthma attack or cot death, and there was also a common belief that antibiotics were required to break up the phlegm (Cornford et al. 1993).

Patients' satisfaction with the consultation depends on both the doctor's clinical and interpersonal skills, and may itself have a positive effect on the pain and other symptoms experienced. For example, a longitudinal study of patients attending neurological clinics for the diagnosis and treatment of severe headache showed that for half the patients seen the main factor related to a reduction in symptom severity appeared to be patients' satisfaction with the initial consultation. Of particular importance was being given information and advice which they felt relevant to their worries and which enabled them to make sense of their symptoms and achieve a sense of control over their illness (Fitzpatrick et al. 1983). Similarly, a series of randomized control trials of patients with diabetes mellitus, hypertension and peptic ulcer, indicated that the amount of emotion (positive or negative) expressed by doctor or patient, and the quality of information sought by patients and given by doctors, formed important influences on patients' functional capacity and physiological measurements on follow-up, and their satisfaction with care (Kaplan et al. 1989). These positive clinical outcomes may have been partly a product of the influence of patients' satisfaction with the consultation on their subsequent adherence with medical advice and treatments. It is known that on average about 50% of people with chronic conditions do not take drugs as prescribed, either taking them irregularly, taking a reduced dose or not taking them at all. Important reasons are that patients often remain worried about possible harmful effects of the drugs, do not understand how they should be taken, or do not think they are appropriate or necessary for their medical problem (Beardon et al. 1993). Another beneficial effect of the social relationship between doctor and patient is what has been termed the 'placebo' effect (which literally means 'I will please'). This is calculated to account for as much as one-third of the success of any drug (Beecher 1955). To take account of this healing effect, trials of new drugs often involve the administration of an inert substance to a control group for comparison.

TYPES OF DOCTOR–PATIENT RELATIONSHIP

The significance of the social relationship between doctor and patient for the clinical, psychosocial and behavioural outcomes of the consultation has resulted in considerable attention being given to the various forms and determinants of this relationship. Whereas Parsons' model identifies general societal expectations which guide the behaviour of doctors and patients, his portrayal of an asymmetrical relationship in which the doctor occupies the dominant position by virtue of his or her specialist knowledge and the patient merely co-operates (a 'paternalistic' relationship), is viewed as only one possible form of relationship. Other forms arise from differences in the relative power and control exercised by doctors and patients (Table 4.2). In reality these different models may not exist in pure form, but nevertheless most consultations tend towards one type.

A **paternalistic** relationship involving high physician control and low patient control describes a situation where the doctor is dominant and acts as a 'parent' figure who is trusted by the patient and decides what he or she believes to be in the patient's best interest. This form of relationship traditionally characterized medical consultations, and at some stages of illness patients derive considerable comfort from being able to rely on the doctor in this way and being relieved of burdens of worry and decision-making. However, medical consultations are now increasingly characterized by greater patient control and relationships based on *mutuality*.

A relationship of **mutuality** is characterized by the active involvement of patients as more equal partners in the consultation. The doctor brings clinical skills and knowledge to the consultation and patients bring their own theories, experiences, expectations and feelings. Both parties thus participate as a joint venture on and engage in an exchange of ideas and sharing of belief systems.

A **consumerist** relationship describes a situation in which power relationships are reversed and the patient takes the active role, whereas the doctor adopts a fairly passive role and accedes

TABLE 4.2 Types of doctor–patient relationship.

	Physician control	
Patient control	Low	High
Low	Default	Paternalism
High	Consumerist	Mutuality

Reprinted with permission from Sage Publications, Inc. from Stewart and Roter (1989) p. 21.

to the patient's requests for a second opinion, referral to hospital, a sick note, etc. Such a relationship mainly occurs in a situation where doctors are dependent on patients' goodwill for their business and financial security.

A relationship of **default** may occur if patients continue to adopt a passive role even though doctors reduce some of their control, with the result that the consultation may lack sufficient direction. This situation may occur if patients are not aware of alternatives to a passive patient role and are timid in adopting a more participative relationship.

Different types of relationship, and particularly those characterized by paternalism and mutuality, can be viewed as appropriate to different conditions and stages of illness. At an acute stage of illness it may be necessary or desirable for the doctor to be dominant, whereas at later stages it may be beneficial for patients to be more actively involved as they are responsible for the everyday management of their condition. For example, patients with diabetes mellitus rely episodically on the doctor's expertise, but are required to assume considerable responsibility for their condition and to monitor their own blood sugar level and alter the dose of insulin or tablets accordingly. Relationships based on mutuality are also of particular importance in a primary care setting, in view of general practitioners' location as the first point of contact for patients and their need to understand the nature of the presenting problem in terms of patients' own beliefs about the causes of their condition, the possible influence of social and emotional factors in exacerbating the condition or triggering a consultation, and patients' particular worries and concerns or expectations of the consultation. However, there is considerable variation in the nature of the relationship between doctor and patient which cannot be explained entirely in terms of the patient's medical condition, but is also influenced by the expectations of doctor and of patient and the structural context of the consultation.

INFLUENCES ON THE DOCTOR–PATIENT RELATIONSHIP

Doctor's orientation and practice style

A major determinant of the nature of the doctor–patient relationship and the extent and forms of communication within the consultation is the doctor's clinical practice style. Byrne and Long (1976), on the basis of tape-recorded interviews of nearly 2500 general practitioner consultations, identified two polar types of consultation style which they termed '*doctor-centred*' and '*patient-centred*'. They found that for three-quarters of the doctors their clinical-practice style tended toward the doctor-centred end of the spectrum. This was characterized by the traditional Parsonian model and *paternalistic* approach, based on the assumption that the doctor is the expert and the patient is merely required to co-operate. Doctors adopting this practice style focused on the physical aspects of the patient's disease and employed tightly controlled interviewing methods aimed at reaching an organic diagnosis as quickly as possible. Questions were thus mainly of a 'closed' nature, such as 'how long have you had the pain?', 'is it sharp or dull?', and aimed to provide information to enable doctors to interpret the patient's illness within their own biomedical disease framework, while providing little opportunity for patients to express their own beliefs and concerns.

At the other end of the continuum were doctors whose consultation style conformed to a patient-centred approach. These doctors adopted a much less authoritarian style and encouraged and facilitated patients' participation in the consultation, thus fostering a relationship character-ized as 'mutuality'. An important feature of this approach was their greater use of 'open' ques-tions, such as 'tell me about the pain', 'how do you feel?', 'what do you think is the cause of the problem?' They also spent more time listening to patients' problems, picking up and responding to patients' cues, encouraging expression of their ideas or feelings and clarifying and interpreting patients' statements.

Byrne and Long found that individual general practitioners could be classified fairly consis-tently as holding either doctor-centred or patient-centred consultations. This suggests that doc-tors develop a particular consulting style which they then employ fairly consistently and do not vary their style significantly in relation to the patient's problems. However, those classified as having a patient-centred style showed the greatest ability to respond to differences in patients' needs or the circumstances of the consultation (Box 4.1).

These differences in communication style reflect not only doctors' communication skills and training but also differences in their attitudes and orientations to the medical task. Doctors who hold a strictly disease-centred model tend to focus almost exclusively on pathophysiological processes, with the aim of reaching a clinical diagnosis as quickly as possible and prescribing appro-priate treatment. In contrast, doctors taking a more patient-oriented approach give greater empha-sis to the importance of people's subjective experience and meanings of illness, recognizing that patients' own beliefs about their condition and its significance for their lives may influence their illness behaviours, expectations of the consultation and subsequent satisfaction and adherence with medical advice and treatment. In some cases stressful events in a person's life may also contribute to physical symptoms, such as abdominal pains, or increase risks of depression, especially if patients lack a strong confiding relationship or other sources of self-esteem and support.

The differences in doctors' orientations and approach to medicine can be illustrated in relation to the task of diagnosing the patient's problem. For doctors adopting a patient-centred approach the task of diagnosis involves not only using clinical skills to identify the patient's disease, but also

---

BOX 4.1

CLINICAL PRACTICE STYLES

Patient-centred	Doctor-centred
High use of:	High use of:
listening	analysing
reflecting	
probing	
silence	active information gathering
clarifying	
facilitating	
interpreting	

eliciting the patient's illness framework in terms of their beliefs about the causes and seriousness of their problem (Fig. 4.1). This approach is also frequently accompanied by greater attention to the psychosocial aspects of illness, in terms of the possible psychosocial origins of the patient's problem, and their experience of anxiety, depression and other emotional problems, as well as a greater recognition of the impact of chronic and disabling illness on the patient's self-concept and everyday activities. Diagnosis and management of the patient's problem may thus require the integration of two forms of knowledge represented by the medical disease framework and the patient's illness framework. Moreover, whereas the doctor as the medical expert traditionally made treatment choices on behalf of patients, doctors characterized by a more patient-centred approach often adopt a participative style, recognizing that the benefits of different forms of treatment may depend on the patient's own evaluations and life circumstances. In situations when various options exist these are therefore frequently presented and discussed with patients, although patients may often choose to be guided by the doctor.

Fig. 4.1 *The patient-centred clinical interview. (Reproduced with permission from Sage Publications from Levenstein et al., 1989.)*

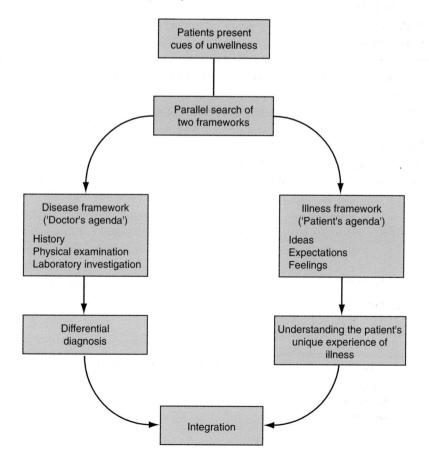

Medical training is now giving increasing emphasis to a whole-person approach to medicine which takes account of patients' beliefs, meanings and experiences and the social context of their illness experience rather than focusing exclusively on a disease-centred model. However, this orientation and an accompanying patient-centred practice style is currently most common among younger doctors, and especially in general practice.

Influence of time

Doctors frequently identify a shortage of time as the major constraint on adopting a patient-oriented approach, with general practice consultations averaging about 6 minutes, although this obscures wide variations in the actual length of consultations, which range from about 2 minutes to over 20 minutes. Pressures of time encourage a more tightly controlled doctor-centred (or 'paternalistic') consultation with less attention paid to the social and psychological aspects of a patient's illness, fewer psychological problems identified and more prescriptions issued (Howie et al. 1992). However, the doctor's own approach to medicine and practice style has been shown to exert a more important influence on the content of consultations than the time available. This was demonstrated by an experiment in general practice in which the time available for consultations was increased to 10 minutes. As a result all doctors asked more questions. However, other skills, such as facilitating patients' participation and explaining the nature of their medical problem, were employed more frequently only by those doctors who already emphasized these aspects of communication. Doctors who usually employed these behaviours least frequently did not necessarily change their practice with the longer booking intervals. Rather than remedying any deficits and changing their style of communication, these doctors tended to increase what they already did and asked more questions, and many did not take advantage of the extended consultation time available (Ridsdale et al. 1992). It has also been shown that general practitioners with a more patient-oriented approach often prefer to run over time, and possibly keep other patients waiting, if they feel it is necessary to spend additional time with a particular patient. These doctors may also deliberately restrict their list size, so that they are able to provide what they regard as good-quality care. As a result, the length of time available for consultations is itself partly a function of practice style, as well as pressures of time serving to constrain the consultation. However, although a more participative patient-centred consultation does require rather greater time, giving sufficient time to listen and respond to patients' worries and concerns may reduce the number of return visits and hence the total consultation time for an episode of illness, as well as often reducing stress levels and increasing job satisfaction for doctors (Wilson et al. 1991).

Influence of structural context

An important aspect of general practice is the continuity of care, with the opportunity for doctors and patients to know each other over a long period. Consultations thus often draw on prior knowledge of the patient's circumstances, past history and concerns rather than forming an isolated encounter. As a result much information is already shared and the consultation takes place in this familiar context.

The content of consultations is also influenced by the system of financing of health care, with consultations financed on a fee-for-service basis generally being longer and doctors' practice style more patient-oriented than when they are paid on a per capita or salaried basis. This is because a fee-for-service payment is often associated with a greater availability of resources and greater priority being given to pleasing the patient; and patients themselves feel they have greater rights to ask questions and have their desires for information met. However, a recent change associated with the introduction of the provider market in the NHS and the Patient's Charter has been the development of a more consumer-oriented approach to medical care, with greater emphasis given to improving the organizational aspects of care (waiting times, facilities, etc.), and providing patients with increased verbal and written information and involvement in treatment decisions.

Patients' expectations and participation

Patients' expectation of a more equal or *mutualistic* relationship with doctors is greater among younger people than among the elderly age group, and generally increases over the course of an illness as patients gain more knowledge and understanding of the condition. This is illustrated by a study of the diagnosis and management of childhood epilepsy which showed that during the initial consultation patients were passive, uncritical and appeared satisfied. However, by the third consultation parents had moved from a situation of low to high control and had begun to initiate questions themselves and to force information out of the doctor. They were also more critical and less satisfied with the doctor, and in some cases this led to a threatened rejection of the doctor's authority and expertise (West 1976).

Patients with a high social and educational level also tend to participate more in the consultation in terms of asking questions and asking for explanations and clarification, compared with patients from a lower socioeconomic background and educational level. This possibly reflects their greater knowledge and confidence and the smaller status gap between doctor and patient. The influence of socioeconomic position was demonstrated in a study of 1470 general practice consultations, which showed that only 27% of working-class patients sought clarification from the doctor about what he had said compared with 45% of middle-class patients. This request for information by patients in turn led to fuller explanations being given by doctors and a rather longer consultation (Tuckett et al. 1985). There is also evidence that doctors volunteer more explanations to some groups of patients, including more educated patients and male patients, even when the explanation is not explicitly requested by the patient, reflecting doctors' own assumptions of the interests of different patient groups (Street 1991). Some patients may therefore be doubly disadvantaged, because of both their passive communication styles and doctors' (mis)perceptions of their informational needs and desires.

A particular set of problems may arise when doctors themselves become patients, as they often experience role ambiguity which constrains their ability to behave like 'typical' patients. This arises because they possess specialized medical knowledge and may be in a position to make informed choices about treatment options and challenge the treating doctor. Such factors may also influence the performance of treating doctors, who may wish to involve the patient–colleague in the consultation more than they might a lay patient. This may be out of deference to the doctor–patient's status and knowledge, or out of a feeling that their own competence is under scrutiny. A study of recently sick doctors found that some doctor–patients complained that they were not given information about their illness or were not appropriately counselled. This is because it was assumed that the doctor–patient was already adequately informed, whereas they felt a need to occupy a more usual patient role and for the treating doctor to pro-vide relevant clinical information and discuss the patient's 'illness.' Other doctor–patients thought they were too involved in decision-making and management of the illness because the treating doctor was unable to take control of the consultation. Some also commented that their doctor seemed embarrassed to treat them, with these problems being most common where the treating doctor was of a lower grade or younger than the patient. Most doctors commented that they found it instructive to experience the doctor–patient encounter from the patient's perspective and some suggested that this transformed their professional sympathy into empathy (McKevitt et al. 1995).

Conflicts in the doctor–patient relationship

Conflicts between doctors and patients rarely become overt. However, in some situations where disagreement occurs about the appropriate course of action each may try to persuade the other of the merits of their own point of view. Patients may therefore present particular aspects of their own case which they believe justifies their request for a referral, more urgent treatment or other action, while doctors may try to convince patients that their approach is best. This may involve overwhelming patients with evidence in the form of laboratory tests or their own previous ex-perience in treating patients with similar types of conditions, perhaps accompanied by a warning of the likely consequences of neglecting their advice.

In some situations either the doctor or patient manages to achieve their desired outcome, but often a compromise or temporary agreement is reached. For example, Waissman (1990) describes the process of negotiating to reconcile doctors' and patients' choices regarding the use of home or hospital dialysis for children with renal disease. She also shows how the doctors' deci-sion and choice of home dialysis was later re-negotiated by parents and other arrangements made if they continued to have difficulty in managing the dialysis at home. Although patients some-times successfully negotiate their treatment and other aspects of their medical care, except in sit-uations characterized by a strong consumerist relationship the doctor retains ultimate control of the consultation as a result of their professional status and specialist knowledge and their greater experience in managing the encounter. Moreover, patients generally display a deferential man-ner in the consulting room, reflecting the traditional expectations of the patient role. As a result, they rarely express dissatisfaction or tell the doctor when they disagree with advice or have no intention of following it. Indeed some patients regularly attend general practitioners for repeat prescriptions even if they do not take the medication or take it only irregularly, in order to keep up the appearance of being a good patient (Morgan and Watkins 1988).

DOCTORS' COMMUNICATION SKILLS

Communication in the consultation is influenced by both doctors' perception of the medical task and consequent practice style and their skills in the technical aspects of communication. The lat-ter involves techniques for providing information and explanations to patients in a manner which will promote their understanding and recall, and ways of eliciting information from patients and facilitating their accounts (Ley 1988).

Communication involves both verbal and non-verbal behaviours. Non-verbal communication contributes to the rapport between doctor and patient and influences the amount of information exchanged. For example, by maintaining eye contact, looking attentive, nodding encouragingly and other gestures doctors can provide positive feedback to patients. In contrast, continued riffling through notes, twiddling with pens, or failing to look directly at patients, may convey disinterest and result in patients failing to describe their problems or seek information and explanation. Indeed it is estimated that in a normal two-person conversation the verbal component carries less than 35% of the social meaning of the situation, and 65% or more is carried by the non-verbal component such as eye contact, gaze, facial expressions and posture (Pietroni 1976) (Box 4.2). Patients are regarded as particularly sensitive to and observant of the non-verbal communications conveyed by their doctors. This is because of the expectations surrounding the relationship, which means that both parties are generally reluctant to express negative sentiments, and because illness usually involves emotions such as fear, anxiety and emotional uncertainty. As a consequence, patients often look for clues to assess the situation and are active in searching for information about different aspects of their disease.

Interaction is also influenced by physical proximity and the relative positions of doctor and patient in the consulting room. Seating of equal height and the lack of a physical barrier between participants encourages communication. This was demonstrated by an experiment in which a cardiologist removed the desk from his clinic on alternate days. When the desk was removed 50% of the patients sat back in their chair and in at-ease positions, whereas only 10% did so when he was sitting behind his desk, with a corresponding decline in the amount of communication by patients (Pietroni 1976).

There are differences not only in the success of doctors in eliciting information but also in ensuring that patients understand their advice and explanations. The failure of patients to understand and their forgetting information given in the medical consultation is common and has been attributed to: (1) doctors' failure to elicit and respond to patients' illness frameworks which may lead to a process of reinterpretation so that the message received by patients differs from the

---

BOX 4.2

STRATEGIES FOR CONTROLLING THE CONSULTATION

Verbal:

- Persuasion
- Negotiation and bargaining

Non verbal:

- 'Body language' (e.g. facial expressions, gestures, posture)
- Behaviours (e.g. standing up, reaching for prescription pad)

original one; (2) patients' lack of understanding of medical terminology; and (3) problems of memory and recall. Promoting greater patient understanding and recall thus requires changes both in doctors' clinical practice style and the adoption of good techniques of oral communication (Box 4.3). This may also be supplemented and reinforced by the use of well-designed information booklets and leaflets to aid remembering and enable patients to acquire information outside the pressures of the consulting room.

Particular problems of communication and demands on doctors arise in disclosing a diagnosis of cancer and giving other 'sad or bad news'. Traditionally doctors withheld such information for as long as possible. This was justified as being in the patients' own interest, although maintaining patients' uncertainty once the diagnosis was firmly based may also have been functional for doctors in protecting them from the stress associated with such disclosures. A more open approach is now generally adopted, supported by patients' desire to be informed and the positive effects that this can have in reducing uncertainty and promoting positive coping (Ong et al. 1995). For example, Blanchard et al. (1988) found that 92% of hospitalized adult cancer patients interviewed desired all the information about their disease, good and bad, although only 69% preferred to participate in treatment-related decisions. However, the giving of such information must be handled sensitively and may involve not only the presentation of factual medical details (e.g. the diagnosis and prognosis, the stage of disease and recommended treatment), but also doctors should elicit and respond to patients' personal worries, such as the pain they may experience, the side effects of treatment, how they will feel and what they will be able to do (Fallowfield 1993). The difficulties experienced by doctors in coping with patients' emotional responses also means that they often develop routinized forms of disclosure to inform patients about the diagnosis of a terminal condition, rather than responding to individual patients' needs.

BOX 4.3

COMMUNICATION TECHNIQUES FOR INCREASING PATIENT UNDERSTANDING AND RECALL

1. Use of primacy effect – give instructions and advice before other information

2. Emphasis – stress the importance of particular content

3. Simplification – use of short words and sentences

4. Explicit categorization – tell patients what categories of information are to be provided and then present information category by category

5. Repetition (by doctor or patient)

6. Give specific information (e.g. 'you need to lose 12 kilos,' rather than 'you need to lose weight')

7. Provide additional written information – booklets, leaflets

Reproduced with permission from Ley (1988) pp. 89–93.

CHANGES IN THE DOCTOR–PATIENT RELATIONSHIP

The NHS reforms introduced in 1991 created a framework in which providers compete for patients in terms both of the cost and quality of services provided (see Chapter 14), and, together with the Patient's Charter introduced in 1992, heralded an increased emphasis on consumerism in health policy. Patients thus came to be seen as making demands and having needs which the Health Service should strive to meet, rather than being more passive recipients of services. This has been accompanied by increased rights, including patients' right of access to their medical records, specified maximum hospital waiting times, and an easier process for changing their general practitioner. Increased emphasis is also given to providing written information about services and procedures, and conducting consumer satisfaction surveys to ensure the quality of health care. Meetings between doctors and patients thus occur within a more consumerist health care system and involve increasingly medically knowledgeable patients, with higher expectations of services and a greater desire to be informed and participate in the consultation and in medical decision-making.

Paralleling changes in patients' expectations is the more widespread adoption of a patient-oriented perspective among doctors. This reflects the influence of new training programmes and greater emphasis on communication skills, the greater prevalence of chronic conditions requiring long-term management and the increased involvement of doctors in counselling, health education and other activities requiring more active involvement by patients. However, despite these changes, problems of communication are identified by patients as their main source of dissatisfaction with medical care (Williams and Calnan 1991). This often appears to be due to patients feeling that they have not been listened to, or that their particular worries and concerns have been inadequately addressed. For example, it has been observed that even among breast cancer patients involved in a trial where a substantial amount of information was provided, about 50% of patients later stated that they did not feel information received at hospital was adequate, and information presented to cancer patients in simple structured formats has been shown to improve later recall but had little effect on levels of dissatisfaction with communication (Steptoe et al. 1991). Educational packages developed for asthma patients have also been shown to increase knowledge of asthma and the actions of the different drug treatments, but to have little effect on adherence with treatment (Hilton et al. 1986). An alternative strategy is to adopt a more participative approach, with the joint development of therapeutic plans becoming increasingly common. This involves patients in each of the three stages of the identification of treatment goals, the choice of treatment options, and the monitoring of symptoms and evaluating regimes (Chewning and Sleath 1996).

Other changes arise from the greater numbers of professional groups who are now members of the primary health care team. The doctor–patient relationship is therefore increasingly complemented by a nurse–patient relationship and meetings with health visitors, counsellors or psychologists who all tend to adopt a patient-centred orientation and practice style. In addition, consultants now frequently provide outreach sessions in a primary care setting, thus blurring the traditional primary/secondary care divide.

An important technological development with implications for the doctor–patient relationship is the increasing use of computers in the consultation. Their effects have been found to be influenced by whether patients are seated in a position to have access to the computer screen, and the doctors' ability to maintain their personal touch in terms of their verbal skills and eye contact with patients (Ridsdale and Hudd 1994). Also of increasing importance with greater computerization is the need to assure the confidentiality of patient data, thus maintaining the essential trust between doctor and patient.

REFERENCES

Beardon, P.H.G., McGilchrist, M.M., McKendrick, A.D., McDevitt, D.G. & MacDonald, T.M.   (1993) Primary non-compliance with prescribed medication in primary care. *Br. Med. J.*, **307**, 846–8.

Beecher, R.   (1955) The powerful placebo. *J. Am. Med. Assoc.*, **159**, 602–6.

Blanchard, C.G., Labrecque, M.S., Ruckdeschel, J.C. & Blanchard, E.B.   (1988) Information and decision-making preferences of hospitalised adult cancer patients. *Soc. Sci. Med.*, **27**, 1139–45.

Byrne, P.S. & Long, B.L.   (1976) *Doctors Talking to Patients*. London: HMSO.

Chewning, B. & Sleath, B.   (1996) Medication decision-making and management: a client-centred model. *Soc. Sci. Med.*, **42**, 389–98.

Cornford, C., Morgan, M. & Risdale, L.   (1993) Why do mothers consult when their children cough? *Fam. Pract.*, **10**, 193–6.

Fallowfield, L.   (1993) Giving sad and bad news. *Lancet*, **391**, 476–8.

Fitzpatrick, R.M., Hopkins, A.P. & Howard-Watts, O.   (1983) Social dimensions of healing. *Soc. Sci. Med.*, **17**, 501–10.

Hilton, S., Sibbald, B., Anderson, H.R. & Freeling, P.   (1986) Controlled evaluation of the effect of patient education on asthma morbidity in general practice. *Lancet*, **i**, 26–9.

Howie, J.G.R., Hopton, J.L., Heaney, D.L. & Porter, A.M.D.   (1992) Attitudes to medical care, the organisation of work, and stress among general practitioners. *Br. J. Gen. Pract.*, **42**, 181–5.

Kaplan, S.H., Greenfield, S. & Ware, J.E.   (1989) Assessing the effects of patient–physician interactions on the outcomes of chronic disease. *Med. Care*, **27**, S 110–27.

Levenstein, J.H., Brown, J.B., Weston, W.W. et al.   (1989) Patient centred clinical interviewing. In: *Communication with Medical Patients*, ed. M. Stewart & D. Roter. New York: Sage Publications.

Ley, P.   (1988) *Communicating with Patients*. London: Croom Helm.

Lockwood, M. (ed.)   (1985) *Moral Dilemmas in Modern Medicine*. Oxford: Oxford University Press.

McKevitt, C., Morgan, M., Simpson, J. & Holland, W.W.   (1995) *Doctors' Health and Needs for Services*. London: Nuffield Provincial Hospitals Trust.

Morgan, M. & Watkins, C.   (1988) Managing hypertension: beliefs and responses among cultural groups. *Sociol. Health Illness*, **10**, 561–78.

Myerscough, P.R.   (1992) *Talking with Patients: A Basic Clinical Skill*. Oxford: Oxford Medical Publications.

Ong, C.M., de Hoes, J.C.J.M., Hoos, A.M. & Lammes, F.B. (1995) Doctor–patient communication: a review of the literature. *Soc. Sci. Med.*, **40**, 903–18.

Parsons, T.   (1951). *The Social System*. Glencoe, IL: Free Press.

Pietroni, P.   (1976) Language and communication in general practice. In: *Communication in the General Practice Surgery*, ed. B. Tanner. London: Hodder & Stoughton.

Ridsdale, C. & Hudd, S.   (1994) Computers in the consultation: the patient's view. *Br. J. Gen. Pract.*, **44**, 367–9.

Ridsdale, L., Morgan, M. & Morris, R.   (1992) Doctors' interviewing technique and its response to different booking time. *Fam. Pract.*, **9**, 57–60.

Steptoe, A., Sutcliffe, I., Allen, B. & Coombes, C.   (1991) Satisfaction with communication, medical knowledge and coping style in patients with metastic cancer. *Soc. Sci. Med.*, **32**, 627–32.

Stewart, M. & Roter, D. (eds)   (1989) *Communicating with Medical Patients*. London: Sage.

Street, R.   (1991) Information-giving in medical consultations: the influence of patients' communicative styles and personal characteristics. *Soc. Sci. Med.*, **32**, 541–8.

Tuckett, D., Boulton, M., Oban, C. & Williams, A.   (1985) *Meetings Between Experts: An Approach to Sharing Ideas in Medical Consultations*. London: Tavistock Publications.

Underwood, M.J. & Bailey, J.S.   (1993) Should smokers be offered coronary bypass surgery? *Br. Med. J.*, **306**, 1047–50.

Waissman, R.   (1990) An analysis of doctor–patient interactions in the case of paediatric renal failure: the choice of home dialysis. *Soc. Health Illness*, **4**, 432–51.

West, P.   (1976) The physician and the management of childhood epilepsy. In: *Studies of Everyday Medical Life*, ed. M. Wadsworth & D. Robinson. London: Martin Robertson.

Williams, S.J. & Calnan, M.   (1991) Key determinants of consumer satisfaction with general practice. *Fam. Pract.*, **8**, 237–42.

Wilson, A., McDonald, P., Hays, L. & Cooney, J.   (1991) Longer booking intervals in general practice: effects on doctor's stress and arousal. *Br. J. Gen. Pract.*, **41**, 184–7.

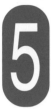

Hospitals, Doctors and Patient Care

MYFANWY MORGAN

Hospitals are typically large institutions with a diversity of activities. Many not only engage in patient care but also serve as centres of education and training for doctors, nurses and other health workers, and provide a setting for research. The patient admitted to hospital thus enters a complex organization with a variety of goals, and with a well-developed system of rules and procedures for co-ordinating the different activities and the large numbers and categories of staff. This chapter examines patients' experiences of hospital care and the changing patterns of hospital use. It also considers the influence of the culture of medicine and demands of medical work on doctors' attitudes and responses to their own ill health, and identifies the changing relationships between doctors, managers and other health professionals.

DOCTORS IN A HOSPITAL SETTING

Hospitals form a major centre for medical work and training. They employed 43 801 medical staff (whole time equivalents) in England in 1993, with a further 28 460 doctors working in primary care. Approximately 35% of hospital doctors are consultants and 8% senior registrars, with the majority occupying junior training grades.

Professional socialization and medical culture

The training of doctors within a hospital environment involves not only the formal training and acquisition of clinical skills but also the experience of professional socialization. This refers to the process by which new members acquire the values, beliefs, expectations and culture of the group to which they will belong, including its ideals and how to conduct themselves (see Chapter 15).

Professional socialization is influenced by the common experiences and demands on junior doctors, which encourage the adoption of common strategies and responses (Box 5.1).

BOX 5.1

DEMANDS ON CLINICAL STUDENTS AND JUNIOR DOCTORS

- Cope with workload and hours
- Cope with uncertainty
- Acquire clinical skills and fulfil the expectations of seniors
- Cope with stressful situations and events

A shared experience of junior doctors is their heavy workload and long hours of work. This has traditionally been justified in terms of their need to gain a wide range of clinical experience and skills. As a result, an inability to cope with these demands is regarded as identifying a lack of suitability and fitness for the profession. Clinical students and junior doctors are therefore often unwilling to admit to stress and health problems, and are also reluctant to take time off for sickness. The need to 'get through' the workload also leads to the development of common strategies. These include concentrating on the technical aspects of medicine, and giving less emphasis to the psychosocial aspects of care that traditionally have been less highly valued within the profession.

Another common experience of junior doctors is the need to cope with uncertainties in fulfilling their clinical role. This involves problems of personal uncertainty due to their own incomplete mastery of medical knowledge, and increasing recognition of the gaps and inadequacies in medical knowledge itself. A third problem arises from the difficulties often experienced in distinguishing between these two sources of uncertainty. One way junior doctors cope with uncertainty is to be over-cautious. For example, they frequently order unnecessary tests as a failure of omission attracts considerable censure, whereas performing unnecessary procedures is generally viewed by clinicians as of much less significance. Similarly, junior doctors are often reluctant to make the decision to discharge a patient from outpatient follow-up, which produces high levels of unnecessary repeat attendances.

At an interpersonal level, clinical students and junior doctors often experience difficulties in coping with relationships with patients, and especially with chronically sick and dying patients. One response, which is first acquired at the initial dissection of cadavers in anatomy, is to develop a 'detached concern' or perspective of objectivity in dealing with death, disease and the human body. Detachment protects medical staff from strain. It is also functional in enabling doctors to conduct physical examinations in situations that would otherwise cause embarrassment to both doctors and patients. However, this approach may also contribute to the inappropriate depersonalization of patients and insufficient attention being given to their identity and feelings. This frequently occurs on ward rounds, where the medical or surgical team may talk about a patient in the third person as 'a case of X', as if the patient was invisible. More generally, the treatment of the patient as 'a case' rather than 'a person' neglects the psychosocial dimensions of care. This frequently contributes to patients' anxiety and their view of hospital doctors as cold, offhand and uncommunicative (Scott et al. 1995).

Another characteristic of the medical culture is the informal evaluation of patients by medical staff. One common distinction is between '*interesting*' and '*routine*' cases. Interesting cases consist of patients whose condition is unusual or complex, requiring a high degree of medical skill, whereas routine cases add little to doctors' professional development. A second dimension relates to the social evaluation of patients as '*good*' patients or '*problem*' patients. Good patients are intelligent, although not questioning the doctors' judgement, and are seen as helpful and co-operative. Problem patients are those who are regarded as difficult to manage and as making unnecessary demands on staff time, or who have social problems that make discharge difficult and time consuming to organize (Mizrahi 1986). This informal evaluation and categorizing of patients has been studied most often in accident and emergency (A&E) departments. These departments operate on an open access basis, and thus cater for a large proportion of patients with medically trivial or 'routine' conditions with little scope for developing clinical skills. The clientele also includes drunks, homeless people and other stigmatized groups, whose demands on hospital A&E services are often viewed by staff as unnecessary, troublesome or inappropriate (Roberts 1992).

The expectations and attitudes that comprise the medical culture not only influence the approach of doctors to their work and patient care, but also affect their attitudes and responses to problems of their own health.

Work stress, health and sickness absence

The all-cause mortality rate of doctors is relatively low compared with the general population and is comparable to that for social class I. However, for certain causes of death, including suicide and accidental poisoning (drugs and other substances), cirrhosis and chronic liver disease, their standardized mortality ratios (SMRs) are particularly high (OPCS 1986). For example, doctors are among the ten highest risk occupations for suicide, with women doctors and those who have recently qualified being at greatest risk (Baldwin and Rudge 1995).

The measurement of morbidity is complex. However, a large number of surveys indicate that medical students and doctors experience high levels of emotional distress and depression. A major study of medical students from three British universities found that during their fourth year in training nearly a third (31.2%) were assessed as experiencing emotional disturbance, defined as a score of 3 or more on the 12 item General Health Questionnaire (GHQ) (Firth 1986). This was similar to levels of emotional disturbance reported among medical students in the US, but considerably higher than for other groups of young people in the general population (Firth 1986). The same cohort of students, as junior house officers in their preregistration year, identified continuing high levels of emotional disturbance with half achieving a score of 4 or more on the 30 item GHQ. At this stage there was also a difference between the sexes, with overall levels of emotional distress higher for women than for men. This compared with the classification of 36% of men and 34% of women executive Civil Servants as emotionally disturbed (Firth-Cozens 1987).

Stress is highly correlated with GHQ scores for junior doctors, with aspects of work rated as particularly stressful including overwork, talking to distressed relatives, the effects of the demands of work on their personal lives and serious treatment failures (Table 5.1). Problems with sleep patterns and the amount of sleep in the last 48 hours also contributed to stress, and one-fifth of junior doctors reported bouts of heavy drinking (Firth–Cozens and Morrison 1989). Sources of stress identified as of greater significance for women are conflicts between career and personal life, sexual harassment at work, a lack of female role models, prejudice from patients and discrimination by senior doctors (Firth–Cozens 1990).

TABLE 5.1 *Sources of stress in junior house officers.*

Source	No. (%)	Perceived stress[a] (Mean)
Dealing with death and dying	31 (18.6)	2.90
Relationships with senior doctors	26 (15.6)	2.85
Making mistakes	21 (12.6)	2.72
Overwork	19 (11.4)	3.11
Relationships with ward staff	16 (9.6)	2.75
A lack of skills	11 (6.6)	2.73
Dealing with patients' relatives	9 (5.4)	3.00
Career decisions	6 (3.6)	2.33
No answer	8 (4.8)	—

Reprinted by permission of John Wiley & Sons Ltd from Firth–Cozens & Morrison (1989).
[a] Items rated on a 4-point scale from 'not stressful' to 'extremely stressful'.

Problems of stress and emotional disturbance are not confined to junior doctors. For example, Caplan (1994) found that 47% of a group of hospital doctors, general practitioners and managers achieved a score of over 5 on the GHQ (28 item version). Similarly, 23% of consultants and 30% of both general practitioners (GPs) and managers were rated as displaying anxiety (anxiety scores of over 10 on the Hospital Anxiety and Depression scale). Another study compared the levels of stress experienced by doctors with company 'fee-earners' (accountants and management consultants) who also work under considerable pressure. Altogether 72% of GPs, 50% of hospital doctors (48% juniors and 62% consultants), and 58% of management consultants rated their job as 'often' or 'always' stressful. Important stresses for all groups were the pressure of work and the effects of work on home life. Organizational changes following the introduction of the provider-market were identified as a particular source of stress for senior hospital doctors, whereas for many general practitioners the introduction of general practice fund-holding and new conditions of work in primary care were perceived as stressful (McKevitt et al. 1996).

Although doctors experience considerable emotional disturbance and depression they are often reluctant to acknowledge health problems in themselves or their colleagues, and may resort to alcohol or drug abuse. There is also a general expectation of 'working through' illness and not taking time off work for routine sickness. A recent study found that 47% of hospital doctors and 35% of GPs had taken sick leave in the last year, compared with 71% of management consultants. These differences held after adjusting for age and sex, and were mainly due to doctors taking fewer short periods of sickness absence for minor illness (3 days or less) (McKevitt et al. 1996).

The reluctance of doctors to acknowledge health problems and their greater tendency to 'work through' illness partly reflects a medical culture in which admitting such problems may be seen as indicating an individual's inability to cope with the job. This cultural attitude may stem from the responsibility of senior doctors to ensure that doctors are fit to practise. Thus the GMC places a duty on doctors to protect patients when they believe a colleague's conduct, performance or health is a threat to them, and if necessary, to inform the employing authority or regulatory body. However, within the medical culture there is a reluctance to 'inform' on colleagues who are neglecting health problems, thus leading to a culture of the non-recognition of illness (Nuffield Provincial Hospitals Trust 1996). Organizational aspects of medical work also have implications for the acknowledgement of minor illness and sickness absence, and particularly the lack of flexibility of medical work and shortage of locum cover. Doctors' sickness absence therefore places additional demands on already busy colleagues and may involve cancelling clinic sessions, whereas the work of other professional groups is generally more flexible and under a greater degree of individual control (McKevitt et al. 1996) (Box 5.2).

A number of recent developments have implications for doctors' health. Of particular significance are the changes in the conditions of medical work introduced by the new contract signed in 1991, referred to as the 'New Deal,'. This set a timetable for the reduction of working hours, and limited the average number of contracted working hours to 56 per week. It also set standards for other aspects of working conditions, including minimum standards for accommodation and catering, and requirements for job descriptions, induction courses and complaints procedures.

Other preventive strategies have focused on reducing risks of stress and emotional distress among medical students and doctors, through the development of mentoring schemes, personal learning programmes, career guidance and specific courses in time management. In addition, a

---

BOX 5.2

CAUSES OF DOCTORS' RELUCTANCE TO ACKNOWLEDGE ILL HEALTH AND TAKE SICK LEAVE

- Problems of time and access to GP for junior doctors
- General expectation that doctors do not succumb to ill health and are able to cope with stresses
- Expectations of seniors
- Problems of increased workload on colleagues
- Problems of cancelling clinics

number of support networks have developed in general practice, such as Young Principals Groups and Trainers Groups. These developments have been complemented by national and local initiatives concerned with the provision of services to respond to problems of stress and addictive behaviours among doctors including telephone help-lines, stress management training, counselling services, and various self-help groups. However, use of these services is often limited by the reluctance of doctors to acknowledge health problems and to seek appropriate help and support at an early stage. This identifies the importance of changing attitudes to achieve changes in illness behaviour.

Relationships among hospital staff

A major difference between hospitals and other large-scale organizations is that they were traditionally characterized by two lines of authority and accountability, with the professional authority structure of medicine being relatively autonomous and distinct from the managerial authority structure. The managerial authority structure was primarily concerned with the non-medical staff, and was responsible for budgets, organizational arrangements, and the 'hotel' aspects of hospital care. Doctors were a distinct and separate group, accountable to their own profession. They were also concerned almost entirely with individual patient care, and did not allow resource issues to explicitly intrude into clinical decisions. However, various changes designed to promote the efficiency and effectiveness of medical services have had the effect of increasing the accountability of individual hospital consultants and reducing the divide between managerial and professional control within hospitals (Box 5.3).

One set of changes has centred on the introduction of standards and guidelines for clinical practice with the aim of developing an evidence-based approach and promoting the more rapid adoption of proven techniques and practices. Guidelines are generally developed under the auspices of the Royal Colleges or speciality groups, and may be modified locally to take account of local conditions (Woolf 1992). This has been accompanied by the introduction of medical audit

---

BOX 5.3

STRATEGIES FOR MANAGING CLINICAL ACTIVITY

1. Raising professional standards (minimal intervention)
   - Medical audit
   - Standards and guidelines
   - Accreditation

2. Involving doctors in management
   - Budgets for doctors
   - Resource management initiative
   - Doctor-managers

3. External management control of doctors (maximal intervention)
   - Managing medical work
   - Changing doctors' contracts
   - Extending provider competition

Reproduced with permission from Benzeval et al. (1994).

as part of the 1991 NHS reforms (Secretaries of State for Health, 1989). Medical audit involves 'the systematic, critical analysis of the quality of medical care, including diagnostic and treatment procedures, the use of resources, and the resulting clinical outcomes and quality of life for the patient.' This is undertaken through a four stage process (the audit 'cycle') – defining standards that should be practised; comparing practices with these standards; where different, implementing changes; and finally, re-observing practice. Participation in medical audit, although required of all hospital doctors, is designed as an internal quality review mechanism with managerial involvement being limited to ensuring that these activities take place. However, the existence of medical audit and standards against which clinical care may be judged serve to reduce individual clinician's autonomy and the associated variations in practice styles.

A second change relates to the increasing involvement of doctors in management, with responsibility for speciality budgets and the planning and organization of clinical services. This was firmly established with the resource management initiative introduced by the 1983 Griffiths Report (see Chapter 14). However, following the 1991 reforms the involvement of doctors in management was strengthened with the grouping of specialities into clinical directorates. These are managed by a medically qualified clinical director, assisted by a small management team involving a nurse director and administrator. The clinical director has freedom to manage the speciality, but is responsible to the hospital general manager as budget holder for the directorate (Harrison and Pollitt 1994).

A third change is the increased role and responsibility given to hospital (Trust) managers in relation to clinical staff and clinical care. A major change in managerial control occurred in response to the introduction of a system of contracting for services under the 1991 NHS reforms. This had the effect of moving from a provider-led service in which hospital consultants were responsible for their caseload and practices, to one in which managers are required to negotiate to provide services to external purchasers (health authorities). In this situation, managers need to ensure that consultants deliver those services to an acceptable standard and price. For example, contracts negotiated with purchasers may include requirements for day surgery/inpatient care and follow-up outpatient attendance, or specifications regarding types of treatment and procedures of proven effectiveness (see Chapter 14). To achieve this, managers have been granted increased control over clinicians. This has involved more detailed specification of consultants' contracts of employment, and managers' involvement in consultant appointments and in decisions regarding 'C' grade merit awards. In addition, systems of external performance review, such as comparative league tables for hospitals in terms of waiting times, deaths following surgery, cancelled operations, etc., provide a form of external monitoring and management control. Thus the work of hospital doctors is now much more likely to be costed, audited, subjected to explicit budgetary control, and the subject of managerial and consumer evaluations. However, this increased accountability is not unique to doctors, and reflects a more general experience of professional groups.

Another general change is in relationships that exist between hospital doctors and other health professionals. The work of nurses, midwives, physiotherapists and other groups within the hospital was traditionally controlled by doctors. However, these groups are now becoming autonomous practitioners with specific expertise and responsibilities for patient care. This is reflected in their new training and career structures and the increased emphasis given to the development of a collaborative multiprofessional approach to patient care, with the team leader drawn from any of the health professionals or involving a non-medical co-ordinator. The Department of Health has encouraged the development of multiprofessional 'clinical' audit to replace uniprofessional 'medical' audit to accelerate the development of this new model of team-work based on a co-ordinated multiprofessional approach. However, clinical audit is still in its infancy in most specialities (Humphris and Littlejohns 1995).

PATIENTS' EXPERIENCE OF HOSPITAL CARE

Changing patterns of hospital use

The past 30 years has been characterized by increasing rates of hospital admission despite a reduction in the total numbers of hospital beds, as illustrated by data for the period 1984–94 (Table 5.2). This situation has been made possible as a result of the substantial reductions in length of stay which have occurred across all specialities, age groups and diagnoses. For example, patients admitted for myocardial infarction stayed in hospital in the 1940s for 5–7 weeks compared with 5–7 days today. Similarly, groin hernia repair required a length of stay of about 6 weeks in the 1940s; this was reduced to an average of 4.9 days in 1985, and today involves either one night in hospital or is performed as day surgery. In addition, whereas psychiatric patients formerly spent many years in hospital care, they are now generally discharged within one month and many patients are admitted for much shorter periods of diagnosis and treatment.

TABLE 5.2 Changes in hospital beds and activity, England 1984–94.

	1994/95 (thousands)	Change since 1984 (%)
General and acute[a]		
Beds available	145	–25
Cases treated	6210	+18
Outpatient attendances	34932	+10
Day cases	2439	+180
Psychiatric		
Beds available	55	–55
Cases treated	288	–14
Outpatient attendances	2067	+14

Crown copyright is reproduced with the permission of the Controller of HMSO from Department of Health (1996) Table 5.12.
[a] *General and acute = total acute (excluding well babies) plus geriatric medicine.*

Explaining patterns of hospital use

General hospital patients   Changes in hospital use reflect the interaction and outcome of several factors. One important influence has been the changing medical views regarding the need for bed rest for recovery following surgery or major illness, with the emphasis now on encouraging patients to become mobile as soon as possible. In addition, shorter stays and the use of out-patient or day surgery as an alternative to inpatient care is viewed as beneficial in reducing the stress of hospitalization, especially among children. Secondly, patients' needs for hospital care have reduced as a result of clinical developments. These include more effective pain control and new and less-invasive medical technologies and surgical procedures such as laprascopic tech-niques and the use of lasers and lithotripsy to replace conventional open surgery. Thirdly, eco-nomic changes in terms of new ways of financing hospital services have provided incentives to reduce lengths of stay and increase the throughput of patients. Previously hospitals received a global budget to cover their activity and therefore had little incentive to increase throughput. Indeed higher levels of activity could lead to risks of a budget overspend resulting in the so called 'efficiency trap'. However, in a provider-market the increased levels of throughput achieved through greater efficiency and reduced lengths of stay have the effect of putting a hospital at a competitive advantage by reducing costs per case, with the revenue received being related to the volume of activity and contracts for services.

Psychiatric patients   The changing pattern of psychiatric care from long-term custodial care to the use of hospitals for short periods of diagnosis and treatment began in the 1950s with a shift from long-term care within institutions to a policy of 'community care'. This has been accompanied by the gradual run-down and closure of large psychiatric hospitals which often catered for over 1000 patients. Thus care for psychiatric patients now primarily occurs outside the hospital, with short periods of admission to psychiatric beds in general hospitals if required for diagnosis and treatment. This change in policy and provision has again been attributed to a variety of attitudinal, clinical and economic factors. Some people regard the introduction of the major tranquillizers from the mid 1950s as the key factor making community care possible by enabling people to be treated and aggressive behaviour controlled outside the hospital. However, others argue that this exaggerates the therapeutic achievement these drugs represented. They suggest that a more important factor was the prior change in ideas regarding mentally ill people who were no longer viewed as violent and dangerous and requiring long-term custody and care. In particular they point to several hospitals that adopted the policy of early discharge well before the new drugs were introduced.

A third major reason advanced to explain the new emphasis on community care was the increasing recognition of the harmful effects on patients of large psychiatric hospitals. A book by Erving Goffman (1961), based on his own observational study of a large psychiatric hospital in the USA, was particularly influential in drawing attention to the adverse effects of the organiza-tion of care in psychiatric hospitals. Goffman identified in these hospitals an 'institutionalization' among patients in response to their organizational environment. This condition is characterized at a psychological level by patients' lack of interest in leaving the institution, general apathy and a lack of concern about what is going on around them. Institutionalized patients also demon-strate an inability to make choices and decisions, to plan activities or to undertake simple every-day tasks. They may also lose interest in and neglect their own appearance and develop mumbled speech and a characteristic shuffling gait. Such institutions were thus seen as performing a dis-abling function, and as actually promoting disturbed and regressive behaviour. This was mainly attributed to the high level of depersonalization that occurred in the interests of organizational efficiency. Thus patients were subjected to 'batch processing', in which they were all treated alike, and performed activities such as getting up, bathing and eating according to an institutional schedule with little scope for individual choices, preferences and decision-making. Personal possessions were also kept to a minimum to make it easier for staff to cope with large numbers of patients, and there was often little regard for privacy. As a result of these pressures patients frequently lost their self-identity, took on a passive role and became dependent on the institution. These institutional pressures were particularly strong for patients who experienced long lengths of stay and lost contact with the outside world. Recognition of the harmful effects of the institutional environment, together with a number of scandals regarding the neglect and ill treatment of patients in psychiatric hospitals and other long-stay institutions, thus provided an important pressure towards a policy of deinstitutionalization on humanitarian grounds. In addition, economic factors are identified as playing a significant role in promoting the policy of community care (Scull 1984). This centred on the need to renovate the large psychiatric institutions built in the Victorian era and their considerable running costs. Thus a policy of community care was regarded as reducing costs to the health service, although the overall costs of community care are dependent on the level of service provision (see Chapter 16).

In terms of the provision of hospitals for chronically ill patients, the studies by Goffman and others emphasized the importance of achieving an individualized approach. Key requirements in achieving this are the availability of staff in sufficient numbers and the acceptance by staff of the importance of providing personal care and of encouraging independence. This means that talking with patients (or residents), providing choices, encouraging participation in everyday activities, encouraging visitors and keeping routines flexible need to be viewed as important by staff at all levels in achieving the goal of rehabilitation. These tasks may sometimes conflict with and require greater priority than the achievement of 'efficient' management, which involves the completion of tasks on schedule.

Whereas the recent trend has been towards reducing lengths of hospital stay and unnecessary hospital use, increasing emphasis is now given to ensuring that the quality of care and favourable clinical outcomes are achieved with the new patterns of patient care. This partly depends on good patient communication and the appropriateness of discharge decisions and the efficient co-ordination of services and follow-up in the community where necessary. There is also a need to monitor clinical complications and needs for readmission, and to examine the causes of instances of violent and aggressive behaviour among psychiatric patients living in the community.

Stress and anxiety among hospital patients

Currently about 8% of men and 12% of women in the population are admitted to hospitals each year. Although a patient's admission is routine for hospital staff, it forms a major event in people's lives and is often a source of considerable anxiety and stress. The fact that 'something is wrong,' requiring diagnosis, treatment or both, often forms a source of anxiety in itself. For some patients there are further uncertainties about whether they may be cured, left with a physical disability or faced with an early death. As well as these worries about the outcome of treatment, patients are frequently apprehensive about the discomfort and pain they may experience in undergoing diagnostic or operative procedures, and may worry about having an anaesthetic. The actual experience of being a patient in hospital is often also found to be stressful. Particular sources of stress include the lack of privacy, a lack of familiarity with the different categories of staff and with the general routines of the ward, problems of being disturbed on the ward and not being able to sleep, and not being given sufficient information about their medical condition or treatment. Patients about to be discharged may also worry about how they will manage at home.

Recognition of the high level of stress often experienced by hospital patients has led to greater emphasis on preparing patients for admission, by providing booklets and other written information to explain their treatment and hospital stay. This has positive effects on pain and distress as well as increasing patients' satisfaction and reducing stress. For example, one study compared a group of women undergoing hysterectomy who had received a booklet about how to survive in hospital and cope with anxiety, with a control group who did not receive the booklet. This indicated that the intervention group experienced less postoperative pain and distress and were discharged from hospital more quickly than the controls (Young and Humphrey 1985). Written and oral communication to prepare patients is particularly important for day surgery, which requires that patients are admitted and discharged the same day and manage their recovery at home. Increasing use is also now made of audio tapes and cassettes to provide patients with information about their condition and treatment options.

Patients' evaluations of acute hospital care

Some hospitals and specialist units place considerable emphasis on providing patients with booklets and leaflets prior to admission to explain about their condition, its treatment and their hospital stay, and how to manage at home after discharge. However, surveys of hospital patients' evaluations of their care continue to identify a lack of information and problems of communication as major causes of concern. For example, a survey conducted in 1992/93 (based on a random sample of 36 of the 278 acute hospitals in England with 200 beds or more), identified the principal problems reported by patients as relating to communication, pain management and discharge planning. Patients frequently felt that they were not given important information about the hospital and its routine, their condition or treatment. When given this information they also frequently felt that it had been provided in an upsetting way or with little respect for privacy. Of the 61% of patients who suffered pain, 33% were in pain all or most of the time and 87% had severe or moderate pain. Many patients had been discharged with no information about how to help their recovery, and 5% had problems getting home (Bruster et al. 1994).

Patients' dissatisfaction with communication in the hospital setting arises partly from a discrepancy between patients' needs for information and doctors' views of what patients need to know. Other important influences are time constraints, patients' difficulties in requesting information and making their needs known and the organization of work which, unlike in the outpatient sector, provides little opportunity for personal contact between doctor and hospital inpatient (Meredith 1993). However, an important change within hospitals is that increasingly the nursing profession is emphasizing its function in the psychosocial aspects of care. It is, therefore, redefining the nurse–patient relationship in terms of a partnership or relationship of 'mutuality' and adopting a patient-centred approach (see Chapter 4). One aspect of this is the development of primary nursing which frequently takes place in day surgical units. Primary nursing involves continuity of care by the same nurse for the same group of patients from admission to discharge, with beneficial effects for both nurses' job satisfaction and patients' anxiety and satisfaction with care (Morgan and Reynolds 1991). Secondly, the introduction of the Patient's Charter in 1992 identified explicit rights and expectations (standards of care). For hospital patients this includes patients' right of access to their own health records, and to have a clear expectation of the treatment provided including the risks and options, and the expectations that they will have a named nurse in charge of their care (Box 5.4).

BOX 5.4

PATIENT'S CHARTER RIGHTS AND STANDARDS IN NHS HOSPITALS

Patients have a right to:

- A clear explanation of the treatment proposed, including risks involved and any alternatives clearly explained before deciding whether to agree to it

- Access to health records and for records to be kept confidential

- Have any complaint about NHS services investigated and to get a quick, full written reply from the relevant chief executive or general manager

- Choosing whether they wish to take part in medical research or medical student training

- Be guaranteed admission within 18 months of being on the waiting list (and expect treatment within 1 year for coronary artery by-pass)

National Charter standards:

- To be given a specific appointment time for outpatient clinics and to be seen within 30 minutes of that time

- To be seen immediately at A&E department or have need for treatment assessed

- If admitted through an A&E department can expect a bed as soon as possible and within 2 hours

- To have a qualified nurse, midwife or health visitor responsible for care and be told their name

- To have single-sex washing and toilet facilities (and to be told before admission whether planned to be cared for in a mixed-sex ward)

- To respect privacy, dignity, religious and cultural beliefs

- If agreed, relatives and friends kept up to date with progress of treatment

Reproduced by the permission of the Controller of HMSO from Department of Health (1996).

CHANGING ROLE OF THE HOSPITAL

Hospitals, like any large organizations, are in a continuous process of evolution and change. They were founded as institutions for the care of the sick poor who were removed from the community because of infectious disease. However, they became the major site of clinical practice and the location of technologies for diagnosis and treatment. Recent changes in patient care have involved new forms of organization within the hospital. This includes the need for a higher staff:patient ratio, as the reduction in lengths of stay has meant that patients are receiving more active care requiring greater staff input. There has also been greater emphasis on pooled resources as a means of achieving greater efficiency. Thus whereas hospital beds were formerly designated as the responsibility and resource of individual consultants they are now generally controlled by a bed manager or senior nurse with this responsibility. This allows greater flexibility, and avoids situations in which consultants might retain patients until they were ready for a new admission to their firm's beds or junior doctors spent considerable time locating beds (Green and Armstrong 1993).

A second type of change is the current trend for care to move outside the hospital. This is exemplified by the expansion in minor surgery undertaken by general practitioners, the availability of home dialysis and fetal monitoring, developments in consultant outreach sessions, the substantial increases in day surgery, and the emphasis on community-based care for psychiatric patients. These changes have been accompanied by increasing numbers of nurses, physiotherapists, midwives and other health professionals working in the community, with some hospital consultants holding specialist outreach sessions for diabetes, ophthalmology and other conditions. The future evolution of the hospital is unclear. However, current trends suggest that the hospital will become the centre of a vertically integrated system where acute beds play only a modest role. This change in function and blurring of the primary/secondary interface has implications for clinical training and medical work, as well as for patients' experiences of medical care (Stoeckle 1995). A key question is whether the co-ordination of services will be undertaken by the hospital, giving rise to the notion of a 'boundaryless' hospital, or whether this function will be increasingly performed from a primary care base.

REFERENCES

Baldwin, D.S. & Rudge, S.E.   (1995) Depression and suicide in doctors and medical students. In: *Health Risks to the Health Care Professional*, ed. P. Litchfield. London: Royal College of Physicians.
Benzeval, M.   (1994) *Society and Health*. Issue No. 1, London: International Centre for Health and Society/Kings Fund Institute.
Bruster, S., Jarman, B., Bosanquet, N., Weston, D., Erens, R & Delbanco, T.L.   (1994) National survey of hospital patients. *Br. Med. J.*, **309**, 1542–6.
Caplan R.   (1994) Stress, anxiety and depression in hospital consultants, general practitioners and senior health service managers. *Br. Med. J.*, **309**, 1261–3.
Department of Health   (1991) *The Patient's Charter*, London: HMSO.
Department of Health   (1994) *Health and Personal Social Services Statistics for England, 1994*. London: HMSO.
Department of Health   (1996) *Health and Personal Social Services Statistics for England*. London: The Stationery Office.
Firth, J.   (1986) Levels and sources of stress in medical students. *Br. Med. J.*, **292**, 1177–80.
Firth-Cozens, J.   (1987) Emotional distress in junior house officers. *Br. Med. J.*, **381**, 89–91.
Firth-Cozens, J.   (1990) Sources of stress in women junior house officers. *Br. Med. J.*, **301**, 89–91.
Firth-Cozens, J. & Morrison, L.   (1989) Sources of stress and ways of coping in junior house officers. *Stress Med.*, **5**, 121–6.
Goffman, E.   (1961) *Asylums*. New York: Doubleday.

Green, J. & Armstrong, D. (1993) Controlling the 'bed state': negotiating hospital organisation. *Sociol. Health Illness*, **15**, 337–52.

Ham, C.J. & Hunter, D.J. (1988) *Managing Clinical Activity in the NHS*. Briefing Paper No. 8, London: Kings Fund Institute.

Harrison, S. & Pollitt, C. (1994) *Controlling Health Professionals; the Future of Work and Organisation in the NHS*. Buckingham: Open University Press.

Humphris, D. & Littlejohns, P. (1995) Multiprofessional audit and clinical guidelines. *J. Interprofessional Care*, **9**: 207–19.

McKevitt, C., Morgan, M., Simpson, J. & Holland, W.W. (1996) *Doctors' Health and Needs for Services*. London: Nuffield Provincial Hospitals Trust.

Meredith, P. (1993) Patient satisfaction with communication in general surgery: problems of measurement and improvement. *Soc. Sci. Med.*, **37**, 591–602.

Mizrahi, T. (1986) *Getting Rid of Patients*. New Brunswick, N.J.: Rutgers University Press.

Morgan, M. & Reynolds, A. (1991) Day surgery units: are they attractive to nurses? *J. Adv. Health Nurs. Care*, **1**(2), 59–74.

Nuffield Provincial Hospitals Trust (1996) Taking care of doctors' health: Report of a Working Party. London: Nuffield Provincial Hospitals Trust.

OPCS (1986) *Occupational Health: Decennial Supplement*, Series DS no. 10. London: HMSO.

Roberts, H. (1992) Professionals' and parents' perception of A&E use in a children's hospital. *Social. Rev.*, **40**, 109–131.

Scott, R.A., Aiken, C.H., Mechanic, D. & Moravisik, J. (1995) Organisational aspects of caring. *Millbank Q.*, **73**, 77–95.

Scull, A.T. (1984) *Decarceration: Community Treatment and the Deviant – a Radical View*, 2nd edn. Cambridge: Polity Press.

Secretaries of State for Health (1989) Working for Patients. Cmd 555. London: HMSO.

Stoeckle, J.D. (1995) The citadel cannot hold: technologies go outside the hospital, patients and doctors too. *Milbank Q.*, **73**, 3–17.

Woolf, S.H. (1992) Practice guidelines: a new reality in medicine. Methods of developing guidelines. *Arch. Intern. Med.*, **152**, 946–52.

Young, L. & Humphrey, M. (1985) Cognitive methods of preparing women for hysterectomy: does a booklet help? *Br. J. Clin. Psychol.*, **24**, 303–4.

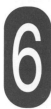

Living with Chronic Illness

DAVID LOCKER

Since the early 1970s sociologists have increasingly turned their attention to the issues and challenges involved in chronic illness and disability. Studies of people with disabilities were common before this time, but were predominantly concerned with psychological factors and their role in the rehabilitation process.

During the 1970s considerable effort was invested in developing appropriate measures of chronic illness and disability, estimating the prevalence and severity of disability, assessing the needs of people with disabilities and identifying gaps in service provision for these individuals and the families who cared for them. In the 1980s more attention was paid to the experience of living with chronic illness and disability (Conrad 1987; Anderson and Bury 1988). A growing number of studies have begun to describe in some detail what it is like for individuals and families to live with a long-term, disabling disorder. The rationale underlying this work is that 'a sound, effective and ethical approach to chronic illness must lie in awareness of and attention to the experiences, values, priorities and expectations of (these people) and their families' (Anderson and Bury 1988). This means that a detailed understanding of the impact of chronic illness and disability on daily life is necessary for the providers of medical and social services to offer appropriate care and support.

This recent emphasis on chronic illness reflects the fact that chronic disabling disorders, rather than acute infectious diseases, are the major cause of mortality in industrial societies and present a significant challenge to the medical-care system (see Chapter 1). Even where chronic conditions are not fatal, they are major sources of suffering for individuals and families. As Verbrugge and Jette (1994) indicate, people mostly live with rather than die from chronic conditions. Given that the populations of western societies are ageing (see Chapter 11), it is predicted that the proportion of consultations in medical practice devoted to the psychosocial and other problems of daily living associated with chronic illness will increase. As a result, there will be a fundamental shift in medical practice from 'cure' to 'care' (Williams 1989).

The emergence of an interest in chronic illness also coincided with an increase in government provision for people with disabling disorders. In the UK, 1970 saw the passing of the Chronically Sick and Disabled Persons Act, which made it mandatory for local authorities to identify people with disabilities, to determine their needs and to provide services to meet those needs (Topliss 1979). In 1974, a Minister for the Disabled was appointed with specific responsibilities for the group. These developments led to an increase in services and financial benefits for people with disabilities and those who cared for them, although these were somewhat eroded during the late 1980s.

A further development which stimulated a greater awareness of the needs and priorities of people living with chronic illness was the emergence of the 'disability movement' (Conrad 1987). This consisted of groups dedicated to self-help and political action. The former offered help and support through the sharing of individual experience, while the latter used the political process to secure fundamental rights and to promote independent living. The aim here was to ensure that people with chronic disabling disorders would themselves define their needs and the most appropriate way of providing for them, rather than having these imposed by putative 'experts' and professionals.

CHARACTERISTICS OF CHRONIC ILLNESS

The term 'chronic illness' encompasses a wide range of conditions affecting almost all body systems. Cancer, stroke, end-stage renal disease, poliomyelitis, multiple sclerosis, rheumatoid arthritis, psoriasis, epilepsy and chronic obstructive airways disease are common examples. The most fundamental characteristic of chronic illnesses is that they are long-term and have a profound influence on the lives of sufferers. Some are fatal and some are not; some are stable with a certain prognosis, others may show great variation in terms of their day-to-day manifestations and their long-term course and outcome. In the majority of cases medical intervention is palliative; it seeks to control symptoms but cannot offer a cure. Consequently, maximizing the welfare of these individuals and their families means maintaining or improving the quality of daily life rather than attempting to eradicate the disease process itself.

Some of the problems encountered by people with a chronic disabling disorder stem directly from the symptomatic character of their illness. In this respect, every chronic condition is somewhat distinct. For example, the person with rheumatoid arthritis must cope with chronic pain, the person with respiratory disease must live with breathlessness and an inadequate oxygen supply, and the person with end-stage renal failure must cope with the demands of a dialysis machine. In other respects the problems faced by people with chronic illness may be common to all, irrespective of the nature of their condition. Unemployment or reduced career prospects, social isolation and estrangement from family and friends, loss of important roles, changed physical appearance and problems with self-esteem and identity are experienced by many such individuals. Another fundamental characteristic of chronic conditions is that these assaults on the body, daily activities (encompassing home, work and leisure) and social relationships (including relationships with self and others) must be managed in the course of everyday life. When chronic illness becomes severe, daily life may be entirely consumed in coping with its symptoms, the medical regimens intended to control it and its social consequences (Locker 1983).

Prevalence of chronic illness and disability

A number of surveys of national and local populations have been undertaken in order to estimate the prevalence of disability. These have produced somewhat different results, largely because different definitions and measures of disability have been employed. The most recent study, the Survey of Disability in Great Britain undertaken in 1985 by the Office of Population Censuses and Surveys (OPCS), found that 14.2% of the adult population were disabled (OPCS 1988). Rates increased substantially with age and were higher among women than men. Other studies have reported that the most common causes of significant disability are neurological, musculoskeletal and respiratory diseases such as stroke, multiple sclerosis, Parkinson's disease and rheumatoid arthritis. Similarly, it has been estimated that about 35 million Americans, or one in seven, have disabling conditions sufficiently severe to interfere with daily life. One factor increasing the prevalence of disability is medicine's increasing success at averting the death of many people with developmental abnormalities such as spina bifida and the consequences of accidents such as spinal cord resection.

Studies of disability probably underestimate the prevalence of chronic illness. Conditions such as diabetes, psoriasis and epilepsy may not be identified by conventional measures of disability. Consequently, the percentage of the population living with a chronic condition is likely to be higher than the 14.2% identified by the OPCS survey. One estimate derived from work by the Royal College of Physicians suggested that just over one-fifth of the population was subject to some type of chronic illness.

Impairment, disability and handicap

A systematic approach to thinking about chronic illness is to be found in the International Classification of Impairments, Disabilities or Handicaps (ICIDH), a manual which classifies the consequences of disease (Wood 1980; Badley 1993). In order to better understand these consequences, it offers three concepts: impairment, disability and handicap. Impairment is concerned with abnormalities in the structure or functioning of the body or its parts, disability with the performance of activities, and handicap with the broader social and psychological consequences of living with impairment and disability. Because it is dependent on the social context in which it occurs, handicap can best be understood by sociological enquiry. Formal definitions of these terms are given in Box 6.1.

The three concepts are also organized into a model or theoretical framework which relates these dimensions of experience to each other (Fig. 6.1).

This model has caused some confusion, especially since some have interpreted the arrows to indicate time; so that an individual with a chronic condition moves along the sequence and inevitably becomes handicapped. In fact, the arrows mean 'may or may not lead to'. Disability may result from impairment and handicap may result from disability, but this is not necessarily

---

BOX 6.1

ICIDH DEFINITIONS

Impairment: an impairment is any loss or abnormality of psychological, physiological or anatomical structure or function.

Disability: a disability is a restriction or lack (resulting from an impairment) of ability to perform an activity in a manner or within the range considered normal for a human being.

Handicap: a handicap is a disadvantage for a given individual, resulting from an impairment or a disability, that limits or prevents the fulfilment of a role that is normal (depending on age, sex and social and cultural factors) for that individual.

Fig. 6.1 *Linear model of disease and its consequences.*

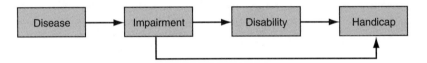

so. The examples given in Box 6.2 illustrate this point. Moreover, there is no necessary relationship between the severity of impairment and the severity of disability and/or handicap that results. For example, a study of people with multiple sclerosis found that the psychosocial handicaps they suffered were not related to the severity of the underlying disease (Harper et al. 1986). Similarly, a study of individuals with chronic respiratory disease found that clinical measures of lung function were not good predictors of disability, and there was considerable variability in the extent of handicap associated with a given level of disability (Williams and Bury 1989a,b).

Although the ICIDH scheme has been widely used it has been subject to some criticism, particularly in the US, where alternative schemes have been developed and adopted (Verbrugge and Jette 1993; Nagi 1991). At the heart of the problem is the use of the term handicap and the way in which is has been defined. In the US the term handicapped has been used to describe people in a pejorative way and is now generally avoided. In addition, the term carries the implication that the problems people experience are intrinsic, that is, the product of personal deficiencies and failings. Finally, because the definition of handicap uses the word 'role', which generally refers to activities and tasks, some have found the distinction between disability and handicap unclear.

One way around these difficulties is to think of handicap in terms of disadvantage and deprivation. For example, an individual who uses a wheelchair may be at a disadvantage in seeking work compared to the able-bodied simply because many workplaces have steps, stairs and washrooms or other facilities inaccessible to a wheelchair. As a consequence individuals may be deprived of jobs commensurate with their education and skills, or may become unemployed and deprived of the income, social contacts and other benefits that accrue from work. Even less-

---

BOX 6.2

INTERRELATIONS OF IMPAIRMENT, DISABILITY AND HANDICAP

An individual with arthritis (**disease**) will have pain and swelling in involved joints which will be stiff and limited in their range of motion (**impairment**). Consequently, there may be difficulty in carrying out activities such as walking or climbing stairs (**disability**). This may disadvantage the individual in terms of mobility around the community or finding a job, which in turn may lead to social isolation of relative poverty (**handicap**).

People with extreme short sight or diabetes are **impaired** but because these conditions can be corrected with devices or drugs, they would not necessarily be **disabled** in terms of any limitations in the activities they perform. However, in certain circumstances they may be **handicapped** by their conditions. For example, short sight may prevent access to certain occupations and diabetes may impose a burden on the individual because of dietary restrictions and the need for regular insulin injections.

A person with a severe facial disfigurement which is present at birth or the result of an accident would be **impaired**. They would not experience any limitations in the tasks or activities of daily life and would not be **disabled**. However, they may be **handicapped** in the sense that social attitudes towards physical attractiveness could lead to low self-esteem and difficulty in forming romantic relationships.

A person with cerebral palsy may have a range of **impairments** including problems with speech or use of the limbs. These could lead to **disabilities** in many activities including mobility around the community, difficulties with self-care and difficulties with communication. As a result, the individual could be **handicapped** in a number of areas of life. Alternatively, recognition of the person's intellectual abilities could open opportunities for a high status professional career with a high income. In turn, this would facilitate autonomy and choice.

Adapted from Badley, 1995.

---

tangible problems such as the mental burden and low self-esteem that may accompany chronic illness can be understood in these terms: the individual is deprived of peace of mind and a sense of self-worth.

This example highlights a crucial aspect of handicap. It does not stem from the individual but from the environments in which he/she must live. An alternative definition which makes this explicit states that handicap consists of 'the opportunities that a person has missed because of barriers in the environment' (Halbertsma 1989). In fact, a review of recent definitions of handicap found that they all contained reference to the environment (Badley 1995). In this context, environment refers not only to the physical, but also to material, social and attitudinal environments.

THE MEANING OF CHRONIC ILLNESS

From a sociological point of view and from the point of view of those living with a chronic illness, handicap is the most important consideration. This is because it is closely allied with the quality of life. Arguably, within the right environments, the quality of life of people with impairments and disabilities would not be much different from that of those without.

Because of its significance, two issues concerning handicap warrant further attention: first, its multidimensional character and second, its genesis in the interaction of individuals with their environments.

Dimensions of handicap

Whereas early sociological approaches to chronic illness and disability drew on the theory of the sick role (Parsons 1951) (see Chapter 4), labelling theory (Lemert 1967) and Goffman's analysis of stigma (Goffman 1963) (see Chapter 13), more contemporary approaches have used detailed case studies to understand what it means to live with a chronic disabling disorder. This 'experience of illness' perspective is to be found in numerous books and scholarly papers published over the last 10 years and all have handicap and quality of life as their central concern.

The meaning of chronic illness is to be found in its practical and symbolic consequences (Blaxter 1976; Bury 1988). These consequences take the form of problems which chronically sick people and their families must solve if they are to attain a quality of life of minimal tolerability.

One study of people with rheumatoid arthritis found that all faced the following: problems managing the symptoms of the disease and the medical treatments designed to control them; problems with the practical matters of everyday living, such as self-care, household management and mobility around the home and community; problems with respect to finding work or maintaining a meaningful role in the work-force; economic problems following unemployment; and problems in social relationships and family life (Locker 1983). The emotional burden of being chronically ill, its psychological consequences in the form of depression and frustration and feelings of vulnerability were prominent among this group of people, as was the necessity of adapting to a more limited life. The subjects in this study also encountered what might be termed cognitive problems. That is, they were faced with the task of making sense of the onset of chronic illness and sought answers to the unanswerable question 'Why me?'. In addition, they were constantly engaged in efforts to make sense of the day-to-day variation in levels of pain and stiffness in an attempt to establish order in their world and render their unpredictable existence predictable. As many studies have revealed, a significant aspect of being or caring for a person with a disability is the 'daily grind'; the never-ending and unrewarded practical and psychological work involved in coping with these problems on a daily basis. A more detailed account of some of these issues is presented below.

The genesis of handicap

An early modification to the ICIDH model emphasized the need to view handicap as emerging out of external factors which interact with disease/impairment/disability. One attempt to describe these factors made reference to the physical environment, the social situation of the person and the resources available to them (Badley 1987). In a more recent contribution, Verbrugge and Jette (1994) provided a more elaborate classification, including both personal and environmental factors in the process which links impairment/disability and their outcomes (Box 6.3).

BOX 6.3

FACTORS INFLUENCING THE DISABLEMENT PROCESS

Extra-individual factors

- Medical care and rehabilitation (surgery, physical therapy, speech therapy, counselling, health education, job retraining, etc.)

- Medication and other therapeutic regimens (drugs, recreational therapy, aquatic exercise, biofeedback meditation, rest/energy conservation, etc.)

- External supports (personal assistance, special equipment and devices, day care, respite care, meals-on-wheels, etc.)

- Build, physical and social environment (structural modifications at home/job, access to buildings and public transport, health insurance and access to medical care, laws and regulations, employment legislation, social attitudes, etc.)

Intra-individual factors

- Life-style and behaviour changes (overt changes to alter disease activity and impact)

- Psychosocial attributes and coping (positive affect, emotional vigour, locus of control, cognitive adaptation to disability, personal support, peer support groups, etc.)

- Activity accommodations (changes in kinds of activities, ways of doing them, frequency or length of time doing them)

Reprinted with kind permission from Elsevier Science Ltd from Verbrugge and Jette (1994).

The importance of these factors is that they provide avenues for interventions which aim to improve the quality of life of persons so affected.

A crucial factor which has an influence on how, and the extent to which, the problems associated with chronic illness and disability are managed is the resources to which individuals have access. These resources may take many forms; time, energy, money, social support, appropriate housing, formal services which foster independence rather than exacerbate dependence and knowledge and information are perhaps the most important. Psychological resources and dispositions are also important. The magnitude and range of resources available to individuals and families, and the coping strategies of which they form a part, influence how well the consequences of chronic conditions are managed.

In a sense, the fact that personal and social resources must be allocated to solving mundane practical matters is part of the handicap that flows from chronic illness. Money may have to be used to pay someone to clean the house and do the shopping rather than being used to make life more enjoyable. As chronic illness progresses, it is sometimes the case that available resources shrink. Physical resources may decline as a result of the worsening of the disease, money may decline when the individual becomes unemployed and his/her spouse gives up work to adopt a full-time caring role, and social support may be eroded as friendship networks or families collapse under the strain of chronic illness. In these instances, life becomes nothing more than the work and effort of solving illness-related problems and getting through the day.

The concept of resources is a crucial one. On the one hand, it provides one of the mechanisms which link disability and handicap; while on the other, it draws attention to the unequal distribution of resources in society and the ability/inability of individuals from different socio-economic groups to maintain a satisfactory existence in the face of chronic illness. In this way, it links personal concerns with wider social and political issues. People from working-class backgrounds, women, ethnic minorities and those who live in deprived urban communities are the most vulnerable in the face of chronic illness.

It is also the case that the illness experience can vary with historical period and culture. As Bury (1988) has indicated, chronic illness has two levels of meaning. One is to be found in the kinds of problems described above. The other is to be found in the significance or connotations that particular conditions carry, and the extent to which a given condition renders an individual culturally incompetent, that is, unable to perform ordinary activities in socially appropriate ways. The extent to which an individual is devalued by chronic illness will also be influenced by what the illness means in its particular cultural environment. For example, chronic obstructive airways disease is 'linked in the public mind to smoking (so) that the image of a wheezing, coughing, breathless old man is often greeted with little sympathy' (Williams and Bury 1989b: 609). This lack of sympathy may reflect a lack of attention to, and resources invested in, those suffering from the disease. Similarly, AIDS is closely allied in public thinking to devalued and socially stigmatized groups such as male homosexuals and i.v. drug users and behaviours which predispose the person to disease transmission. In this sense, AIDS constitutes a major assault on privacy. To reveal AIDS does not just reveal the presence of a disease, it reveals much more about identity and life-style. In this way, the handicapping nature of chronic illness flows also directly from social and cultural values.

MAJOR THEMES IN RESEARCH ON THE EXPERIENCE OF ILLNESS

It is not possible to convey the realities of living with chronic illness within the confines of a short chapter such as this. However, some impression can be gained of its pervasive effects by a brief discussion of some of the major themes evident in research on the experience of illness. Conrad (1987) has identified a number of such themes. Five are mentioned here; another, stigma, is the subject of Chapter 13.

Uncertainty

Many chronic conditions are surrounded by uncertainty. This may begin at the time when the individual first notices that something is wrong and may continue throughout the entire course of the illness. Many chronic illnesses have a slow and insidious onset and emerge in the form of vague symptoms which persist for years before diagnosis (prediagnostic uncertainty). With multiple sclerosis the delay between appearance of symptoms and diagnosis may be as long as 15 years (Robinson 1988). During this time sufferers are convinced that something is wrong, but often find their complaints dismissed by medical practitioners as trivial or as evidence of malingering or hypochondria. This can be a very trying time for the individual and his/her family. When a diagnosis is finally obtained, it often comes as a relief; it legitimates the person's complaints and experiences and brings to an end conflicts with others over the reality of the symptoms (Robinson 1988).

However, uncertainty may follow the diagnosis itself. This is often so with respect to predicting the course and outcome of the disease (trajectory uncertainty). Coupled with the uncertainty which can surround day-to-day fluctuations in symptoms (symptomatic uncertainty), this can severely disrupt family life. It makes both short- and long-term planning impossible and often means that living arrangements have to be constantly revised. Managing this uncertainty by whatever means available can become a major component of daily life.

A good example of uncertainty is provided by rheumatoid arthritis (RA). The symptoms of this disease, joint pain and stiffness, are highly unpredictable. The location and severity of the pain varies from day to day, and may even change during the course of a day. What seems to be a 'good day' in the morning may become a 'bad day' by the afternoon. This variability and unpredictability means that people with RA find it difficult to make sense of their symptoms and to contain them within acceptable boundaries. Many attempt to impose a degree of certainty on their existence by trying to identify events which precede acute phases or particularly painful days. Cold or damp weather and physical and emotional stress are frequently seen as the cause of pain and avoided as far as possible. However, a 'bad day' for which no apparent reason can be found leaves sufferers confused and adds to their distress (Locker 1983).

Family relations

There is clear evidence that chronic illness can place intolerable strains on families. This can arise because of the necessity to provide high levels of care and support, the emotional connotations of giving and receiving help and changes in family roles and relationships. Even where families are able and willing to provide help, the person with a chronic disabling condition may feel that he or she is a burden and may refuse the assistance that is needed. It is also the case that particularly distressing symptoms, such as chronic pain, may lead the individual to withdraw from family life altogether. In some instances, both individual and family become isolated from the wider world. Marital breakdown is not uncommon in these instances.

MacDonald (1988) provides insights into the effects of chronic illness on marital and family relationships in her study of people living with the sequelae of rectal cancer. Two-thirds of the people she interviewed had a colostomy, with the remainder having been treated by excision of the cancer and anastomosis. Most of the individuals reported a loss of sexual capacity and a decline in the quality of the marital relationship. This was partly due to the physical effects of surgery and partly due to feelings of shame and embarrassment. These feelings of stigma were most marked among younger men, who reported that the consequences of surgery and fears for the future had created a barrier between them and their wives.

The consequences of surgery also had a profound effect on social relationships in general. Again, shame and embarrassment about noise and odours from the stoma, worries about offending others and feelings of self-disgust caused many to avoid social contacts and to lead a far more restricted life.

Biographical work and the reconstitution of self

All chronic disabling conditions pose a threat to identity and self-concept. One of the reasons for this is that the onset of chronic illness constitutes a 'biographical disruption' (Bury 1982) and calls into question both past and future. It necessitates a fundamental rethinking of both biography and self-concept. Williams (1984) argues that people with chronic illness must indulge in a process he calls 'narrative reconstruction', in which the individual's biography is reorganized in order to account for the onset of illness. This identification of cause, which draws on lay theories concerning the aetiology of illness, is part of the process of coming to terms with chronic illness. It gives meaning and order to the individual's world.

Charmaz (1987) has described how chronically sick people are involved in a constant struggle to lead valued lives and maintain definitions of self which are positive and worthwhile. This can be difficult; cultural definitions of disability devalue the individual and interactions with others may constantly undermine the individual's sense of self-worth. Charmaz (1987) considers the 'loss of self' to be a powerful form of suffering experienced by the chronically ill.

Managing medical regimens

People with chronic disabling disorders must learn to manage their symptoms and manifestations during everyday life. The person with rheumatoid arthritis, for example, rapidly learns how much activity is possible before pain rises to intolerable levels. Daily life is then planned and organized in ways which allow the individual to accomplish a few valued activities before pain intercedes and he or she is forced to rest. The individual must also learn to manage the medical regimens prescribed to control symptoms. These can include diet, drugs or the use of advanced technologies such as a dialysis machine. In some instances the treatment can be as bad as the disease, consuming time, energy and financial resources and requiring hard work (Jobling 1988). The whole life of the chronically sick person can become organized around treatment.

An illuminating example is provided by a study of people with postpolio respiratory impairment, whose capacity to breathe had deteriorated to such an extent that permanent connection to a positive-pressure ventilator by means of a tracheostomy became necessary (Locker and Kaufert 1988). This highly efficient form of mechanical ventilation substantially improved physical and psychological health, allowed for far greater mobility than older technologies and transformed the quality of everyday life. However, the use of this machine meant that the individual concerned, and those providing care and support, had to learn a wide range of skills in order to manage the machine, including recharging batteries, suctioning tubing and maintaining the humidification system. Because this machinery often malfunctioned, usually without warning, it had to be carefully monitored and strategies had to be developed to cope with sudden failure. The potential for respiratory crises left both sufferers and family members feeling vulnerable and insecure. As a consequence, the machine, and tending to the needs of the machine, became a central focus of everyday life.

A less dramatic example is provided by a study of people with psoriasis, a disfiguring skin disease (Jobling 1988).

'Treatment' involves strict conformity over weeks, months or even years, to a programme of repetitious daily bathing, rubbing and scrubbing. This is followed by anointment with oils, creams, pastes or ointments, some of which may involve a subjectively noxious smell. Regular exposure to the sun's rays, or at least an equivalent produced by a machine, is another component. All of this may take up several hours a day.

It is often the case that any prescribed regimen is substantially altered by the person concerned. This allows them to exert control over their illness and to maximize their well-being by avoiding some of the negative aspects of medical treatments.

Information, awareness and sharing

For the chronically ill, information is a significant resource for managing their lives. It reduces uncertainty, helps the individual to come to terms with the illness and allows for the development of strategies for managing the illness in everyday life. Nevertheless, many people with chronic conditions express dissatisfaction with the amount of information they are able to obtain about their disorder. Difficulty with communication is a major problem in the relationships between people with chronic illnesses and their doctors. Many rectal cancer patients interviewed by MacDonald (1988) were dissatisfied with what they were told about their operation, and some felt inadequately prepared for dealing with the colostomy and its effects. Some reported not knowing what a colostomy was, even at the time of surgery, and many complained of inadequate follow-up care from their family doctor.

Given these problems in communication, information may be culled from a variety of sources: from books and publications, from self-help groups or from others with the same or similar illnesses. This information provides the basis for action and the feeling that it is possible to do something about and have some control over the illness.

THE DOCTOR–PATIENT RELATIONSHIP IN CHRONIC ILLNESS

Patients with chronic disabling disorders can be difficult for a medical practitioner to manage successfully. This is only partly due to the fact that medicine has relatively few interventions which make a real difference to the patient's condition. It also arises because the medical gaze is frequently a narrow one, concerned predominantly with disease to the exclusion of its social and emotional consequences for patients and families.

Anderson and Bury (1988) indicate the need for 'a reorientation of the focus for care from repairing damage caused by disease to education and understanding for living with chronic illness'. In this sense, information, advice and support are among the most important interventions a doctor has to offer, their goal being to help the patient live as normal and satisfying a life as possible within family and community. Such help needs to be approached with care and sensitivity; patients need to be offered choices, not have them made by others on their behalves. This means ensuring that individuals are helped to be independent and not encouraged into dependency.

By giving due attention to the particular handicaps associated with a chronic condition, the care that is offered to both the sufferer and the family can be made more appropriate and relevant to their social and emotional concerns. This presupposes that the professional is fully aware of the many meanings of chronic illness, the burdens carried by the individual and those who provide informal support, and the contextual factors which shape these meanings and burdens.

This, in turn, highlights the issues of communication and information (see Chapter 4) and the importance of a free exchange of information between doctors and those with a chronic illness. Each has much to teach the other in working together to maximize the patient's quality of life.

REFERENCES

Anderson, R. & Bury, M. (eds)   (1988) *Living With Chronic Illness: The Experiences of Patients and Their Families*. London: Hyman Unwin.

Badley, E.   (1993) An introduction to the concepts and classifications of the international classification of impairments, disabilities and handicaps. *Disabil. Rehab.*, **15**, 161–78.

Badley, E.   (1995) The genesis of handicap: definition, models of disablement and role of external factors. *Disabil. Rehab.*, **15**, 53–62.

Badley, E.M.   (1987) The ICIDH: format, application in different settings, and distinction between disability and handicap. *International Disability Studies*. **9**, 122–8.

Blaxter, M.   (1976) *The Meaning of Disability*. London: Heinemann.

Bury, M.   (1982) Chronic illness as biographical disruption. *Soc. Health Illness*, **4**, 167–82.

Bury, M.   (1988) Meanings at risk: the experience of arthritis. In: *Living With Chronic Illness: The Experiences of Patients and Their Families*, ed. R. Anderson & M. Bury. London: Hyman Unwin.

Charmaz, K.   (1987) Struggling for a self: identity levels of the chronically ill. *Res. Soc. Health Care*, **6**, 283–321.

Conrad, P.   (1987) The experience of illness: recent and new directions. *Res. Soc. Health Care*, **6**, 1–31.

Goffman, E.   (1963) *Stigma*. Englewood Cliffs, NJ: Prentice Hall.

Halbertsma, J. (1989) The ICIDH: A study of how it is used and evaluated. A review of the application of a classification relating to the consequences of disease. Zoetermeer: WCC Standing Committee on Classification and Terminology of the National Council of Public Health.

Harper, A., Harper, D., Chambers, L., Cino, P. & Singer, J.   (1986) An epidemiological description of physical, social and psychological problems in multiple sclerosis. *J. Chron. Dis.*, **39**, 305–10.

Jobling, R.   (1988) The experience of psoriasis under treatment. In: *Living With Chronic Illness: The Experiences of Patients and Their Families*, ed. R. Anderson & M. Bury. London: Hyman Unwin.

Lemert, E.   (1967) *Human Deviance, Social Problems and Social Control*. Englewood Cliffs, NJ: Prentice-Hall.

Locker, D.   (1983) *Disability and Disadvantage: the Consequences of Chronic Illness*. London: Tavistock.

Locker, D. & Kaufert, J.   (1988) The breath of life: medical technology and the careers of people with post-respiratory poliomyelitis. *Soc. Health Illness*, **10**, 24–40.

MacDonald, L. (1988) The experience of stigma: living with rectal cancer. In: *Living With Chronic Illness: The Experiences of Patients and Their Families*, ed. R. Anderson & M. Bury. London: Hyman Unwin.

Nagi S.   (1991) Disability concepts revisited: implications for prevention. In: *Disability in America: Toward a National Agenda for Prevention*, ed A. Pope & A. Tarlov. Washington DC: National Academy Press.

Office of Population Censuses and Surveys   (1988) *OPCS Surveys of Disability in Great Britain: The Prevalence of Disability Among Adults*. London: HMSO.

Parsons, T.   (1951) *The Social System*. New York: Free Press.

Robinson, I.   (1988) Reconstructing lives: negotiating the meaning of multiple sclerosis. In: *Living With Chronic Illness: The Experiences of Patients and Their Families*, ed. R. Anderson & M. Bury. London: Hyman Unwin.

Topliss, E.   (1979) *Provision for the Disabled*. London: Martin Robertson.

Verbrugge, L. & Jette, A.   (1994) The disablement process. *Soc. Sci. Med.*, **38**, 1–14.

Williams, G.   (1984) The genesis of chronic illness: narrative reconstruction. *Soc. Health Illness*, **6**, 175–200.

Williams, S.   (1989) Chronic respiratory illness and disability: a critical review of the psychosocial literature. *Soc. Sci. Med.*, **28**, 791–803.

Williams, S. & Bury, M.   (1989a) Breathtaking: the consequences of chronic respiratory disorder. Unpublished paper.

Williams, S. & Bury, M.   (1989b) Impairment, disability and handicap in chronic respiratory illness. *Soc. Sci. Med.*, **29**, 609–16.

Wood, P.   (1980) The language of disablement: a glossary relating to disease and its consequences. *Int. Rehabil. Med.*, **2**, 86–92.

7

Dying, Death and Bereavement

GRAHAM SCAMBLER

The inescapable fact of death provides one of the principal parameters of the human condition. As Lofland (1978) writes, 'it can neither be "believed" nor "magicked" nor "scienced" away'. Increasingly in the twentieth century physicians and other health workers have been called upon to give treatment and support to the terminally ill and their first-degree relatives. This chapter focuses on problems of communication about dying between health workers, patients and relatives; various 'stages' of dying; alternative facilities for the care of the terminally ill in Britain; aspects of the treatment of dying persons; and processes of bereavement.

TALKING ABOUT DEATH

In the final quarter of the twentieth century a higher proportion of people than ever before experience 'slow' as opposed to 'quick' dying, that is, dying has typically become a more protracted process. The reasons for this have been well documented and are summarized in Box 7.1. For obvious reasons this change has enhanced the salience of communication around death. It is ironic, therefore, that many historians have maintained that death over the last 100 years or so has become more and more 'unmentionable'. Aries (1983) characterizes modern – demytholo-gized and secularized – death as invisible death: 'we ignore the existence of a scandal that we have been unable to prevent; we act as if it did not exist, and thus mercilessly force the bereaved to say nothing. A heavy silence has fallen over the subject of death'. According to Aries, death has grown fearful again, imbued with all its 'old savagery'.

Countering this view that the denial of death is now ubiquitous, however, Seale (1995) has pointed to evidence that 'scripts' for proclaiming 'heroic self-identity in the face of death' are currently being promoted by many professional 'experts' and appropriated by growing numbers of lay people. His contention is that these scripts, less 'masculine' and more 'feminine' in

BOX 7.1

CONDITIONS FACILITATING 'QUICK DYING' IN THE PRE-MODERN ERA AND 'SLOW DYING' IN THE MODERN ERA

Conditions facilitating quick dying	Conditions facilitating slow dying
Low level of medical technology	High level of medical technology
Late detection of disease- or fatality-producing conditions	Early detection of disease- or fatality-producing conditions
Simple definition of death (e.g. cessation of heart beat)	Complex definition of death (e.g. irreversible cessation of higher brain activity)
High incidence of mortality from acute disease	High incidence of mortality from chronic or degenerative disease
High incidence of fatality-producing injuries	Low incidence of fatality-producing injuries
Customary killing or suicide of, or fatal passivity towards, the person once he or she has entered the 'dying' category	Customary curative and activist orientation toward the dying with a high value placed on the prolongation of life

Reproduced with permission of Sage Publications Inc. from Lofland (1978).

orientation than their predecessors, re-define 'heroic death' as involving a struggle to gain knowledge, opportunities to demonstrate courage, and a state of emotional calm or equilibrium in which dying people and carers alike participate. The emphasis is on care, concern and emotional expression. Some deaths, Seale admits, cannot be written into such scripts; for example, those of the very old, the mentally confused and sudden unexpected deaths. And there are rival scripts: there are those, for example, who prefer the benefits of continuing the everyday project of the self oblivious of oncoming death, with others sharing the burden of awareness in an attempt to protect the dying person from the strain of knowing. But Seale conjectures that what he terms scripts of heroic death are gaining ground.

Independently of differences between writers like Aries and Seale, it is not surprising that deciding whether or not to tell someone he or she is dying continues to be regarded as problematic for health workers. When asked, most people anticipate that they would want to be told if they were dying; physicians are themselves unexceptional in this respect. But how much credibility should be attached to such responses? Can young, healthy individuals accurately predict how they will feel as death approaches?

Cartwright et al. (1973), who interviewed relatives of a national sample of people who had died in the preceding year in Britain, were told by relatives that 37% of those dying knew as much, and a further 20% 'half knew'. Nearly three-quarters of the relatives felt they had them-selves known. It was also apparent from this study that the relatives received more information from all sources than did the people who were dying. If death occurred in a hospital less information was forthcoming than if it occurred at home; in both contexts, however, the general practitioner was the key informant. Herd (1990), in a study of terminal care in a semirural part of Britain, also found principal lay carers to be less aware and knowledgeable about what was happening if death took place in hospital than if it took place in the home. A more recent study by Seale and Cartwright (1994), however, suggests a changing picture. In 250 accounts from lay relatives, friends and others who knew people in a random national sample of adult deaths, 54% reported that both parties had been aware that the person was dying. In 36% of situations the respondent knew, but the dying person did not; in 8% neither knew; and in 1% the respondent did not know, although the deceased did.

Awareness of dying

Glaser and Strauss (1965) found there to be four common types of 'awareness contexts' in rela-tion to the dying. They define 'awareness context' as: 'what each interacting person knows of the patient's defined status, along with his recognition of others' awareness of his own defini-tion'. The four types are summarized in Box 7.2. Some commentators, as has been noted, have assumed that 'closed', 'suspected' and 'mutual pretence' awareness contexts are intrinsically undesirable and that health workers, especially physicians, are exclusively to blame for the fact that they frequently exist. As a study by McIntosh (1977) suggests, however, such assumptions can be naive and misleading. McIntosh interviewed both patients and physicians. Most patients he spoke to suspected malignancy. The majority sought information from members of the hos-pital team but, according to McIntosh's estimate, two out of every three did not 'really' want their diagnostic suspicions confirmed and fewer still 'really' wanted to know their prognosis. They sought exclusively information which would reinforce an optimistic conception of their condition: uncertainty afforded hope. Most patients also felt – somewhat unrealistically, given

---

BOX 7.2

'AWARENESS CONTEXTS' IN RELATION TO DYING

1. *Closed awareness:* the situation in which the patient does not recognize his impend-ing death even though everyone else does.

2. *Suspected awareness:* the situation when the patient suspects what others know and attempts either to confirm or to invalidate his suspicions.

3. *Mutual pretence awareness:* the situation where each party defines the patient as dying but each 'pretends' that the other has not done so.

4. *Open awareness:* the situation where health workers and patient are each aware that the latter is dying, and where they act on this awareness fairly openly.

Reproduced with permission of Aldine Press from Glaser and Strauss (1965).

McIntosh's documentation of physicians' predisposition *not* to disclose – that they would be told everything if they asked.

Timmermans (1994) has suggested that Glaser and Strauss' 'open awareness context' requires refinement 'to include the diversity of viewpoints of family members and patients'. He delineates three types of open awareness. The context of 'suspended open awareness' occurs when patients and their relatives simply ignore or 'deny' the information. This can arise in three sets of circumstances. First, it can be a transitory feature after the disclosure of the terminal condition and prognosis. Disbelief here is an initial reaction to cope with the shock of disclosure – 'the open awareness context is nascent: the news has been given but its radical consequences have not been fully assimilated'. Second, disbelief can become a permanent and preferred state, with even the reality of the underlying condition being called into question. And third, patients can come to question or doubt the outcomes of their conditions in situations of unexpected deterioration or improvement. The context of 'uncertain open awareness' occurs when patients and relatives do not dismiss the possibility of death, but 'prefer the uncertainty of not understanding exactly what is going on'. The context of 'active open awareness' occurs when hope for recovery is abandoned and patients and their families understand the full ramifications of the impending death and try to find ways of coming to terms with it.

As McIntosh found, physicians are not always ready to communicate openly. In a Canadian study of 118 encounters during which 17 male surgeons disclosed the results of biopsies to women with breast cancer, Taylor (1988) found that each surgeon appeared to have adopted a favoured 'strategy' which he used routinely, thus 'bypassing the individuality of each case'. Four techniques were discerned. The first, *communication*, was deployed by some surgeons when they were in a position to make a reasonable and definite prognosis of the condition in terms comprehensible to the patient. Many surgeons claimed to use this technique, but in fact few did. Only 10% of the 118 disclosures were of this type. The second, *admission of uncertainty*, was used by a small minority of surgeons when no clinical prognosis was justified; 15% of the disclosures took this form. The third technique, *dissimulation*, or the pronouncement of a prognosis which could not be clinically substantiated, occurred when surgeons were reluctant to share the extent of their uncertainty with their patients; 30% of the disclosures fell into this category. The final technique, *evasion*, or 'the failure to communicate a clinically substantiated prognosis', was used by a number of surgeons who preferred not to respond directly to patients' questions. 'For those surgeons whose patients asked direct questions to which the appropriate technical response might reveal a low chance of long-term survival, repressing information was a favoured policy.' Not infrequently, replies to specific questions drew on general statistics not easily applicable to the individual case. In 45% of disclosures surgeons used evasion as a means of coping with direct questions posed by women.

If one thing is clear it is that there is no easy, general answer to the question 'To tell or not to tell?'. Hinton (1967) offers physicians the following counsel:

> *Although it is not an infallible guide as to how much the dying patient should be told, his apparent wishes and questions do point the way. This means that the manner in which he puts his views should be closely attended to – the intonations and the exact wording may be very revealing. It also means that*

he must be given ample opportunity to express his ideas and ask his questions. If the questions are sincere, however, then why not give quite straight answers to the patient's questions about his illness and the outcome? It makes for beneficial trust.

A study by Hinton (1980) highlights the importance of giving dying patients the opportunity to talk. He interviewed 80 patients with terminal cancer at a mean of 10 weeks before death; 66% told him that they recognized they might or would soon die, 8% were non-committal, and 26% spoke only of improvement. Some patients spoke of dying to either their spouse or the staff and not to the interviewer, but they tended to say less to their spouse than to the interviewer and less still to members of the staff. This tendency is illustrated in Fig. 7.1. Hinton concludes that people are often ready to share their awareness if someone is prepared to listen.

Fig. 7.1 *Awareness of the possibility of dying as shown by different people by 80 patients with terminal cancer. The square represents the 80 patients and the three shaded circles their communicated awareness to staff, spouse and interviewer. Reproduced with permission from Hinton (1980).*

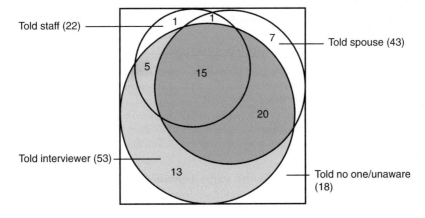

Stages of dying

How people come to terms with the prospect of imminent death depends on many factors (Hinton 1984). Of obvious importance is the nature of the physical and mental distress experienced. In a randomized national survey of terminal illness, Cartwright et al. (1973) reported the following symptoms occurring to a 'very distressing degree' during the last year of life: pain 42%, breathing troubles 28%, vomiting 17%, sleeplessness 17%, loss of both bladder and bowel control 12%, loss of appetite 11%, and mental confusion 10%. It has regularly been found that, when compared with lay carers, health workers tend to underestimate patients' symptoms and to overestimate the success of treatment (Herd 1990).

Among the many factors which can influence how individuals cope with terminal illness are age, family intimacy and support, and religious convictions. There is enormous individual variation and hence unpredictability in any given case. Kubler-Ross (1970) has claimed, however, that people who know they are dying typically pass through five 'stages' (Box 7.3).

BOX 7.3

'STAGES OF DYING'

First stage: denial and isolation

Many people, on being told they are dying, experience a temporary state of shock. When the numbness disappears, a common response is: 'No, it can't be me'. One's own death is all but inconceivable. 'Denial' is usually a temporary defence, but some take it further, perhaps 'shopping around' for a more amenable clinical opinion (only three of the 200 patients in Kubler-Ross' study attempted to deny the approach of death to the very end). A deep feeling of 'isolation' is normal at this stage.

Second stage: anger

When the initial stage of denial can no longer be maintained, it is often replaced by feelings of anger, rage, envy and resentment. The question 'Why me?' is posed. The anger can be displaced and at times projected onto the environment almost at random (although it can of course be justified as well as unjustified). The hospital team, especially the nursing staff, frequently bear the brunt of these outbursts.

Third stage: bargaining

The third stage of 'bargaining', Kubler-Ross argues, has only rarely been acknowledged. The point is that terminally ill people will sometimes negotiate – openly with health workers or secretly with God – to postpone death: postponement will be the reward for a promise of good behaviour. For example, many patients in the study promised to donate parts of their bodies to medical science if the physicians undertook to use their knowledge of science to extend their lives.

Fourth stage: depression

When terminally ill patients can no longer deny their illness, when they are compelled to endure more surgery, when they grow weaker, the numbness or stoicism or anger gives way to a sense of great loss. This 'depression' may be *reactive*, for example a woman with cancer of the uterus may feel she is no longer a woman, or what Kubler-Ross calls *preparatory*, that is, based on impending losses associated with death itself.

Fifth stage: acceptance

The final stage of 'acceptance' is one in which dying patients commonly find a sort of peace, a peace which is largely a function of weakness and a diminished interest in the world. 'It is as if the pain has gone, the struggle is over . . .'. Kubler-Ross adds that this is also the time during which the family usually needs more help, understanding and support than the patient.

Reproduced with permission of Tavistock Publications from Kubler-Ross (1970).

Several writers have criticized Kubler-Ross' specification of discrete stages of dying, usually on the grounds that it represents an over-generalization based on subjective data. Certainly Kubler-Ross' stages should not be regarded either as unidirectional or as sequential.

PLACE OF DEATH

Those like Aries who argue that death has become increasingly invisible during the twentieth century attach considerable significance to the fact that, since the 1930s and 1940s, death has been substantially removed from the community or 'hospitalized'. In the hospital, according to this thesis, death is no longer an occasion of ritual ceremony over which the dying person and his or her kin and friends hold sway. The physicians and hospital team are the new 'masters of death', of its moment as well as its circumstances. This interpretation of changing events is once again open to criticism, but there is no doubt that the hospitalization of death has continued. In 1990 23% of deaths occurred in people's own homes, and 72% in institutions: 54% in hospitals, 4% in hospices and 14% in nursing or residential homes (OPCS 1992).

There is a growing feeling that the hospital is too frequently an inappropriate place in which to die. In his essay on *The Loneliness of Dying*, Elias (1985), who is fully aware of how emotionally taxing, as well as rewarding, a death in the family home can be, nevertheless stresses that in modern hospitals 'dying people can be cared for in accordance with the latest biophysical specialist knowledge, but often neutrally as regards feeling; they may die in total isolation'. Most hospitals are designed to provide for acute illness, and terminally ill people in acute wards can both disturb other patients and members of ward staff and be disturbed by them; most hospitals do not set aside a whole or part of a ward for dying patients because they are anxious to avoid the stigma of a 'death ward'. Several alternative locations exist in Britain, including special units within conventional hospitals, but the most discussed are the home and the hospice.

The home

For many health workers and lay persons alike, despite the statistical trend to hospitalization, the home remains the 'natural' and 'proper' place in which to die. As Bowling and Cartwright (1982) discovered, however, the care of dying people at home imposes severe physical, financial and psychological strains on relatives. In Herd's (1990) study, 74% of lay carers (four out of every five of them female relatives) mentioned 'emotional strain' as a problem, and 51% mentioned 'physical strain'. Table 7.1 ranks those aspects of home care that Herd's lay carers defined as 'worrying'. Lay carers are also likely to find their own activities restricted: Bowling and Cartwright report 26% describing their activities as 'severely restricted' and a further 19% as 'fairly restricted'. The extent to which professional and other support is at hand is likely to be contingent upon ad hoc factors affecting local planning and provision. Currently in Britain hospitalization is typically a function of the absence of local planning and provision. There are shortages of helpers ranging from Macmillan nurses to home helps and providers of meals-on-wheels.

The hospice

The hospice movement was founded in the mid-nineteenth century and was largely pioneered in Britain, although inpatient hospices still deal with only 4% of dying people and generally with

TABLE 7.1 *Worrying aspects of home care identified by lay carers.*

	Number (%) of respondents
Anxiety about medication	26 (49)
Inability to leave patient unattended	22 (42)
Not knowing what to expect	18 (34)
Inability to help	15 (28)
Fear of being alone when death took place	11 (21)
Anxiety about what to do when death took place	5 (9)
Anxiety about calling the doctor	3 (6)
Other	5 (9)

Reproduced with permission from Herd (1990).

those dying from cancer. The favoured pattern in Britain is to build small units in the grounds of general hospitals, using their facilities but remaining administratively independent. The range of care provided in a hospice is intermediate between that of a long-stay hospital and that of an acute hospital. The staffing ratios are similar to those of an acute hospital, but the call for diagnostic and other 'support' services is much less. The average length of stay is also closer to that of patients in an acute hospital than that of patients in a long-stay hospital, and costs are in keeping with this.

Central to the philosophy of the hospice is the view that the whole professional caring team should work in unison to develop the skills the dying person needs. Dramatic improvements in care have originated in hospices in the last quarter of the twentieth century, for example in standards of palliative medicine; hospice teams have reduced levels of uncontrolled pain to 8% and less (Parkes 1984). It should not be assumed, however, that, given the choice, everybody would opt for death in a hospice. In one study the care given in four radiotherapy wards of an acute hospital, in a Foundation Home visited by two general practitioners and in a hospice were compared (Hinton 1979).

Little difference was found between the acute hospital and the Foundation Home, but there was some evidence that patients were less depressed and anxious in the hospice and preferred the more frank communication available there. It was also found, however, that patients gave most praise to the outpatient system of care, despite experiencing more anxiety or irritability at home. The author concluded: 'treatment cannot be judged solely by the mental quiet it brings; freedom or hope may be preferred even if they bring worry'. It has been found that home-centred patients tend to experience more pain than hospital-centred patients, and their relatives more stress; but it does not follow that, even knowing this, patients and their relatives would necessarily choose to leave home. It should not be concluded that because adequate support for home care is rarely available the hospitalization of death should be accelerated.

Fig. 7.2 summarizes the sources of help available to people who are dying in Britain.

Fig. 7.2 *Sources of help for people who are dying. Reproduced with permission of Open University Press from Field and James (1993).*

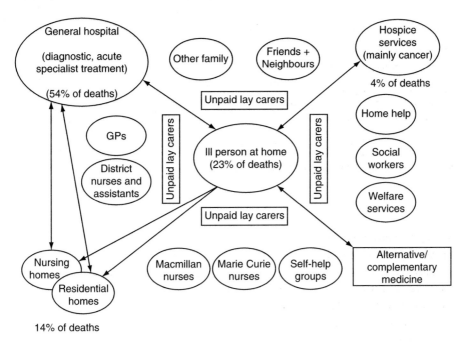

PATTERNS OF DEATH AND BEREAVEMENT

Sudnow (1967) has drawn a distinction between biological and social death. The problem of how to define biological death has been resolved by the medical profession for the time being in favour of the irreversible cessation of higher brain activity. Sudnow uses the term 'social death' in a general sense to refer to how organizations deal with different modes of dying and death. More specifically, social death is marked, within the hospital setting, by that point at which a patient is treated essentially as a corpse, although still perhaps biologically alive. He gives an example of social death preceding biological death. A nurse on duty with a woman she explained was 'dying' was observed to spend two or three minutes trying to close the woman's eyelids. After several unsuccessful attempts she managed to shut them and said, with a sigh of relief, 'Now they're right'. When questioned, she said that a patient's eyes must be closed after death, so that the body will resemble a sleeping person. It was more difficult to accomplish this, she explained, after the muscles and skin had begun to stiffen. She always tried to close them before death. This made for greater efficiency when the time came for ward personnel to wrap the body. It was a matter of consideration toward those workers who preferred to handle dead bodies as little as possible.

Mulkay (1993) interprets the concept of social death more broadly. Social death may precede biological death, as in Sudnow's example, or, alternatively, social existence may continue long after death, 'for example, when distraught parents visit the grave of a dead child and talk and write to that child about their previous life together and about the reunion to come' (Clegg 1988). The defining feature of social death, then, is the cessation of the individual person as an active agent in others' lives. Mulkay argues that the profile of social death has changed considerably over the last century due to people's collective responses to changes in the social distribution of biological death, changes in the social setting of death, and changes in the clinical nature of death. Consider the elderly for example. Mulkay suggests that the start of the 'death sequence' in our society occurs, particularly for men, at the time of retirement from work. This is a key transition, when people's participation in social life significantly diminishes – independently of personal variations in state of health – owing to the socially recognized approach of death. From retirement on, elderly people in Britain are typically channelled away from the principal arenas of social activity and their ties with the wider society progressively weakened in anticipation of their biological end (Williams 1990). With admission to a hospital or, increasingly, a residential or nursing home, where the bureaucratic 'neglect of the patient as a person' (Field 1989) converges with the physical, emotional and communicative withdrawal of the living from those on the death sequence, the death sequence of society at large is repeated in microcosm.

Trajectories of dying

Glaser and Strauss (1968) distinguish seven 'critical junctures' in what is sometimes called the 'career' of the dying patient:

1. the definition of the patient as dying;
2. staff and family then make their preparations for the patient's death, as the patient may do if he or she knows that death is near;
3. at some point there seems to be 'nothing more to do' to prevent death;
4. the final descent, which may take weeks, days or merely hours;
5. the 'last hours';
6. the death watch;
7. death itself.

When these critical junctures occur as expected – as it were, on schedule – then all those involved, including sometimes the patient, are prepared for them. When, however, critical junctures occur unexpectedly, hospital staff and the patient's family alike may be unprepared. If a patient is expected to die quite soon, for example, but vacillates sufficiently often, then both staff and family are likely to find the experience stressful.

Predictability, then, makes the work of hospital teams easier. Miscalculations in forecasting can play havoc with the organization of work. When crises do occur, the staff attempt to regain control as quickly as possible, but sometimes the disruption of work is accompanied by a shattering of what Glaser and Strauss (1965) have called a ward's characteristic 'sentimental mood' or order. They cite an example: 'in an intensive care unit where cardiac patients die frequently, the mood is relatively unaffected by one more speedy expected death; but if a hopeless patient lingers on and on, or if his wife, perhaps, refuses to accept his dying and causes "scenes", then both mood and work itself are profoundly affected'.

Glaser and Strauss (1968) differentiate between a number of patterns of death, 'dying trajectories', paying special attention to the distinction noted earlier between 'quick' and 'slow' dying. Quick dying, they claim, may take three forms: 'the expected quick death'; 'unexpected quick dying, but expected to die'; and 'unexpected quick dying, not expected to die'. They report that, in general, unexpected quick deaths are more disturbing for staff and families than expected quick deaths. Even expected quick deaths, however, can give rise to distinctive difficulties. Glaser and Strauss focus on staff–family interaction and note, for example, that the likely presence of the family at the bedside when death occurs requires careful handling by the staff, since a 'scene' will disrupt ward order and worry other patients. Slow dying 'is fraught with both hazard and opportunity'. On the one hand, the dying may take 'too long', be unexpectedly painful or unpleasant, and so on; on the other hand, a slow decline may allow time for wills to be made or families to come together, and may provide the setting for quiet and dignified endings. All these consequences are less likely to occur with quick dying.

Bereavement and mourning

Just as experiences of impending death vary from person to person, so does the experience of losing a relative or friend. Much depends on the nature of the relationship. However, a sudden, unexpected death is often harder to get over than one where there was time to grieve before the occurrence of death: this is known as 'anticipatory' or 'pre-bereavement mourning'.

In his anthropological study of death in Britain, Gorer (1965) argues that mourners typically pass through three stages:

1. a short period of shock, usually lasting from death until the disposal of the body;
2. a period of intense mourning, accompanied by withdrawal of attention and affect from the external world and by physiological changes like disturbed sleep, vivid dreams, failure of appetite and loss of weight; and
3. a final period of re-established social and physical homeostasis, with sleep and weight stabilized and interest again directed outwards.

Gorer's principal thesis is that, in an increasingly secular Britain, only the first of these three periods is socially acknowledged and surrounded by ceremony and ritual. After the funeral or postfuneral meal mourners are frequently abandoned to cope alone. To counter this social isolation during a time of continuing need for succour and support (periods 2 and 3) he advocates the creation of new secular rituals to replace now defunct religious ones.

Kamerman (1988) suggests that this twentieth-century process of 'deritualization' has been accompanied by a process of 'rationalization'. By this he means that death has increasingly come to be subsumed under conventions or routines which render it non-intrusive. Responses to death have become more 'business-like'. Both deritualization and rationalization are epitomized by the growing preference for cremation over burial. Approximately two-thirds of bodies are now cremated in Britain.

As if in affirmation of the need for continuing support after the funeral, several studies have shown elevated rates of morbidity and mortality and of visits to general practitioners among samples of recently bereaved persons.

It remains the case that many health students and workers receive minimal preparation for coping with terminal care and bereavement. Glaser and Strauss argue that much non-technical conduct in relation to the dying and bereaved is influenced by common-sense assumptions, 'essentially untouched by professional considerations or by current knowledge from the behavioural sciences'. The argument for the provision of a good grounding in those aspects of care – psychological, social, organizational and ethical – which are now relatively neglected is a strong one.

REFERENCES

Aries, P.   (1983) *The Hour of our Death*. London: Penguin.
Bowling, A. & Cartwright, A.   (1982) *Life After Death: A Study of the Elderly Widowed*. London: Tavistock.
Cartwright, A., Hockey, L. & Anderson, J.   (1973) *Life Before Death*. London: Routledge & Kegan Paul.
Clegg, F.   (1988) *Decisions at a Time of Grief*. Cambridge: Cambridge University Press.
Elias, N.   (1985) *The Loneliness of Dying*. Oxford: Basil Blackwell.
Field, D.   (1989) *Nursing the Dying*. London: Tavistock/Routledge.
Field, D. & James, N.   (1993) Where and how people die. In: *The Future for Palliative Care*, ed. D. Clark. Milton Keynes: Open University Press.
Glaser, B. & Strauss, A.   (1965) *Awareness of Dying*. Chicago, IL: Aldine.
Glaser, B. & Strauss, A.   (1968) *Time For Dying*. Chicago, IL: Aldine.
Gorer, G.   (1965) *Death, Grief and Mourning in Contemporary Britain*. London: Cresset Press.
Herd, E.   (1990) Terminal care in a semi-rural area. *Br. J. Gen. Pract.*, **40**, 248–51.
Hinton, J.   (1967) *Dying*. London: Penguin.
Hinton, J.   (1979) Comparison of places and policies for terminal care. *Lancet*, **ii**, 29–32.
Hinton, J.   (1980) Whom do dying patients tell? *Br. Med. J.*, **281**, 1328–30.
Hinton, J.   (1984) Coping with terminal illness. In: *The Experience of Illness*, ed. R. Fitzpatrick, J. Hinton, S. Newman, G. Scambler & J. Thompson. London: Tavistock.
Kamerman, J.   (1988) *Death in the Midst of Life: Social and Cultural Influences on Death, Grief and Mourning*. Englewood Cliffs, NJ: Prentice Hall.
Kubler-Ross, E.   (1970) *On Death and Dying*. London: Tavistock.
Lofland, L.   (1978) *The Craft of Dying: The Modern Face of Death*. Beverly Hills, CA: Sage Publications.
McIntosh, J.   (1977) *Communication and Awareness in a Cancer Ward*. London: Croom Helm.
Mulkay, M.   (1993) Social death in Britain. In: *The Sociology of Death*, ed. D. Clark. Oxford: Blackwell.
OPCS   (1992) Mortality statistics: general review of the registrar general on death in England and Wales. London: HMSO.
Parkes, C.   (1984) 'Hospice' versus 'hospital' care: a re-evaluation after 10 years as seen by surviving spouses. *Postgrad. Med. J.*, **50**, 120–4.
Seale, C.   (1995) Heroic Death. *Soc. Health Illness*, **29**, 597–613.
Seale, C. & Cartwright, A.   (1994) *The Year Before Death*. Aldershot: Averbery.
Sudnow, D.   (1967) *Passing On: The Social Organization of Dying*. New York: Prentice Hall.
Taylor, K.   (1988) 'Telling bad news': physicians and the disclosure of undesirable information. *Soc. Health Illness*, **10**, 109–32.
Timmermans, S.   (1994) Dying of awareness: the theory awareness contexts revisited. *Soc. Health Illness*, **16**, 322–39.
Williams, R.   (1990) *A Protestant Legacy: Attitudes to Death and Illness among Older Aberdonians*. Oxford: Clarendon Press.

SOCIAL STRUCTURE AND HEALTH

8 Inequality and Social Class

DAVID BLANE

In Bethnal Green in the year 1839 the average age of death in the several classes was as follows: 'Gentlemen and persons engaged in professions, and their families . . . 45 years; tradesmen and their families . . . 26 years; Mechanics, servants and labourers, and their families . . . 16 years' (Chadwick 1842). The average age of deaths in these social classes was found to vary somewhat from area to area, but similar differences between the classes were found in all areas of Britain.

Although 'the average age of death' would be criticized today as a measure which is oversensitive to high childhood mortality, Chadwick's study provided some of the first evidence that health varies with social class. The population's general level of health has improved dramatically since the first half of the nineteenth century, but subsequent investigations have shown that a relationship between mortality rates and social class remains. This has been repeatedly confirmed and shown to apply equally to morbidity (DHSS 1980). It is important, therefore, to understand both what is meant by 'social class' and why it should be related to health indicators of many kinds. With this in mind, this chapter starts with details of some modern inequalities and of different ways of accounting for them, the most influential of which draws on concepts of social class. It then goes on to examine the relationship between social class and health.

BOX 8.1

HEALTH INEQUALITIES IN BRITAIN

- There would be 42 000 fewer deaths each year for people aged 16–74 if the death rate of manual workers was the same as for non-manual.

- The majority of causes of death are more common in manual classes than non-manual; 65 out of the 78 main causes of death among men are more common in manual than non-manual classes, as are 62 out of the 82 main causes of death among women.

- Socioeconomic gradients exist for the commonest causes of long-standing illness and disability – musculoskeletal, heart and circulatory and respiratory conditions – with the highest rates among manual workers.

- A child from an unskilled manual family is twice as likely to die before the age of 15 as a child from a professional family.

- If the whole population had experienced the same death rate as the non-manual classes, in 1988 there would have been 700 fewer still births and 1500 fewer infant deaths.

Reproduced with permission from International Centre for Health and Society with King's Fund Institute. Society and Health No. 1. June 1994. London: King's Fund Institute.

SOME DIMENSIONS OF INEQUALITY IN THE UK

Wealth and income

Wealth, defined in terms of marketable assets, is very unequally distributed. In 1985 the richest 1% of the population aged 18 or over owned 20% of the country's total personal wealth, and the richest 10% over half. The poorest 75% of the population owned approximately the same as the richest 1% (Central Statistical Office (CSO) 1989). The form of this wealth varied with its distribution. Some two-thirds of the wealth of those owning £50 000–100 000 in 1984 consisted of homes and life insurance policies, whereas land and company shares contributed a mere 6%. In contrast, land and company shares accounted for 50% of the wealth of those owning more than £300 000, and homes and life-insurance policies 17% (Board of Inland Revenue 1989). It can be argued that the wealth which is owned by the majority of the population is used in an attempt to guarantee the necessities of life, whereas the wealth of the rich also brings with it social power, in the sense of ownership of land and voting rights in the decisions of financial and industrial corporations.

Income, which mainly consists of earnings from employment but also includes investment income and the various state benefits, is more equally distributed than wealth. After income tax had been deducted, the top 10% of 'taxable units' (married couples are counted as one unit) received over one-quarter of total personal income in 1985, and the top 50% nearly three-quarters. The bottom 50% of taxable units received approximately the same as the top 10%

(CSO 1989). Access to state facilities such as the education system and health service can also be seen as part of income, as can benefits in kind which are received on top of earnings from employment. Although those on low incomes derive marginally greater benefit from the former, benefits in kind disproportionately go to those with high incomes and tend to be greatest for those with the highest salaries. Thus, large inequalities in income remain despite the redistribution achieved by mechanisms such as income tax, state benefits and access to state facilities.

Living conditions

As would be expected in a market economy, the differences in income and wealth result in differences in such things as diet, possessions and housing. Compared to that of the better paid, the diet of the low paid contains far less fresh fruit, significantly less fresh vegetables, fresh fish and cheese, and more white bread, potatoes, sugar, lard and margarine (MAFF 1989). A car was owned by 92% of households whose weekly income in 1988 exceeded £350, central heating by 87%, a washing machine by 94% and a telephone by 95%; in contrast, a car was owned by only 34% of households receiving less than £100 per week, central heating by 67%, a washing machine by 80% and a telephone by 78% (CSO 1990). In 1986, 2.9 million dwellings in England, or 15% of the total stock, were inadequate in one or more of the following respects: unfit for habitation (0.9 million); lack of basic hygienic amenities (0.45 million); in need of urgent repairs costing more than £1000 (2.4 million). Living in poor housing was strongly related to income. Households with an annual income of less than £6000 accounted for 69% of dwellings which were unfit for habitation, 76% of those which lacked basic hygienic amenities and 55% of dwellings in poor repair; the comparable figures for households with an annual income of over £15 000 were 2%, 1% and 4%, respectively (Department of the Environment 1988). In addition, the homes of families on low incomes were more likely to be in areas where the air was polluted with industrial waste and, lacking gardens, their children were more likely to have to play in an already overcrowded flat, or in the street.

Working conditions

An individual's income is strongly tied to the nature of their work. About 60% of male manual workers were paid a basic hourly rate of £5 or less in 1989, compared with 20% of non-manual workers, and virtually no manual workers were paid more than £11 per hour, compared with 20% of non-manual workers. For a number of reasons the difference in total weekly pay is not as great as the difference in the hourly rate. Manual workers work a greater number of hours per week, with three-quarters in 1989 having a basic working week of more than 38 h, compared with one-quarter of non-manual workers, and 60% working overtime compared with 25% of non-manual workers. Manual workers are also more likely to work shifts, which attract additional payment, and to be paid some form of production bonus. Approximately one-third of manual workers' earnings are derived from overtime, shift payments and production bonuses and, in 1989, if these had been removed, the proportion of manual workers earning less than £200 per week would have increased from half to four-fifths (Department of Employment 1989). As these additional sources of income are likely to vary from week to week, it is more difficult for manual workers and their families to make financially sound plans, a disadvantage which is reinforced by manual workers' greater likelihood of being made redundant. Of considerable financial importance after retirement, manual workers are less likely to be members of an occupational pension scheme than non-manual workers; in 1987, 80% of professional workers were members of such schemes, compared with less than 50% of manual workers (OPCS 1989).

Manual work is usually more physically demanding, noisier and more dangerous than non-manual work (Hunter 1975), as well as being more likely to involve the physical and social disruption of shift work. Despite its more hazardous nature, manual work lasts longer than non-manual work. Manual workers enter the work-force at an earlier age and, as has been noted, their basic working week is likely to be longer and they are more likely to work overtime. In addition, their holidays are shorter, with non-manual workers being more likely to receive in excess of 5 weeks holiday per year. Manual work is also more likely to be repetitive than the work of professionals and managers, to offer little autonomy and to be experienced as boring. Perhaps as a result, manual workers are subject to closer supervision and tighter discipline; most have to clock in to work, automatically lose money when late for work, face dismissal if continually late, and many need a supervisor's permission to use the lavatory or obtain a drink outside of the set work-breaks.

POVERTY

The inequalities so far documented have been illustrated in terms of manual compared with non-manual, professional compared with unskilled, and so on. Such comparisons are useful because they indicate the direction and size of the general trends, but they can create the misleading impression that the work-force is divided into homogeneous blocks whose members share the same income and living and working conditions and that these, in turn, are clearly higher or lower than those of the next block. In reality there is considerable variation in income and conditions within each block and considerable overlap between them. As a result there is always room for debate about where it is appropriate to draw lines on this continuous distribution in order to identify specific groups. This problem complicates the definition of poverty, and attempts to identify those who are exposed to poverty first need to be clear about the sense in which the term is being used.

The term 'poverty' has been used in two ways. **Absolute poverty** refers to a standard of living which is incapable of sustaining life. When the term is used in this sense it could describe, for example, destitute people in the drought-stricken areas of the Sahel. One problem with this definition, however, is its failure to specify how long people can live before their standard of living is judged incapable of sustaining life. As the experience of hunger-strikers demonstrates, no standard of living is so low as to kill instantaneously, and low-grade malnutrition may only influence mortality after many years. In addition, because very few people in the rich countries of the world are starving, using the term poverty in its absolute sense fails to address the hardships which are endured by many members of these societies.

Relative poverty refers to a standard of living below that which is considered normal or acceptable by the members of a particular society. 'The resources (of those in relative poverty) are so seriously below those commanded by the average individual or family that they are, in effect, excluded from ordinary living patterns, customs and activities' (Townsend 1979). Using the term in this relative sense allows the concept of poverty to be applied to rich societies such as Britain, although for research purposes it does pose the problem of how to establish empirically what is considered normal or acceptable in a particular society. This relative 'poverty line' can be established by means of surveys. A less expensive method, which is frequently used in research, is to equate relative poverty with an income below the level of eligibility for the various State benefits (at present, Income Support, Income Credit and Housing Benefit).

The most recent classic study of poverty in the UK found that 7% of households, containing 3.3 million people, received an income below the State benefits level, and that a further 24% of households which contained 11.9 million people were on the margins of poverty, defined as an income less than 40% above the state benefits level. When those in poverty were analysed according to their labour market, personal and other characteristics, the three largest groups were those employed on low wages or in casual work, the disabled and long-term sick and the elderly retired, with the unemployed and one-parent families being the next largest groups (Townsend 1979). Since this survey the numbers living in poverty have probably increased and the relative importance of unemployment has certainly increased, but there is no reason to believe that the characteristics of those who are most vulnerable to poverty have changed.

A potential shortcoming of such cross-sectional data is the extent to which they obscure the association between poverty and certain phases of the life cycle. In societies where incomes are primarily derived from the labour market and where human reproduction predominantly occurs within nuclear families, there is an in-built tendency for an individual's standard of living to be lowest during childhood, active parenthood and old age, and to be highest during the intervening phases. This longitudinal approach has certain advantages: it draws attention to the association between poverty and childhood; it reminds us that those who are not currently living in poverty may have experienced it in the past or may realistically expect to experience it in the future; and it enables us to see that it is often the same individuals whose standard of living will dip below the poverty line during the low phases of the life cycle. Thus, the child reared in poverty is educationally handicapped and is likely to be an early entrant to the unskilled sector of the labour market, where low wages and insecure employment will make family formation financially difficult and where the lack of an occupational pension scheme will predispose to poverty after retirement. Some idea of the proportion of the population which is likely to experience relative poverty at some stage during their lives is given by combining those who were found to be in poverty with those who were on its margins in the study quoted earlier; that is, 31% of households or 15 million people. Rather than being a marginal problem, therefore, poverty or the realistic fear of it is a fact of life for a substantial proportion of the population.

There is a considerable overlap between medical problems and poverty or the phases of the life cycle where the standard of living tends to dip. The size of this overlap is illustrated by the 75% of prescriptions which are exempt from charges, a figure which can rise to 90% in some areas. The medical consequences of poverty start before birth, with poor maternal nutrition contributing to prematurity and low birth weight. During childhood, poor nutrition inhibits normal growth and development, lack of hygienic facilities predisposes to infestations with scabies, head lice and intestinal worms, damp housing increases the incidence of upper-respiratory-tract infections which may lead to chronic ear disease, partial deafness and a poor educational record, and lack of play facilities hinders psychological development and increases the risk of accidents. During active parenthood the health hazards stem from attempts to maximize income. Men may seek the premiums attached to shift work, or the 'danger money' associated with hazardous jobs, as well as working overtime, taking a second part-time job on top of their main employment or working in the informal economy where poor health-and-safety conditions predominate. Such strategies increase income, but at the cost of physical exhaustion, risk of accidents, disrupted family life and increased vulnerability to depression in the mothers alone at home with their young children. Other, psychological, effects include exhaustion by the ceaseless struggle to 'make ends meet' and low self-esteem because of failure in this struggle, shame because one's children cannot have the same things as other children and fear lest the furniture is repossessed, the gas or electricity is cut off or one is made homeless because of insufficient money to pay hire purchase instalments, energy bills and rent. During old age, the health effects of poverty reflect both immediate problems and the accumulation of past effects. Malnutrition ('tea and toast syndrome') and hypothermia are obvious examples, although the large increase in mortality during the winter compared with the summer months is probably a more important effect.

In summary, relative poverty affects a sizeable proportion of the British population. Because of the relationship between poverty and ill health, an even larger proportion of the patients whom doctors treat are likely to be affected in some way by its associated problems.

SOCIAL STRATIFICATION

Many other aspects of inequality could have been examined, in addition to those already discussed, including education, career prospects and leisure activities (Reid 1989). These inequalities tend to go together, so that an individual who is disadvantaged in one area of life is likely also to be disadvantaged in others. In the same way, someone who is advantaged in one area of life is likely to be similarly advantaged in others. The term 'social stratification' refers generally to this kind of socially structured inequality, and the concept of social class describes the form which social stratification takes in societies such as contemporary Britain. Most societies to date have been hierarchically structured in some way. Historical forms of stratification have included, for example, the Hindu caste system and the various estates of feudal society. Some social theorists, drawing on the work of the early German sociologist Max Weber, consider that the stratification of modern industrial societies involves three main dimensions: social class, social status or honour, and the political power of organized groups. Although class, status and power are usually related, so that, for example, unskilled labourers generally have low social status and little political influence, they are analytically distinct and can vary independently of one another. Although it is generally agreed that social class is the most fundamental dimension of stratification, sociologists often differ in their precise definition and treatment of class and there are a number of competing theories.

The theory most widely used in the general population divides society into two stereotyped groups of roughly equal size. The 'middle class' consists of people who earn monthly salaries in non-manual jobs, borrow money to buy their own homes and encourage their children to get as much formal education as possible. The 'working-class', in contrast, consists of people who earn weekly wages in manual jobs, rent their homes, mainly from a Local Authority, and try to get

---

BOX 8.2

CLASS DIFFERENCES IN HEALTH

Illustrative Data 1981

Adult males:	Social class I	SMR of 66
	V	159.
Adult females:	Social class I	SMR of 68
	V	130.
Male infants:	Social class I	IMR of 9
	V	18.
Female infants:	Social class I	IMR of 7
	V	13.

---

their children started in a good job as soon as they are allowed to leave school. Most of the population appear to have little difficulty in placing themselves in one or other of these two classes. One study which included an unprompted question about self-rated social class found that 40% of the population spontaneously described themselves as middle class and 48% as working class. The study's subjects were found to have made this distinction chiefly on differences in life-style, but they were also influenced by considerations of family background, occupation and wealth (Townsend 1979). Recent social changes may have blurred this distinction somewhat: the downward spread of home ownership, foreign holidays and wine consumption and the upward spread of job insecurity and trade unionism may all have had this effect.

Most academic social scientists tend to favour some version of Weber's class scheme, whereas the lay population, as we have seen, tends to use the working class–middle class distinction. Another approach, derived from the work of Marx, is unusual in having advocates in both camps. It divides society into two main social classes on the basis of ownership and control of the land, industry and financial institutions. The 'working class' in Marx's analysis consists of the overwhelming majority of the population, who own only things they can use and live by selling their mental or physical labour power. Social changes since Marx's death have required considerable, and often disputed, elaboration of his original analysis.

For research purposes a more precise and detailed definition of social class is generally necessary. Many scales have been devised to meet this need, although each of these has its own particular strengths and weaknesses. The Registrar General's classification (Table 8.1) is the most widely used in medical research. It divides the population into five social classes, I–V, with social class III being further subdivided into non-manual (IIIN) and manual (IIIM). This system of classification is based on occupation, and it groups occupations into social classes according to their skill level and general social standing in the community. Men are allocated to a social class on the basis of their own occupation, married women on the basis of their husband's occupation, children on that of their father and the retired and unemployed on that of

TABLE 8.1 *Registrar General's classification of social classes.*

Social class	Description	Examples	% of economically active and retired	
			Males	Females
I	Professional	Accountant Doctor Lawyer	5	1
II	Intermediate	Manager School teacher Nurse	22	21
IIIN	Skilled non-manual	Clerical worker Secretary Shop assistant	12	39
IIIM	Skilled manual	Bus driver Coal-face worker Carpenter	36	9
IV	Semi-skilled manual	Agricultural worker Bus conductor Postman	18	22
V	Unskilled manual	Labourer Cleaner Dock worker	7	7

Reproduced with permission from HarperCollins Publishers Ltd from Reid (1989: Tables 2.6 and 3.1).

their last significant period of employment. Single women are classified on the basis of their own occupation (OPCS 1980).

Certain characteristics of the Registrar General's classification need to be appreciated. Being based on the general social standing of different occupations, it is primarily a measure of status rather than economic class or living standards. As the earlier comments on Weber indicate, however, the link between social status and economic class is sufficiently strong for the classification to act as a reasonable indicator of lifetime earnings and conditions of life. Second, the Registrar General's social classes are not internally homogeneous. Social class II, for example, contains both tenant farmers working a few dozen acres and farmers who own thousands of acres; similarly, it contains both the corner shopkeeper and the senior manager in a multinational company. Third, the Registrar General's classification deals inadequately with women's employment, which among other things weakens its power as an indicator of living standards. Married women are classified by the occupation of their husband, although the standard of living of the family's members can be decisively affected by whether or not she has paid employment. It has been calculated that the number of families living in poverty would double if they were deprived of these earnings. Finally, it is possible to question the relevance of an occupationally based classification to a world of flexible labour markets, job insecurity and high unemployment rates.

Problems such as these have prompted frequent attempts to find a more appropriate alternative, and these efforts continue. In the meantime the classification remains widely used in research. It is convenient to use, having clear decision rules which allow the great majority of the population to be placed into one of the social classes. Its long-standing use in a wide range of research areas facilitates comparison between different studies. It has also proved capable of identifying social differences in most areas of life, although, as the earlier comments on internal homogeneity indicate, it is likely to provide conservative estimates of the size of these differences.

SOCIAL CLASS AND HEALTH

UK data

As the quotation from Chadwick in the opening paragraph of this chapter illustrates, it has long been recognized that the various positions in the social hierarchy are associated with different chances of premature death. Good quality data on the relationship between social class and mortality in England and Wales have been published each decade for most of the twentieth century. The data reproduced in Table 8.2 are the most recent available, but the general pattern which they reveal has been a constant feature of all the earlier reports. The mortality rates increase in a

TABLE 8.2 Social class and deaths due to all causes (England and Wales; 1979–80, 1982–83).

Social class	Still-birth rate[a]	Infant mortality rate[b]	Mortality rate 1–15 years[c]	Standardized mortality ratio[d]
Males				20–64 years
I	5	9	0.3	66
II	6	10	0.2	74
IIIN	6	10	0.3	93
IIIM	7	12	0.3	103
IV	9	15	0.4	114
V	9	18	0.6	159
Females				20–59 years
I	4	7	0.2	68
II	5	8	0.2	76
IIIN	6	8	0.2	86
IIIM	7	9	0.2	97
IV	8	12	0.3	108
V	8	13	0.4	130

Reproduced with permission of the Controller of HMSO and the Office for National Statistics from OPCS (1986, 1988).
[a] *Number of deaths per 1000 live and dead births; rounded to the nearest integer.*
[b] *Number of deaths in the first year of life per 1000 live births; rounded to the nearest integer.*
[c] *Number of deaths per 1000 population aged 1–15 years; rounded to one decimal place.*
[d] *The ratio of the observed mortality rate in a social class to its expected rate from the total population, multiplied by 100.*

step-wise fashion as one moves from the Registrar General's social class I to social class V, with the mortality rate of the latter being approximately twice that of the former. This social class gradient in total deaths due to all causes is found among both males and females and within all age groups, although the differences tend to narrow with increasing age.

The specific causes of death listed in Table 8.3 are the most prevalent for each sex, and they jointly account for some 50% of all deaths in the years of working life. For most causes the mortality rates increase as one moves from social class I to class V, so showing the same gradient as deaths due to all causes combined. There are exceptions, however, which show no social class gradient; breast cancer in women is the most prevalent of these. Also, unlike the gradient for deaths due to all causes, the social class gradient for some causes of death has changed during this century. Coronary heart disease is the most prominent of these; its mortality rate was highest in social class I and lowest in class V for the first half of the century; this gradient flattened out in the third quarter and reversed in the final quarter so that its mortality rate is now highest in social class V and lowest in class I.

The data presented so far have been mortality rates, and their use as a measure of health has certain advantages. In the vast majority of cases death is an unambiguous event which can be recorded with high reliability. Death is also one of the few times that an individual is legally obliged to be seen by a doctor, with the result that the recording of death is virtually complete. Mortality rates, therefore, are reliable and complete measures. Nevertheless, they are not perfect measures of health. The term 'health' implies the absence of disease as well as the absence of

TABLE 8.3 Social class and main causes of death (England and Wales; 1979–80, 1982–83): standardized mortality ratios.

Cause of death	Social class					
	I	II	IIIN	IIIM	IV	V
Males 20–64 years						
Ischaemic heart disease	69	81	102	106	110	137
Lung cancer	42	62	78	117	125	175
Cerebrovascular disease	61	70	88	105	114	171
Bronchitis	34	49	84	109	134	208
Motor-vehicle accidents	64	75	79	101	114	175
Pneumonia	34	49	80	89	121	211
Suicide	86	78	94	84	110	190
Females 20–59 years						
Ischaemic heart disease	41	55	69	106	119	152
Breast cancer	107	103	105	100	99	94
Cerebrovascular disease	58	69	79	105	117	144
Bronchitis	33	54	71	100	119	165
Motor-vehicle accidents	76	89	102	63	94	114
Pneumonia	37	51	67	86	110	140
Suicide	77	81	99	55	76	84

Reproduced with permission of the Controller of HMSO and the Office for National Statistics OPCS (1986).

premature death (see Chapter 18). As a result, attempts to understand the relationship between social class and health have recently begun to examine the way in which morbidity (illness) varies with social class.

For a variety of reasons, the measurement of morbidity is more difficult than that of mortality. Consulting a doctor could be taken as a measure of morbidity. Manual workers consult doctors more frequently than non-manual workers (OPCS 1989), but it should not be assumed that this is solely due to differences in health. Differences in consultation rates result from differences in illness behaviour (Chapter 3) as well as differences in morbidity. Indeed, non-manual workers appear to be the more frequent consulters when 'use/need ratios' are used to relate consultation rates to the prevalence of illness in the various social classes. The illnesses which people report when questioned as part of a representative survey may appear to avoid this problem with consultation rates, so rates of reported illness could be taken as a second measure of morbidity. Manual workers report more illnesses of all types (acute, chronic and limiting long-standing) than non-manual workers, with the differences tending to widen in the older age groups (OPCS 1989). All measures of self-reported morbidity, however, involve subjective judgements about illness and its severity. The observed class differences on these measures may be due to systematic variation in these judgements. The more physically demanding nature of manual occupations, for example, may mean that illness is less easily tolerated and recognized earlier.

Some studies have used clinical measures of morbidity on samples of the whole population. These studies should provide results which are free from possible contamination by illness behaviour and systematic subjective variation. Among middle-aged men in the British Regional Heart Study, manual workers were more likely to have experienced angina than non-manual workers; similar social class differences were found in obesity and, to a lesser extent, in blood pressure (Pocock et al. 1987; Weatherall and Shaper 1988; Shaper et al. 1988). Among men and women of working age in the Health and Lifestyle Survey, manual workers were more likely to experience psychological malaise, to have poorer respiratory function and, to a lesser extent, higher blood pressure than non-manual workers (Cox et al. 1987). Studies of this type are expensive and therefore rare. An additional disadvantage is that they usually concentrate on one specific disease, so they are unable to provide information about social class differences in overall morbidity. Like all surveys, they also suffer from non-responders, so their results are not based on the complete coverage achieved by mortality data.

In summary, for many decades reliable and complete data in Britain have shown a step-wise gradient in mortality across the social classes, with members of social class V having approximately twice the chance of dying at any particular age as members of social class I. Recently, attention has turned to morbidity, which is a more valid measure of health than mortality, but difficult to measure with comparable reliability and completeness. Social class differences have been found in various measures of morbidity. The size of these differences appears to vary considerably. The lack of a close match between social class differences in mortality and in morbidity is not surprising. Some major causes of death, such as accidents and violence, need not be preceded by illness and disease, and some common serious diseases, such as arthritis and depression, rarely cause death.

International data

British data on health inequalities are richer and longer standing than elsewhere. In recent years, however, information on socioeconomic differences in health have become available for many other countries. In most cases these studies have used measures of social position which differ from the Registrar General's occupational social classes. The number of years of formal education and the level of income are the most frequently used. In general these alternative measures of socioeconomic position show the same relationship to health as the Registrar General's classes in Britain. Mortality and morbidity rates are lowest in the most advantaged group, highest in the least advantaged group and, in between, increase along a step-wise gradient.

USA   In 1990 death rates at ages 25−64 years, for males and females combined, were 471 per 100 000 for those who received eight years or less of formal education compared with 264 for those who received 16 years or more (DHHS 1994). In another large-scale study the death rates of white males showed an inverse gradient with the level of median family income. At the extremes of the income distribution, those with a median family income of less than $7500 had a death rate of 81 per 10 000 compared with 39 for those with more than $32 500 (Davey Smith et al. 1992).

European Union   In The Netherlands in 1981−85 the rate of self-reported chronic illness among people aged 16 years or more was over 50% higher in those who left formal education after primary school compared with those who had received a university education (Mackenbach 1993). In Spain in 1987 the prevalence of chronic illness among women aged 20−44 years was nearly 50% higher in the poorest income group compared with the highest income group (Kunst and Mackenbach 1994).

Eastern Europe   In Poland in 1988−89 the death rate among men aged 50−64 years was 22 per 1000 among those who left formal education after primary school compared with 10 per 1000 among those with a university education (Brajczewski and Rogucka 1993). Among women in Russia who received primary school and university education a similar, although smaller, difference in death rates has been reported (Davis et al. 1994).

Socioeconomic differences in health are therefore not confined to Britain. They have been found in every country which has examined the issue and are probably a feature of all industrialized societies. British efforts to understand this phenomenon are now part of an international endeavour.

INTERPRETATION OF THE RELATIONSHIP BETWEEN SOCIAL CLASS AND HEALTH

The association between social class and health shows that death and disease are socially structured, as opposed to randomly distributed throughout the population, and that they vary in line with the differences in living standards which were documented earlier. However, correlation does not imply causation, and the relationship needs to be examined further in order to establish the status and direction of causality. This can best be achieved by using the explanatory framework which was first developed by the Department of Health's Research Working Group on

---

BOX 8.3

TYPES OF EXPLANATION

The Black Report

1. Artefact
   The association between social class and health is an artefact of the way these concepts are measured.

2. Social selection
   Health determines social class through a process of health-related social mobility.

3. Behavioural/cultural
   Social class determines health through social class differences in health-damaging or health-promoting behaviours.

4. Materialist
   Social class determines health through social class differences in the material circumstances of life.

Inequalities in Health (DHSS 1980). This report, which has become known as the Black Report, suggested four types of explanation of social class differences in health: artefact, social selection, behavioural/cultural and materialist.

Artefact

The artefact type of explanation examines the possibility that observed social class differences in mortality may be an artefact of the processes by which these two variables are measured. One example of this type of explanation is numerator–denominator bias. The Black Report relied on mortality rates which had been calculated from two sources. Death registration provided the number of *deaths* in each social class and the Decennial Census the number of *individuals* in each class. It is possible that an individual's occupation might have been described differently at these two events. Any systematic bias towards 'promoting oneself' on the census form would artefactually increase the death rates in classes IV and V. The OPCS longitudinal study has followed a 1% sample of the 1971 census population. It eliminated any numerator–denominator bias by categorizing individuals at death according to their social class at the 1971 census. When used in this way, social class differences in mortality were found to be similar to, although smaller than, those which depend on both death registration and census information (Fox and Goldblatt 1982). Social class differences in mortality are, therefore, not an artefact of registration bias.

The relevance of artefact explanations may lie in the opposite direction. Social class differences in mortality are wider when alternative measures of social class and mortality are used. When social position is measured in terms of employment grade within particular industries, the mortality differences between the top and bottom of the social hierarchy are considerably wider than when the Registrar General's classification is used (Davey Smith et al. 1994). Similarly, when death rates are measured in terms of years of potential life lost, so weighting deaths according to the age at which they occur, the resulting social class differences are wider than when standardized mortality ratios are used (Blane et al. 1990).

Artefact explanations, in summary, do not explain social class differences in mortality, but they do suggest that the differences shown in Table 8.2 are conservative estimates.

Social selection

Social selection explanations argue that health determines social class through a process of health-related social mobility in which the healthy are more likely to move up the social hierarchy and the unhealthy to move down. There is little doubt that chronically sick and disabled people may be additionally disadvantaged in this way. Similarly, those who are taller than average, and in this context height is taken as an indicator of good health, have been found to have a greater than average chance of upward mobility. Health-related social mobility is therefore a real phenomenon. In theory it could explain the *whole* social class gradient. Whether it does so is the relevant question to ask.

The social distribution of mortality, when seen in relation to the Registrar General's classification rules, suggests that the contribution of social mobility is unlikely to be large. First, social class differences in mortality are found where health-related mobility is not possible. The social gradient in childhood mortality is similar to those among adults. The childhood gradient cannot have been created by mobility associated with child health, however, because the Registrar General's scheme classifies children according to their father's occupation. The same reasoning applies to married women. Their mortality gradient is similar to that of adult men. The married women's gradient cannot be due to mobility associated with their own health, because the Registrar General's scheme classifies them according to their husband's occupation.

Second, social class differences in mortality are found where social mobility of any type is not possible. Class gradients after retirement are similar to those during working life. The post-retirement gradients cannot be due to health-related social mobility. The Registrar General's scheme classifies retired people according to their last significant period of employment, which eliminates any subsequent social mobility.

Third, social class differences in mortality due to diseases which kill quickly, such as lung cancer, are similar to those which kill slowly, such as chronic bronchitis and emphysema. If health-related social mobility made an important contribution to social class differences in health, the gradients should be steeper for causes of death which allow time for social mobility between the onset of disease and death.

Fourth, social mobility tends to occur before the serious diseases become prevalent. Social mobility is most frequent, and movement between the working class and middle class most likely, during the early years of working life, particularly between leaving formal education and the mid-twenties age group. Serious disease, which could interfere with performance, does not become widespread until several decades later. Most social mobility takes place when the population is generally healthy and it is comparatively rare in the age groups where serious disease is prevalent.

Finally, incapacitating illness does not inevitably lead to downward mobility. The chronically sick and disabled have other options, including early retirement, unemployment and moving to a similar but less demanding job. All of these alternatives are likely to entail a reduction in income, but none of them involves downward social mobility on the Registrar General's scheme.

Research points to the same conclusion as these more general considerations. An examination of health and social mobility among men aged 45–64 years found no evidence that health-related social mobility systematically contributed to the social class differences in their mortality (Goldblatt 1989). The contribution of health to social mobility during the early years of working life is still uncertain (West 1991), but the weight of evidence indicates that its contribution is small (Wadsworth 1986; Power et al. 1990). Educational achievement, the type of secondary school attended and the material and cultural resources of the family of origin, rather than health, are found to be the main influences on social mobility between formal education and the world of work (Halsey et al. 1980).

Social selection explanations, in summary, are most relevant to the early years of working life and even at these ages the contribution of health-related social mobility to social class differences in health is probably small.

Behavioural/cultural and materialist

The behavioural/cultural and the materialist types of explanation both see health as determined in some way by social class, but they differ in the aspects of social class which they see as responsible. Behavioural/cultural explanations involve class differences in behaviours which are health-damaging or health-promoting and which, at least in principle, are subject to individual choice. Materialist explanations, in contrast, involve hazards which are inherent in the present form of social organization and to which some people have no choice but to be exposed.

Dietary choices, the consumption of drugs like tobacco and alcohol, active leisure-time pursuits and the use of preventive medical services such as immunization, contraception and antenatal surveillance are examples of behaviours which vary with social class and which could account for class differences in health. Considerable weight is given to this type of explanation by the evidence which has accumulated as a result of medicine's long interest in such issues. However, the social and economic context in which these behaviours occur needs to be recognized. Diet is influenced by both cultural preferences and disposable income. The ability of nicotine to maintain a constant mood in situations of stress and monotony may predispose towards cigarette smoking in repetitive and highly supervised occupations. Other evidence cautions against a one-sided emphasis on behavioural factors. Earlier this century cigarette smoking was more prevalent among the middle class than the working class, but class gradients in mortality were similar to the present. Intervention studies have rarely produced the clear-cut improvements in health which would be predicted by the behavioural/cultural approach, despite achieving reduction in the hazardous behaviours.

The Black Report judged that materialist explanations were the most important in accounting for social class differences in health. The health-damaging effects of air pollution and occupational exposure to physicochemical hazards had already been recognized. More recently, local levels of economic and social deprivation have been identified as powerful predictors of mortality and morbidity. The health effects of income distribution and the psychosocial aspects of employment have been demonstrated. Damp housing has been shown to be associated with worse health, particularly with higher rates of respiratory disease in children. Unemployment has been associated with psychological morbidity and raised mortality among unemployed men and their wives. Each of these factors could contribute to class differences in health because they are all more likely to be experienced by working class than middle class people.

There is thus a certain amount of evidence which supports the materialist type of explanation. Nevertheless most medical researchers would probably judge behavioural/cultural factors, and cigarette smoking in particular, to be of greater importance. The primacy assigned to materialist explanations by the Black Report can be defended on the grounds that research so far has ignored the accumulation of advantage or disadvantage which is associated with social class. As the earlier sections of this chapter have indicated, inequalities are found in many spheres of life. Social class is the concept which stresses the likelihood that advantage or disadvantage in one sphere will be associated with advantage or disadvantage in others. Those who experience occupational disadvantage are likely to be the same people who are residentially disadvantaged, and these disadvantages in their various forms are likely to accumulate through childhood and adulthood and into old age. It will not be possible to make a secure judgement about the relative importance of behavioural/cultural and materialist explanations until the effect on health of such combined and accumulating disadvantages has been established.

THE OVERALL PICTURE

The work of social researchers such as Chadwick and Farr made the Victorians aware of the vicious circle of 'poverty causes disease which causes poverty'. Despite the subsequent development of the welfare state, disabled people and those with chronic diseases are still at risk of relative poverty. This side of the Victorians' vicious circle, however, would now appear less important than the side which stresses the effect of material well-being, or the lack of it, on health. The health inequalities of today are primarily due to the combined effect of class differences in exposure to factors which promote health or cause disease.

This was the conclusion reached by the Department of Health Working Group which produced the Black Report. The Report went on to suggest measures for starting to eliminate health inequalities. There are 37 of these recommendations. A few were designed to ensure better information about class differences in health. Most were carefully targeted at a limited number of issues where class differences in health were thought to be widest and most likely to respond to relatively small sums of money. Disability was the subject of six recommendations designed to break its links with poverty. These covered prevention (fetal screening for neural tube defects and Down's syndrome), welfare procedures (a comprehensive disablement allowance), housing (more specialist housing for disabled people) and community-care services (resources shifted towards home-help and nursing services for disabled people). This set of recommendations appears designed to prevent disability where this is presently possible (fetal screening) and, where it is not, to ensure that the lives of working-class people with disabilities are not markedly disadvantaged in terms of income (welfare procedures) and living conditions (housing and community services).

In addition to disability, equally detailed recommendations were made concerning infant and child health, cigarette smoking, occupational health and safety and Local Authority housing. Particular priority was given to the abolition of child poverty by means of a new infant-care allowance, increased child benefit and the provision of free school meals. These recommendations, in common with the rest of the report, were described by the Government as 'unrealistic' and the report was published 'without any commitment by the Government to its proposals'. Nevertheless, subsequent research has greatly increased our understanding of the relationship between social class and health. The Government, through its involvement in the World Health Organization's campaign for 'Health for All by the Year 2000', has also committed itself to narrowing class differences in health by that date. Unfortunately a subsequent authoritative review has pointed out that child poverty, for example, is increasing rather than decreasing and that on present policies the Government is unlikely to meet its target (Whitehead 1987).

REFERENCES

Blane, D., Davey Smith, G. & Bartley, M.   (1990) Social class differences in years of potential life lost: size, trends and principal causes. *Br. Med. J.*, **301**, 429–32.
Board of Inland Revenue   (1989) *Inland Revenue Statistics 1989*. London: HMSO.
Brajczewski, C. & Rogucka, E.   (1993) Social class differences in rates of premature mortality among adults in the city of Wroclaw. *Am. J. Hum. Biol.*, **5**, 461–71.
Central Statistical Office   (1989) *Social Trends 19*. London: HMSO.
Central Statistical Office   (1990) *Family Expenditure Survey 1988*. London: HMSO.
Chadwick, E.   (1842) *Report on the Sanitary Condition of the Labouring Populating of Great Britain 1842*. Edinburgh: Edinburgh University Press, 1965.
Cox, B.D., Blaxter, M., Buckle, A.L.J. et al.   (1987) *The Health and Lifestyle Survey: Preliminary Report*. London: Health Promotion Research Trust.
Davey Smith, G., Neaton, J.D., Wentworth, D. & Stamler, J.   (1992). Income differentials in mortality risk among 305,099 white men. Edinburgh. European Society of Medical Sociology Conference, September 1992 (Abstract).
Davey Smith, G, Blane D. Bartley M.   (1994) Explanations for socio-economic differentials in mortality: evidence from Britain and elsewhere. *Eur. J. Public Health*, **4**, 131–44.
Davis, C.E., Deev, A.D., Shestov, D.B., Perova, N.V. et al.   (1994) Correlates of mortality in Russian and US women: the Lipid Research Clinics Program. *Am. J. Epidemiol.*, **139**, 369–79.
Department of Employment   (1989) *New Earnings Survey 1989*. London: HMSO.
Department of the Environment   (1988) *English House Condition Survey 1986*. London: HMSO.
Department of Health and Human Services (DHHS)   (1994). *Health United States 1993*. Hyattsville, MD: National Centre for Health Statistics.
Department of Health and Social Security   (DHSS) (1980) *Inequalities in Health: Report of a Research Working Group* (The Black Report). London: HMSO.
Fox, A.J. & Goldblatt, P.O.   (1982) *Longitudinal Study: Socio-demographic Mortality Differentials*. London: HMSO.
Goldblatt, P.O.   (1989) Mortality by social class 1971–85. *Popul. Trends*, **56**, 6–15.
Halsey, A.H., Heath, A.F. & Ridge, J.M.   (1980) *Origins and Destinations: Family, Class and Education in Modern Britain*. Oxford: Clarendon Press.
Hunter, D.   (1975) *The Diseases of Occupations*, 5th edn. London: English Universities Press.
Kunst, A.E. & Mackenbach, J.P.   (1994) *Measuring Socio-economic Inequalities in Health*. Copenhagen: WHO Regional Office for Europe.
Mackenbach, J.P.   (1993) Inequalities in health in The Netherlands according to age, gender, marital status, level of education, degree of urbanisation and region. *Eur. J. Public Health*, **3**, 112–18.
Ministry of Agriculture, Fisheries and Food (MAFF)   (1989) *Household Food Consumption and Expenditure 1988* London: HMSO.
Office of Population Censuses and Surveys   (1980) *Classification of Occupations 1980*. London: ¹
Office of Population Censuses and Surveys   (1986) *Occupational Mortality: Decennial St* 1982–83. London: HMSO.
Office of Population Censuses and Surveys   (1988) *Occupational Mortality: Childhood Su* 1982–83. London: HMSO.
Office of Population Censuses and Surveys   (1989) *General Household Survey 1987*. Lond
Pocock, S.J., Cook, D.G., Shaper, A.G. et al.   (1987) Social class differences in ischaemic h British men. *Lancet*, **ii**, 197–201.
Power, C., Manor, O. & Fox, A.J.   (1990) *Health and Class: the Early Years*. London: Chapma
Reid, I.   (1989) *Social Class Differences in Britain*, 3rd edn. London: Fontana Press.

Shaper, A.G., Ashby, D. & Pocock, S.J.   (1988) Blood pressure and hypertension in middle-aged British men. *J. Hypertens.*, **6**, 367–74.

Townsend, P.   (1979) *Poverty in the United Kingdom*. London: Penguin.

Wadsworth, M.E.J.   (1986) Serious illness in childhood and its association with later-life achievement. In: *Class and Health: Research and Longitudinal Data*, ed. R.G. Wilkinson. London: Tavistock, pp. 50–74.

Weatherall, R. & Shaper, A.G.   (1988) Overweight and obesity in middle-aged British men. *J. Clin. Nutr.*, **42**, 221–31.

West, P.   (1991) Rethinking the health selection explanation for health inequalities. *Soc. Sci. Med.*, **32**, 373–84.

Whitehead, M. (1987) *The Health Divide: Inequalities in Health in the 1980s*. London: Health Education Council.

9

Women as Patients and Providers

SHEILA HILLIER AND GRAHAM SCAMBLER

The special issues surrounding women's health are important for several reasons: first, epidemiological evidence shows that there are differences in the disease patterns of women and men; second, female symptomatology and what is defined as illness in women are particularly good examples of the introduction of social definitions into what are often thought of as the purely scientific exercises of diagnosis and treatment; third, looking at the way women are treated as patients is informative not only about how medical practices incorporate many of the socially derived stereotypes of sex and gender, but also how this helps to confine women to certain limited and limiting roles in society; fourth, women form the major part of the health-care labour force, although they are under-represented in the higher echelons of the medical and administrative hierarchies.

THE HEALTH OF WOMEN

Mortality

In modern industrialized societies like Britain or the USA, women live longer than men and at every age there is an excess of male over female mortality. Life expectancy for both males and females has steadily increased over the last 100 years, but the average life expectancy of women is longer: at present in the UK it is 82 years for females and 77 years for males.

These differences appear to be related to social factors. For example, in less-developed countries female life expectancy is lower than that of males, and women are more likely to be malnourished and to have less access to health care. Moreover, there is little difference in female and male rates of death from the epidemics which afflict developing societies or which have occurred in the past in developed ones. The major change affecting the mortality of women over the last 100 years in Britain has been the change in patterns of child bearing and the consequent decline in maternal mortality. The average woman married in 1880 would expect to bear about five live children, whereas a woman married in the 1990s will probably have only two. The other side of the coin, the excess of male mortality, seems to be related, at least partly, to the different living patterns of men and women. Typically, men are more likely to engage in activities which are injurious to health, both at work and during leisure activities: they drink more, smoke more, drive faster and work in more physically hazardous occupations than women (Waldron 1976). Men are more likely to commit suicide and to murder. In trying to live up to a stereotyped self-image of one's own sex, vulnerability to certain causes of death are increased, for example cirrhosis of the liver due to excessive drinking.

The excess of male over female mortality might be even greater were it not that a considerable number of women die of cancers of the breast, cervix and uterus. About 39% of deaths in women aged 25–44 years are from cancer, a third of these being malignant cancers of the breast. Even after the age of 44 years, when diseases of the circulatory system take over as the major cause of death in women as in men, breast cancer accounts for one in ten female deaths.

One important development needs to be noted, however. Since 1970, mortality/sex ratios have remained virtually unchanged and the advantage that females have over males has become stabilized and is not increasing. This does not represent a deterioration in the health of women, but a marked improvement in the rate of decline in mortality for men.

Women have not modified their smoking habits as dramatically as men. Whereas more men (28%) than women (26%) smoke, there was a 24% drop in the number of male smokers between 1972 and 1994, but only a 15% drop among women (CSO 1996). Those most likely to smoke are aged 20–24, in which group about two-fifths of both men and women now smoke. As increasing numbers of women smokers enter the older age groups, when most smoking-related diseases occur, the lung-cancer deaths among women will rise. Whereas male death rates from lung cancer nearly halved between 1971 and 1992, female rates actually increased by 16% over the same period (CSO 1995). A quarter of all female deaths are from lung cancer. In the UK, women in social class V are one and a half times as likely to smoke as those in social class I.

There has been an increase in the number of mental-hospital admissions for alcoholism among women (OPCS 1984), but this may merely reflect a decline in the stigma associated with the condition. There is no evidence overall that women's drinking patterns are converging with those of men, but there is an increase in the number of women who are moderate to heavy drinkers. In 1994/5, one in four men, compared with one in eight women drank over 'sensible levels' (i.e. 21 and 14 units per week, respectively). In the 18–24 age-group, over a third of men and a fifth of women exceeded these levels. About 6% of men, compared with 2% of women, drank to a 'medically dangerous level' (i.e. in excess of 50 and 35 units per week, respectively) (CSO 1996). Single females drink more than married, divorced, widowed or separated women.

There are also iatrogenic risks of disease for women, and perhaps the most well known is that associated with the oral contraceptive pill, with dangers of cardiovascular disease being greatest for women over 40 years who are also heavy smokers. The administration of postmenopausal oestrogens also carries risks, as do hysterectomies.

It has been suggested that the mortality patterns of women will come to resemble those of men as differences in life-styles diminish, and this is particularly related to the growing participation of women in the labour market and their entry into a 'man's world'. By 1995, 38% of women were employed full-time (71% men), 28% part-time (5% men), 5% were defined as unemployed (9% men), and 29% were economically inactive (15% men). Between 1987 and 1995, the number of women in full-time employment has increased by 8%, compared with a decline of 2% for men; over the same period, the number of women in part-time employment has increased by 12% (to 5.2 million), compared with an increase of more than half for men (but only to 1.2 million) (CSO 1996). In addition to entering the work-force most women are doing two jobs, inside and outside the home, for sharing all domestic tasks equally between males and females is still unusual (OPCS 1984). It is estimated that, internationally, women work on average some 80 hours per week compared with their husbands' 50 hours per week and a recent survey showed that even when parents work full time the woman still takes on most of the child-care and household tasks (Jowell et al. 1988).

Occupational stress is thought to be a contributory factor in coronary heart disease and rates continue to rise in the UK. Women are hormonally protected prior to menopause. A study of women working inside and outside the home showed no difference in incidence between them and the rates remained lower than those for men (Haynes and Feinleb 1980). One particular group, however, were at greater risk – clerical and non-manual workers with children in a traditional female work role. It seems clear that it is not working as such that is a risk factor – women in high status work have fewer problems. It is rather the multiple stresses of relatively low status jobs, role expectations at work (e.g. pliability, submissiveness and suppression of anger) and heavy domestic burdens which are a source of danger.

A recent publication summarizing occupational risks to women indicates that most of the occupations which women have traditionally undertaken – nursing, sales, secretarial and clerical work – all carry environmental risks, but interest in improving occupational health has concentrated mainly on the risks associated with conception and pregnancy. Environmental factors, as well as behaviour and situations related to employment, are all in some sense 'toxic', and these problems are most likely to occur among women manual workers and those in traditional female occupations (Denning 1984).

Overall, however, women still enjoy a more favourable mortality experience than men and social changes have, on the whole, been beneficial to them. Men, on the other hand, largely for cultural and social reasons, are less fortunate. However, the class dimension should not be ignored: men of social class I still have a lower overall mortality than women of social class V.

Morbidity

Much illness and suffering is occasioned by diseases which do not in themselves kill, but are often chronic and disabling. Because women live longer than men they are likely to experience the greater morbidity associated with age. It has long been maintained too that at almost every age more women than men report more limiting long-standing illness. Recently, however, this conventional wisdom has been challenged. Using data from the West of Scotland Twenty-07 Study and the Health and Lifestyles Survey, MacIntyre et al. (1996) have suggested a more complex

TABLE 9.1 *Self-reported long-standing illness or disability by sex and age, England 1993.*

Age (years)	Self-reported illness/disability (%)	
	Men	Women
16–44	26.2	26.7
45–64	46.3	47.3
65+	63.4	62.7
All, aged 16 or over	39.1	40.3

Adapted from CSO (1996).

picture. They contend that female excess is only found consistently across the life span for psychological distress, and is much less apparent, or reversed, for a number of physical symptoms and conditions. Table 9.1 lends some support to this view.

Statistics from general practice indicate that women are more likely than men to consult their doctors: on average women visit their general practitioners six times per year, men four times (General Household Survey 1987). The average for both sexes has been rising, with the current average for men now approaching that for women of 10 years ago. Working women have a slightly lower consultation rate than housewives. These visits cannot be regarded as a true measure of illness, however, since not every symptom leads to a consultation (see Chapter 3). Contrary to the view that it is somehow 'easier' for a housewife to visit the doctor, there could equally be under-reporting of female morbidity because of women's domestic responsibilities. Data suggest that, as a group, housewives are less likely to regard themselves as being 'in excellent health' (Waldron 1976). It may be culturally more acceptable for women than for men to admit 'weakness' and seek help from others, which would suggest an under-reporting of male morbidity. It remains likely that the various statistics on morbidity do not afford a complete picture, but rather an approximation of actual sex differences in morbidity.

Because of this, one should beware of drawing too strong conclusions. For example, it is sometimes asserted that women have more mental illness than men. To attribute more to women than to men carries with it greater opportunities for making judgements, often of a stigmatizing kind, about the nature of women. As Standing (1980) says, 'an illness such as "depression" carries a much greater load of [these] messages and judgements than does, say, tonsillitis or malaria'.

If the effects of age and marital status are combined with sex, single males aged 35 years upwards have higher rates of admission to psychiatric hospitals than single women of the same age group. After the age of 65 there are twice as many women as men in psychiatric beds, but this reflects the greater number of women in that age group, as well as the possibility that men are more likely to be cared for by their spouses than women. 'Mental illness' is usually taken to mean psychosis and neurosis. Women are more frequently diagnosed as neurotic than men (although 'neurosis' is a less stable and reliable diagnostic assessment), but not as schizophrenic. If both diagnoses are aggregated – as they usually are – there is a bias in the combination which shows women to have a higher overall prevalence. Mental illness generally does not include alcoholism, personality disorders or acting-out behaviour more often displayed by men.

The causes of mental illness are sometimes attributed to women's social role, which is deemed to be more stressful than that of men, but a study of Camberwell women showed that five times as many working-class women as middle-class women were chronically depressed, so clearly the class factor is important (Brown and Harris 1980). Studies of men's mental illness and social class show a similar concentration of morbidity in the lower social classes.

Some popular stereotypes exist to the effect that women are either intrinsically weaker or less stoical than men and unreasonably fussy about their physical condition. It is plausible, however, to suggest the opposite: that women are more sensitive to and commonsensical about matters of health and sickness, and that there are social pressures on men which lead them to take risks with their health and to fail to protect themselves.

THE SPECIAL PROBLEMS OF WOMEN

Sex and gender

In all known societies assumptions are made about what is appropriate behaviour for men and for women. These assumptions cover not only behaviour but also personal attributes. Social scientists refer to them as sexual stereotypes. Such stereotypes are extremely powerful, deriving much of their strength from the belief that behaviour is biologically based, and that the most fundamental aspect of any person's identity is his or her sex. From this it is but a short step to deduce that the behaviours that men and women are expected to exhibit, for example competitiveness and aggression in men, passivity and nurturance in women, somehow reflect basic differences between the sexes and are biologically determined. Evidence from other cultures, however, shows that the personality traits and behaviour stereotypes attributed to men and women in societies like Britain are not always similarly attributed elsewhere, nor do they necessarily accord with objectively observed behaviour in Britain. Thus it seems that, whatever the ultimate biological basis for the behaviour of males and females may be, the stereotypes result mainly from cultural values.

It may be useful at this stage to distinguish between the biological and the cultural by using the word sex to refer to those elements of the male and female which are indisputably biological, and the term gender to refer to the socially assigned meanings given to sexual differences. For example, differences in sex determine who has menstrual periods and who nocturnal emissions; but it is gender assignment to regard tender loving care as a female characteristic and skill with a surgeon's knife as a male one.

Although it may be easy to realize that gender and sex are not the same thing, it is more difficult to recognize that they may not be coincidental. A biological male may not necessarily be a social male and a biological female a social female (Clarke 1983). One study has shown that 'feminine' social characteristics are associated with poorer mental health and poorer self-asserted physical health than 'masculine' ones – for both male and female subjects (Annandale and Hunt 1990). The strong distinctions between male and female identities result in women being seen as 'other', with normality residing in men, and women as a deviant minority who are judged on the degree to which they approximate 'normality'. This also means that 'women' are falsely regarded as a homogenous group, whose similarities far outweigh their differences.

Some writers would argue that this adds further confirmation to the view that masculine conduct, whether by men or women, has more social power, and is valued more. Bearing these issues in mind, it is appropriate to turn to a discussion of women as patients, and to consider how far the medical management of their illnesses incorporates socially derived sexual stereotypes.

SEXUAL STEREOTYPES IN MEDICAL PRACTICE

One of the commonest stereotypes of women is that they are 'by nature' more delicate and more susceptible to illness because of their reproductive function. This view was often expressed by male doctors in the nineteenth century, who argued that women's physiology made them more prone to hysteria (a term itself derived from the Greek for womb). Some writers have even suggested that doctors contributed to the debate on women's political and legal rights by suggesting that they were biologically unfit to participate in national affairs because of their propensity to 'nervous excitation'. Furthermore, it was argued that women should not be admitted to medical school because they would faint in anatomy lectures and their reproductive organs would be damaged by study, rendering them 'repulsive and useless hybrids'.

Although such ideas would be thought silly today, others possibly as pernicious but less obvious are still around. For example, teaching in medical schools today rarely covers psychosexual development, and recent evidence concerning the nature of female sexuality appears to have had little consideration; lectures tend to limit themselves to female hormonal reactions and the 'mechanisms' of pregnancy and childbirth.

The sexual stereotypes of the woman as potentially sick – the product and prisoner of her reproductive system – and emotionally unstable have militated against a rational approach to women's illnesses. Cystitis, premenstrual tension, pelvic pain, dysmenorrhoea, and menopausal symptoms have sometimes been written off as 'not real' illnesses.

A series of studies in Aberdeen contain some fairly damning evidence of the treatment of 'women's complaints' (Porter 1990). Side-effects of contraceptives were dismissed as minor: patients whose physical complaints could not be explained or satisfactorily treated were labelled as neurotic, and those who could not find a type of contraceptive that suited them as 'unreasonable'.

Labelling women's complaints as 'psychogenic' is sometimes a polite way of saying imaginary. Unfortunately, there has been too little application of accepted scientific methods to the study of disorders of allegedly psychogenic origins. Many of the studies which purport to explain infertility or pregnancy complications were carried out on small groups of patients and lacked controls. They were usually retrospective, or, if prospective, did not assess personality variables before pregnancy (Oakley 1979).

It is useful to remember that many findings are reported in such a way as to create a picture of women that is congruent with social stereotypes of weakness and instability. The consequences of this can be twofold: either symptoms will not be taken seriously, or they will be dealt with in a way which reinforces and reflects women's lack of control over their own health. Some examples might be appropriate here; they relate exclusively to those aspects of women's health which are associated with being female, because it is these aspects, many researchers feel, which demonstrate most clearly the essentially oppressive use of sexual stereotypes.

Pregnancy and childbirth

Over the last 20 years, evidence has continued to accumulate about the lack of control which many women experience over an essentially natural and healthy process – that of giving birth. Many sociologists have written about the 'medicalization' of reproduction (see Chapter 12). Some have argued that the historical shift from female-dominated midwifery to male-dominated obstetrics was related to the largely male medical profession's expansionist tendencies (Oakley 1979), and that this resulted in the transformation of a normal process into a pathological one over which doctors exercise control. Box 9.1 outlines sources of tension or conflict between the ways women and their doctors regard pregnancy and childbirth.

BOX 9.1

DIMENSIONS OF CONFLICT BETWEEN DOCTORS AND PREGNANT WOMEN

1. Most women see pregnancy as a normal healthy process. Doctors tend to treat pregnancy *as if* it were actually or potentially an illness.

2. Most women see themselves as having expert knowledge about what is happening to their bodies and in their lives. Doctors appear to consider that all useful knowledge is medical knowledge. They are the experts.

3. Women express a wish to control what happens to them in childbirth. Doctors usually act as if all decisions are for them to make.

4. Women complain of unsatisfactory communication. Questions are difficult to ask and, if asked, are not answered. Requests for information are interpreted as requests for reassurance. Doctors appear to consider women as anxious rather than wanting information.

Reproduced with permission of Routledge from Graham and Oakley (1981).

Antenatal care   The ceding of control begins with the 'diagnosis' of pregnancy. Women are believed by doctors to be unreliable observers of their menstrual cycles and, therefore, it is the doctor who must make the initial pronouncement of pregnancy (Oakley 1979). Not until this has happened can a woman feel free to communicate the news. Access to antenatal care and confinement is largely controlled by medicine, and it is here that the woman is introduced to a view of childbirth as something that is likely to entail pathology for mother and child. Women will also be given advice on their personal habits, especially smoking, with the warning that smoking can result in a low-birth-weight baby. In one study, few modified their habits, but not because they were unaware of the evidence (Oakley 1990). Women had high levels of anxiety related to previous traumatic births, or after trying to give up smoking experienced serious life events which precipitated a return to the habit. Almost none of this was understood by the staff. One woman described how 'The consultant came down and he said, tut, tut, smoking!, he kept on and on about smoking. That's all he said' (Oakley 1990). And after the initial moral lecture it seemed as if most women were given up as a lost cause.

Antenatal clinics have been criticized for long waiting times, brief examinations, cursory treatment and lack of information (O'Brien and Smith 1981). The 'production line' procedures are such that women's own views and knowledge are ignored. In one absurd, but possibly revealing, consultation (Oakley 1979) the following exchange took place.

> *Doctor (reading case notes): Ah, I see you've got a boy and a girl.*
> *Patient: No, two girls.*
> *Doctor: Are you sure? I thought it said . . . (checks in notes). Oh no, you're quite right, two girls.*

The 'are you sure' could only have been uttered by a doctor who had learned to treat women's experiences as irrelevant and hence not worth listening to. Studies of antenatal consultations in a working-class area of Aberdeen (MacIntyre and Porter 1989) showed that doctors and paramedical workers seemed to have a low opinion of their largely working-class clientele. Women were deemed to be unreliable in keeping appointments, although a follow-up study revealed that very few women failed to turn up, and that those who did not had very good reasons. Only 37% of patients asked questions in antenatal clinics, and those who did were likely to be labelled as 'anxious'. Persistent questioners, or those who seemed to display interest in their routine tests, were likely to be seen as neurotic. Repeated studies in many parts of the UK over 20 years have produced similar findings.

Delivery Today, there is widespread use of technological devices in childbirth. About 98% of births take place in hospital. There has been much criticism of the lack of choice and involvement in decisions over procedures. A particular focus of criticism was the use of induction in labour. Although the rate is now declining, it reached a peak of over 40% in the mid-1970s. It is unpopular with women. One study showed that only 17% of mothers who experienced it would have it again (Cartwright 1977). Intervention in labour remains a contentious issue. In 1985, over 20% of births used forceps, caesarean section or vacuum extraction (OPCS 1988). Although intervention techniques can be of positive benefit, the style in which they are managed is often open to criticism. The long-term consequences of feeling devalued when giving birth are not always considered. Oakley (1979) has shown that having a technologically managed birth is one factor precipitating postnatal depression.

Women may vary in their responses to childbirth, depending on their social class or ethnic group. One of the objections raised to campaigns to improve maternity services was that they were led by 'vocal' white middle-class women. Porter's study of working-class women showed that one of their concerns was time, and that they were less likely to question the medical model of childbirth. But she was unsure, finally, whether or not women simply did not feel it worthwhile to pursue issues or felt unqualified to argue with doctors. In any case, whether concerns are the same or vary between women, usually little attempt is made to establish what these actually are.

New reproductive technologies   In a society which expects that couples should produce children, the realization of infertility is painful for women and men. The number of infertile couples in the UK is estimated at about 10%, and in one-third of cases the husband suffers sterility. Most information on infertility is derived from clinic-based studies, and so only includes those who have come for treatment. It has been suggested that perhaps around 40% of people do not come for treatment. New reproductive technologies (NRT), for example artificial insemination (AID) and *in vitro* fertilization (IVF), seem to offer a way out, but there are social costs as well as benefits. New reproductive technologies are expensive and require elaborate procedures. The service is not widely available and most patients must use the private sector; therefore access is unequal. Furthermore, IVF has a low success rate – many people leave an IVF programme without a baby.

Writers who have looked at the problems, as well as the solutions, posed for women by the NRT usually consider the following issues. First, a proportion of female infertility is due to untreated pelvic inflammatory disease – a condition which is often ignored, overlooked or whose symptoms are described as 'psychosomatic'. If women had appropriate treatment earlier on, infertility problems might be reduced. Secondly, although many women may subscribe to 'marriage-motherhood', not all will. The existence of NRT and the social expectations of women may pressurize them into treatment. Being in an infertility programme is very stressful both physically and mentally. In IVF the woman is exposed to risks like powerful hormonal treatment and surgical intervention.

Thirdly, NRT has legal and ethical implications. For example, when an embryo is fertilized *in vitro* but cannot be replaced in the mother's womb, another woman must carry the baby. This arrangement, known as surrogacy, gave rise to the famous 'baby M' case in 1986, where the surrogate mother refused to give up the baby when she was born. In that case, money had been paid. Commercial surrogacy is outlawed in this country, but the fear exists that poor women might be under commercial pressure to 'womb-lease' or perhaps donate eggs for IVF. Other writers have said that a woman's body is her own to use as she wants, and this should include commercial surrogacy arrangements.

Finally, some writers fear that NRT has the power to subordinate women, and envisage the application of eugenic policies, the rejection of female embryos, and selection of women for breeding. They regard NRT as finally wresting control over reproduction from women. The question as to who controls NRT is seen as central to its potential for good or evil (Arditti et al. 1984).

Abortion

Views about the social role of women as wives and mothers or about their sexuality may be incorporated in judgements about abortion. There are inequalities in the provision of abortion in different parts of the UK which cannot be explained solely in terms of the facilities available. In a study of a clinic which gave antenatal care and also referred patients for abortion, different responses to the pregnancies of single and married women were noted (MacIntyre 1977). For the former, pregnancy was assumed to be a disaster, for the latter a 'happy event'. For single women, abortion was assumed to be the most likely outcome of pregnancy, for married women, childbirth. No attempt was made to verify these assumptions.

The common assumption that there is 'nothing to it' as far as abortion is concerned under-estimates the physical pain and mental distress involved, particularly in second trimester abortions. The belief that women regard the fetus as a nuisance which must be got rid of assumes that grief can attend a miscarriage, but not a legally terminated pregnancy.

Menopause

The menopause marks the end of fertility. Physical changes occur and ovarian functions decline, culminating in the cessation of the menses. However, these physical changes occur in a sociocultural context which reflects how far the value attached to women is associated with their ability to reproduce. This, in turn, shows what the menopause may mean to women in a particular society.

Although there is a clear medical definition of menopause, this is beguiling, because symptoms, including absence of menstruation, are open to different interpretations. Kaufert (1982), writing in a North American context, noted two competing views about menopause. First, the medical view, which characterizes the menopausal woman as relatively wealthy, from a happy conventional home, with time on her hands, succumbing to the temptation to become a hypochondriac. The recommendation is that she takes firm advice from her doctor, who will protect her against over-reaction to her bodily state, will advise her on whether or not she needs hormone replacement, and will monitor for cancer. The potentially pathological character of the menopause and need for medical guidance is emphasized.

Opposed to this view is what Kaufert calls the 'feminist' view, which locates some menopausal symptoms in the suppressed rage that women feel at having given so much of themselves to their families, and so little to themselves. Therapies, somewhat holistic in character, include better diet and exercise, and self-help rather than reliance on doctors is recommended. The use of hormones is usually opposed.

One view sees the woman as passive, the other as active. In one, women's knowledge of their bodies is held to be irrelevant or dangerous, in the other as valuable. There are obvious parallels with the literature on childbirth. However, both agree that the menopause is a problematic life event. How far this is correct remains somewhat questionable. Labelling symptoms as 'menopausal' ignores the fact that some may have a different origin. Research has suggested that depressed mood in middle-aged women is related less to the menopause than to particular life events. No excess of depressive disorder at the menopause has been detected (Gath *et al.*, 1989). Whether menopause is interpreted as dangerous obsolescence or a chance for active new growth and new selfhood, both views have similarities which have the potential of defining women largely in terms of their reproductive capacities and familial relationships, in ignorance of how women from different backgrounds or cultures, single or married, with or without children, may experience this development.

These examples suggest that stereotypes of women's roles and allied beliefs about the causes of women's diseases perhaps serve to divert attention from the serious consideration – as well as the research still needed for a proper understanding – of women's health problems. A change in emphasis which treats the health problems of women as worthy of the same kind of scientific attention as is afforded to the pathological problems which are not confined to women is clearly desirable.

WOMEN AS HEALTH WORKERS

In the National Health Service (NHS), approximately 70% of the work-force are women. There are nurses, doctors, domestics, physiotherapists, occupational therapists, technicians and mid-wives, but the great majority work in the more subordinate positions and are relatively poorly paid. Women have struggled to be allowed to train as doctors and to have nursing recognized as an important and integral aspect of health care. These struggles still continue.

Women doctors

In medieval times, both women and men attended medical schools, but from the late Middle Ages onwards attempts to professionalize medicine by basing it in the universities led to their exclusion. Women were still expected to be skilled in the treatment of minor ailments, and female bonesetters and surgeons continued to practise until their work was outlawed by the professional associations of apothecaries and barber surgeons in the time of Henry VIII. The first woman to be trained at a 'modern' medical school was Elizabeth Blackwell, an American who went to the medical faculty at the University of Geneva and graduated in 1849. During the remainder of that century a tiny number of women were admitted to medical school against enormous opposition. The Medical Press of 1874 stated 'no-one who knows what the course of study of a medical student is can doubt that a woman must be of a very exceptional character if she can pass through those scenes and still remain undimmed in those characteristics that are the beauty and ornament of a woman's life'. It was not until 1944 that it was recommended that women should be admitted to the previously single-sex London medical schools, and not until 1978 that restrictions on the admission of women students were outlawed by the Sex Discrimination Act. Women now form an increasing percentage of medical school entrants.

Much has been made of the problems of 'wastage' of women doctors, although the wastage of male doctors through migration, disability disqualification and death should not be forgotten. A study done in the 1960s showed that only one-fifth of women with young children and one-third of women with older children were working full time (Elliott and Jeffreys 1966). However, most were eager to work and between 1965 and 1976 the proportion of women active in medicine rose from 66% to 83%. Nowadays, women doctors are more likely than other professional women with family responsibilities to continue working. There is still evidence, however, that difficulty in finding suitable part-time work 'forces' a number of women doctors into reluctant unemployment (Rhodes 1990).

One traditional solution for women doctors has been to undertake part-time work which can be combined with family, and the number of part-time doctors in hospitals has increased since 1976, but they comprise a relatively small proportion. Most women doctors in hospital, particularly at the junior levels, are unlikely to be able to pursue their careers as effectively as men, or may be regarded as lacking commitment if they attempt part-time arrangements. For most, it is not an option anyway, since such opportunities are limited below consultant level.

A recent survey of a small number (8%) of female junior hospital doctors showed that, in addition to experiencing the stresses which are reported by all juniors (overwork, long hours and poor relations with consultants), they face additional hazards, including sexual harassment and conflicts between personal or family and work responsibilities. The study found 46% to have scored as clinically depressed (Firth-Cozens 1990). However, there was no comparison made with males.

One particular problem which younger women doctors experience is the lack of women in senior positions who could act as role models. In part, this reflects earlier, discriminatory policies of admission to medical school. The number of women consultants is rising slowly: in 1963, 5.3% of all consultants were women, in 1993 the proportion was 17% (Table 9.2).

At present, only 12% of consultants in general medicine and less than 2% in general surgery are women (Wilson and Allen 1994). Women are still more likely to find consultant posts in the 'shortage' specialities like public-health medicine, mental subnormality or geriatrics. It has been argued that this serves to reinforce the ideas that such specialities are 'second class', and that women, who are seen as 'second class' doctors, are the ones most suitable to work in them. It remains to be seen whether the greater proportion of women entrants to medicine will alter the balance. Certainly in general practice, where 27% of doctors are women, they comprise 40% of those aged under 30 years, compared with 20% in the 40−44 years age group.

TABLE 9.2 *Percentage of women by hospital grade for selected specialities, England and Wales, 1993.*

Speciality	Consultant	Senior Registrar	Registrar	SHO
All	17.0	30.2	27.2	38.1
General medicine	11.9	19.4	20.6	38.5
Cardiology	4.5	9.7	14.7	36.0
Geriatric medicine	13.7	32.5	19.6	40.5
Paediatrics	29.3	52.4	45.6	53.6
General surgery	1.6	6.3	8.8	14.5
Neurosurgery	1.8	3.3	3.0	13.1
Anaesthetics	21.5	30.4	32.7	36.6
Radiology	22.9	31.6	39.8	50.0
Mental illness	24.2	38.7	42.8	48.4
Psychotherapy	34.8	65.6	60.0	50.0
Obstetrics/Gynaecology	14.9	35.0	32.5	48.7

Reproduced with permission of the Controller of HMSO from Wilson and Allen (1994).

Unpaid lay carers

Developments in community care, especially in the care of the elderly, chronically sick or handicapped, are often seen as a better and cheaper alternative to expensive hospital care. However, such care may well have 'hidden costs'. In the absence of trained staff, and where resources are stretched, the unpaid volunteer labour of women who care for sick members of the family on a long-term basis is usually forgotten (see Chapter 16).

Although the proportions of women and men caring for a sick person are not very different (15% women, 12% men), because there are more women than men, about 3.5 million women compared with 2.5 million men are caring for someone who is not a child. Women are more likely to be the main carers, to care for someone outside the home, and to spend longer hours caring. Single women aged 45–64 years carry the heaviest burden. One-quarter of women, compared with only 8% of men, are caring single-handed. Women are also likely to be given less professional help with the job – 66% of men compared with 48% of women were receiving assistance from outside agencies (Green 1985).

Women form the majority of the patients and providers of health care. As patients, they suffer rather than benefit from views which presume their physical and/or psychological weakness. Such views affect not only what will happen to them as patients, but serve to reinforce existing social attitudes towards women. As workers, they suffer from inequality of opportunity, low-status positions and poor pay, for within the health service the distribution of power and the social relationships which exist often mirror the general relationships of inferiority and superiority between women and men in society. The position is slowly changing, however, and it remains to be seen whether increasing numbers of women doctors, coupled with increasing self-confidence on the part of women patients, will fundamentally alter the picture described in this chapter.

REFERENCES

Annandale, E. & Hunt, K.   (1990) Masculinity, feminity and sex: an exploration of their relative contribution to explaining gender differences in health. *Soc. Health Illness*, **12**, 24–47.
Arditti, R., Klein, R. & Minden, S. (eds)   (1984) *Test Tube Women: What Future for Motherhood*? Boston: Pandora Press.
Brown, G. & Harris, T.   (1980) *The Social Origins of Depression*. London: Tavistock.
Cartwright, A.   (1977) Mothers' experiences of induction. *Br. Med. J.*, **2**, 745–9.
Central Statistical Office (CSO)   (1995) *Social Trends 25*. London: HMSO.
Central Statistical Office (CSO)   (1996) *Social Trends 26*. London: HMSO.
Clarke, J.   (1983) Sexism, feminism and medicalisation: a decade review of the literature on gender and illness. *Soc. Health Illness*, **51**, 62–81.
Denning, J.   (1984) *Women's Work and Health Hazards: a Selected Bibliography*. London: Department of Occupational Health, London School of Hygiene and Tropical Medicine.
Department of Health and Social Security   (1987) *Hospital In-patient Inquiry: Hospital Medical Staff*. London: HMSO.
Elliott, P.M. & Jeffreys, M.   (1966) *Women in Medicine*. London: Office of Health Economics.
Firth-Cozens, J.   (1990) Sources of stress in women junior house officers. *Br. Med. J.*, **301**, 89–92.
Gath, D. *et al.*,   (1989) Depression and the menopause. *Br. Med. J.*, **300(12)**, 87–8.
General Household Survey 1987, Morbidity no. 17. London: HMSO.
Godlee, F.   (1990) Stress in women doctors. *Br. Med. J.*, **301**, 76–7.
Graham, H. & Oakley, A.   (1981) Competing ideologies of reproduction, medical and maternal perspectives on pregnancy. In: *Women, Health and Reproduction*, ed. H. Roberts. London: Routledge, pp. 50–75.
Green, H.   (1985) *Informal Carers. OPCS GHS 15*. Supplement A. London: HMSO.
Haynes, S.G. & Feinleb, M.   (1980) Women, work and coronary heart disease: prospective findings from the Framingham heart study. *Am. J. Public Health*, **70**, 137–41.
Jowell, R., Witherspoon, S. & Brook, L. (eds)   (1988) *British Social Attitudes:* the 5th Report. Aldershot: Gower.
Kaufert, P.A.   (1982) Myth and the menopause. *Soc. Health Illness*, **4**, 141–61.
MacIntyre, S.   (1977) *Single and Pregnant*. London: Croom Helm.
MacIntyre, S. & Porter, M.   (1989) Problems and prospects in promoting effective care at the local level. In: *Effective Care in Pregnancy and Childbirth*, ed. M. Enkin, M. Keirse and I. Chalmers. Oxford: Oxford University Press.
MacIntyre, S., Hunt, K. & Sweeting, H.   (1996) Gender differences in health: are things really as simple as they seem? *Soc. Sci. Med.*, **42**, 617–24.
Oakley, A.   (1979) *Becoming a Mother*. London: Martin Robertson.
Oakley, A.   (1990) Smoking in pregnancy: smokescreen or risk factor? Towards a materialist analysis. *Soc. Health Illness*, **11**, 311–35.
O'Brien, M. & Smith, C.   (1981) Women's views and experiences of antenatal care. *Practitioner,* **225,** 123–6.
Office of Population Censuses and Surveys (OPCS)   (1984) *Social Trends: Health*. London: HMSO.
Office of Population Censuses and Surveys (OPCS)   (1988) *Hospital Inpatient Inquiry 1987*. London: HMSO.

Porter, M.   (1990) Professional–client relationship and women's reproductive health care. In: *Readings in Medical Sociology*, ed. S. Cunningham-Burley & N. McKeganey. London: Tavistock Routledge.

Rhodes, P.   (1990) Medical women in the middle: family or career? *Health Trends*, **22,** 33–6.

Standing, H.   (1980) Sickness is a woman's business. In: *Alice Through the Microscope*, ed. L. Birke & S. Best. London: Routledge & Kegan Paul.

Waldron, I.   (1976) Why do women live longer than men? *Soc. Sci. Med.*, **19**, 349.

Wilson, R. & Allen, P.   (1994) Medical and dental staffing prospects in the NHS in England and Wales. *Health Trends*, **26,** 70–9.

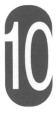

The Health and Health Care of Ethnic Minority Groups

SHEILA HILLIER

Recognizing the needs of ethnic minorities is an important objective of the National Health Service which was explicitly stated as a national policy in the Patient's Charter (Department of Health 1991) with its requirement that the religious and cultural beliefs of ethnic groups should be taken seriously by policy makers and practitioners alike when considering health matters.

NEW DEFINITIONS: WHAT IS ETHNICITY?

There now appears to be a degree of consensus among 'official' bodies like the Department of Health and the National Census as to how ethnicity is to be defined. In the 1982 Census, a question on ethnic origin was omitted since no agreement could be reached as to what categories to use. The term 'ethnic minority' was regarded as contentious since it seemed to imply that there was a homogenous majority somewhere in British society. It also denied variety by using a term like 'Asian' which belies the variety of religious, geographical languages and origins that exist. In preparation for the 1991 Census, field trials were carried out as to what would be the most acceptable question on ethnic origin (Teague 1993). People were given a list of six groups and asked to tick the one to which they belonged.

The data derived from the 1991 Census enabled a much more accurate picture of ethnic groups in Britain to emerge. In contrast with the 1971 Census, which relied on country of birth as a proxy for ethnic origin, the 1991 Census provided information on the increasing numbers of people born in the UK to parents from various ethnic groups. The introduction of ethnic monitoring (noting the ethnic origin of service users) in the NHS should also provide better information on the utilization and access to services.

Problems of coding and categorization have been addressed at a national level, but definitional issues remain. For example, some researchers, especially when trying to identify inherited patterns of disease, use the terms 'race' and 'ethnicity' interchangeably. Yet genetic diseases are not confined to specific 'racial' groups, and within-group genetic variation is far greater than that between the classically defined 'racial' groups or national ones (McKenzie and Crowcroft 1994).

Ethnicity, because it is a socially rather than biologically constructed category, can be fluid, with shifting boundaries. Ethnic identity can change over time, and thus categories need to be revised. It is unlikely that a fixed set of definitions will apply in all places at all times. It is therefore necessary to regard most definitions as 'working' definitions used by researchers and to remember that they may not reflect someone's subjective experience (Box 10.1). Subjective experiences of ethnicity (who people think and feel they 'are') have gone largely unresearched.

BOX 10.1

- **Ethnicity** refers to social groups who often share a cultural heritage with a common language, values, religion, customs and attitudes. The members are aware of sharing a common past, possibly a homeland, and experience a sense of difference.

- **Culture** reflects ethnicity, and refers to habits of thought and beliefs, diet, dress, music, art.

- **Race** is a construct based on phenotypical biological difference (usually skin colour), although social assumptions (often negative) are attributed to biological differences.

- **Racism** deterministically associates inherent biological characteristics with other negatively evaluated features or actions. Racial discrimination is against the law.

The definition of 'ethnicity' is of more than academic significance. Some writers have suggested that it is more useful for groups to unify as having a common 'black' racial identity because they share common experiences of racism. Discussion of 'ethnicity', it is said, merely divides groups, thus preventing effective political action. Such a view is characteristic of the 'anti-racist' school of thought. It is the case that the impact of racism and disadvantage is a common factor which underlies the experience of many groups. Racist murders, and legal measures which impact on ethnic minorities, produce a climate that is hostile. Concentrating on 'ethnicity' and on differences like diet, marriage patterns, family structures or traditional medicine use as causes of ill health among black people, it is argued, obscures the stressful nature of living in a racist society (Ahmad 1995). Other writers have argued that it is important to value as well as describe ethnically different cultural traditions and their supportive and positive aspects to ensure appropriate care and promote understanding. It is important to be aware of these different viewpoints and to realize that all research with 'ethnic minorities', including medical research, has a political dimension.

WHO ARE THE UK'S ETHNIC GROUPS?

The UK has a long history of migration going back to medieval times; Africans were a common sight in eighteenth century London. Large-scale migrations were a feature of the nineteenth and twentieth centuries beginning with post-famine Irish, 'West Indians' in sea ports like Cardiff and Liverpool and people from USA, Canada or Western Europe. After the Second World War an expanding economy recruited in the Caribbean. Migrants were also actively sought from India and Pakistan. Some groups, like Hindu Gujaratis and Sikh Punjabis, came with relatively well off commercial backgrounds. The East African Asians expelled from Kenya and Uganda were also from professional or business families. Some people came to the UK because of war or displacement in their homeland, or rural poverty, like those from the Sylhet provinces of Bangladesh. The 1962 Immigration Act placed restrictions on entry into this country.

The 1991 Census results are given in Table 10.1. The table shows both the resident population as a proportion of the total population, and the proportion of each group who were born in the UK. An analysis of age groups confirms previous findings (OPCS 1991). Three fifths of the ethnic minority population is under the age of 30 compared with two fifths in the population as a whole. About one-third of all ethnic groups are under 16.

Another important general feature is that ethnic minorities are largely, though not exclusively, urban dwellers. The settlement pattern has remained virtually unchanged since the last time data were available some 15 years ago. Over half the ethnic population lives in the south east, forming 20% of the population of Greater London. Ten districts/boroughs in the UK have the highest proportions of minority ethnic population. All except three are in London. In four, ethnic minority population is over 30%. These groups tend to be concentrated in older local authority housing blocks, or, when owner-occupiers, older housing stock. Thus, housing conditions are characterized by overcrowding and dampness.

TABLE 10.1 *Population by ethnic group (%) and percentage born in UK, 1991.*

Ethnic Group	% population	number (000s)	% born in UK
White	94.5	51,584	95
Black Caribbean	0.9	500	54
Black African	0.4	212	36
Black Other	0.3	178	84
Indian	1.5	840	42
Pakistani	0.9	477	50
Bangladeshi	0.3	163	37
Chinese	0.3	157	28
Other Asians	0.4	198	44
Other	0.5	290	

Reproduced with permission of the Controller of HMSO and the Office for National Statistics from OPCS (1991).

People from ethnic minorities earn less for the same work and are nearly twice as likely to be unemployed (Department of Employment 1991). Declining manufacturing in steel and textiles where many ethnic minority people were employed has reduced the number of available jobs. The position of most workers remains much as it was in the 1950s and 1960s, with the majority working in unskilled, low paid occupations where working conditions are poor or dangerous.

Whereas 19% of white males occupy professional or managerial positions, the respective proportion of ethnic minorities are 'West Indian' (5%), Indian (11%) and both Pakistani and Bangladeshi (10%). Only 16% of white males have unskilled jobs, whereas the figure is for West Indians 35%, Indian 42%, Pakistani 43% and Bangladeshi 75% (Ohri and Faruqui 1988). Therefore most members of ethnic minorities are concentrated in social classes IV and V, and to some extent, share the health profiles associated with these classes.

GENERAL HEALTH STATUS OF ETHNIC MINORITIES

Smaje (1995), in a comprehensive review of the evidence, considered two sources, the OPCS study of immigrant mortality 1970–72 (Marmot et al. 1984) and a later OPCS study by Balarajan and Bulusu (1990) of the years 1979–83. Later mortality data are not available at present. These statistics cover only people born abroad, use broad categories like 'Indian subcontinent', and in Marmot's case are over a generation old. However, both sets of data from 25 and 16 years ago are broadly in agreement. Essentially, people who migrate to this country have higher death rates than those born here, but lower death rates than in their home country. It is believed that these figures are because healthier people migrate ('healthy migrant' factor). An exception is the Irish, whose mortality rates in England are raised relative to home and UK populations which suggests that the 'healthy migrant' factor may not fully explain mortality rates. These effects show persistence into the second generation (Raftery et al. 1990). It has been suggested that people bring the risks of mortality of their earlier life with them, and later acquire the risks associated with living in this society, for example cardiovascular risk.

Birth and old age – two ends of the spectrum

Table 10.2 shows that the Pakistani, and to a lesser extent, Caribbean populations appear the most disadvantaged, but it is difficult to sort out the reasons why. Medical factors related to stillbirths and infant deaths are mother's age and parity, the spacing of pregnancies and low birthweight, infectious and congenital abnormalities. Social factors include low socioeconomic status (as measured by social class), consanguineous (marriage with cousins) marriage, and barriers in access to care. Looking at the whole data set, Bangladeshi mothers, who are generally of low economic status, have a high still birth rate but the lowest postneonatal mortality and sudden infant death ('cot death') rates. Although Pakistani and Bangladeshi mothers are almost equally likely to have higher parity than their UK counterparts, perinatal rates were higher for the former than the latter. Pakistani babies also had a higher rate of congenital malformations – these account for one-third of the infant deaths in this group. In contrast, this cause of death was least common in births to Caribbean-born mothers. Marriages between first cousins is common in Pakistani and some other Muslim populations. It serves particular social objectives, the preservation of property, more comfortable in-law relationships and the availability of suitable partners.

TABLE 10.2 *Infant mortality by mother's country of birth per 1000 live births 1982–85 and 1990.*

Place of birth	Infant mortality 1982–85	Perinatal mortality 1982–85	Stillbirths 1990	NMR 80s	NMR 90s	PNMR 80s	PNMR 90s
UK	9.7	10.1	4.4	5.6	4.3	4.1	3.2
Eire	10.1	10.4	5.1	5.9	3.7	4.1	3.4
India	10.1	12.5	5.3	6.1	5.1	3.9	2.2
Bangladesh	9.3	14.3	8.6	6.5	3.9	2.8	1.6
Pakistan	16.6	18.8	9.1	10.2	7.8	6.4	6.4
Caribbean	12.9	13.4	5.7	8.4	8.4	4.5	4.2
East Africa	9.3	12.8	6.9	6.3	5.6	3.0	2.0
West Africa	11.0	12.7	n.k.	8.0	n.k.	3.0	n.k.

Adapted from 1982–85 Balarajan and Raleigh (1992), 1990 Parsons et al. (1993).
Infant mortality rate = deaths in the first year of life per 1000 live births.
Perinatal mortality rate (PMR) = deaths in the first week of life (including still births) per 1000 live and stillbirths.
Neonatal mortality rate (NMR) = deaths in the first 28 days per 1000 live births.
Postneonatal mortality rate (PNMR) = deaths between 28 days and one year per 1000 live births.

Therefore, it is suggested that the social benefits outweigh the risks, which have in any case been exaggerated. Ahmad (1995) argues that the concentration on consanguineous risks, as compared to the effects of poverty, are an example of 'pathologizing culture'.

Recent research has supported the view that material factors are involved. A study of 'Asian' mothers (Muslim and Hindu) who were second generation showed lower perinatal mortality and higher birth weights than a previous cohort, even when other classic risk factors were present.

The elderly

Blakemore and Bonham (1994) have drawn attention to a particular problem that older people in ethnic minorities face. It is often thought that such people will return to their 'homeland' and because there are such small numbers there is no need to plan for the needs of elderly minority people. Stereotyped ideas about the 'Asian extended family' suggest that such needs are adequately cared for in the family setting.

The number of elderly ethnic minority people is still relatively small, estimated at 70 000 (OPCS 1991). They form about 4% of the most commonly listed ethnic minority groups in Britain, but as with the younger members of such groups they are concentrated in the inner cities, chiefly Greater London. In those wards and areas where most of the ethnic minority population live the proportion of elderly will of necessity be higher. Of the major ethnic minority groups the largest number of elderly are African-Caribbean and the lowest are in the Pakistani group who together with the Bangladeshis have a relatively young population. Given that many elderly members of ethnic minority groups worked in manual occupations we would expect them to fall into a group with relatively low incomes in old age.

The position of ethnic elders is sometimes described as that of 'double jeopardy'. Negative views of old age are made worse by racial discrimination. Norman (1985) has added a third strand, that of the inaccessibility and inappropriateness of services.

Patterns of hospitalization at present are roughly the same as the majority UK population. Yet hospital utilization gives only a partial picture of the needs of any group. Surveys of overall health which compare elderly white people with their ethnic minority counterparts show conflicting evidence on a variety of indicators.

Higher rates of stroke and lower risks of heart attack are found among older African–Caribbeans (one group that causes particular concern are older African–Caribbean women) whereas older Asian groups are at a greater risk of experiencing heart attack and stroke when compared to patients born in Britain (Ebrahim et al. 1991). Osteomalacia and rickets, tuberculosis and cataracts all seem to occur with more frequency in elderly ethnic groups. Dental health and problems of ambulation were about the same as those found in white people (Blakemore 1982).

Poorer populations of ethnic minority elders show poorer health compared with a more prosperous group; however, these findings could not be generalized to all disease categories. Even in an economically advantaged group chronic diseases were higher in an Asian Gujarati population, but problems of old age were less likely. There is some evidence to suggest that older African–Caribbean people in this country, despite living in the inner city and in some cases isolated, generally have a network of social support around clubs and churches. Some research has shown greater frequency of contact with friends and relatives which is an important source of social support. However, the comparative research which looks at ethnic minority groups sharing the same social economic and geographical background has not yet been done.

COMMON DISEASES IN ETHNIC MINORITIES (BOX 10.2)

Coronary heart disease

Coronary heart disease (CHD) is a 'Health of the Nation' key area. It is, therefore, of concern to see the raised mortality from coronary heart disease among men and women from the Indian subcontinent. Death rates for males from the Indian subcontinent are 36% higher and for females 46% higher than the population of the UK. For Ireland, males are 14% higher and females 20% higher than the average for the UK population. Men born in the African commonwealth, many of whom originate in the Indian subcontinent, also have high CHD mortality. The lowest rates were among African–Caribbeans (Balarajan and Bulusu 1990). Most importantly those born in the Indian subcontinent are the only ones to have experienced a rise in mortality from coronary heart disease between 1972 and 1983, 8% for men and 14% for women, when rates for the rest of the world were falling (Balarajan 1991). The risk of greater mortality from coronary heart disease for this group is to be found world-wide which suggests that local factors are not primary. Further, an examination of the classical risk factors, like smoking, fat intake, cholesterol levels and hypertension, does not show any great difference between the South Asian population and the rest of the United Kingdom. One factor which has been examined to account for the difference is the insulin resistance hypothesis. The association with insulin resistance has been suggested by the fact that diabetes, a major risk factor for coronary heart disease, is highly prevalent

---

BOX 10.2

MAIN HEALTH ISSUES FOR ETHNIC MINORITY GROUPS

- **Coronary heart disease** – mortality is higher in people from the African commonwealth and Indian subcontinent.

- **Hypertension/stroke** – mortality is higher in people from the African commonwealth, the Caribbean and Indian subcontinent.

- **Perinatal mortality** – mortality is higher in African, Caribbean and South Asians, especially Pakistani babies.

- **Haemoglobinopathies** – sickle cell disease affects people in the Caribbean and African population; thalassaemia affects people from the Mediterranean, the middle East, and some South Asians and Chinese.

- **Mental illness** – the diagnosis rates of schizophrenia are high in African–Caribbeans.

- **Diabetes** – mortality is higher in South Asians, Africans and African Caribbeans.

---

in expatriate South Asian populations. Insulin resistance is particularly associated with certain deposits of bodily fat and the pattern of obesity in South Asian populations shows that they are more likely to have abdominal fat deposition, what is sometimes called an 'apple' shape rather than the 'pear' shaped body characteristic of Europeans. However, the role of insulin resistance remains unclear, and it is suggested that most South Asian people with coronary heart disease do not have diabetes.

A competing explanation is that of social stress and although this is often dismissed by biomedical researchers Williams (1994) regards it as an important cause. The theory basically is that social stress, which is increased for migrant populations because of a likely excess of stressful life events which remain unmediated by any form of social support network is likely to lead to coronary heart disease. The fact that there is not a social class gradient associated with coronary heart disease for the South Asian population might be a generalized effect of stress. On the other hand it may suggest that biomedical factors may form a risk factor common to all members of the South Asian ethnic group. Furthermore, it should be remembered that socioeconomic stresses are likely to be as great if not greater for the Caribbean-born population in which the lowest coronary heart disease rates are observed. The changing gradient of coronary heart disease in South Asian populations may well be related to the ageing of that population, a factor which has not yet been examined. For the Irish, whose mortality rates remain relatively unexamined, the only link that has been made so far is with an excess of smoking.

Hypertension and stroke (cerebrovascular disease)

Cerebrovascular disease (CVD) ranks second after coronary heart disease as a major cause of death among white, South Asian and Caribbean populations in Britain. CVD mortality is very much raised for people from the African and Caribbean commonwealth with African–Caribbean women having the highest standardized mortality rates (110% higher than the average UK population as a whole). Hypertension is a risk factor for CVD mortality but Caribbean and West Africans in Britain do not show raised blood pressure compared to whites. The exception is African–Caribbean women who have a systolic blood pressure 17 mmHg higher than British women. The reasons for the high prevalence of hypertension and high CVD mortality remain to be established.

Diabetes

Non-insulin dependent type 2 diabetes is more common in Asians, Caribbeans and Africans than in whites, and the prevalence for Caribbeans can range from double to three or four times higher than national levels. Mortality from diabetes is three to four times greater in Caribbean-born people, three times greater in Asians and double in African-born people. As noted above, diabetes is a risk factor for coronary heart disease, which makes the low rates of coronary heart disease, despite the prevalence of diabetes in African–Caribbeans, something of a mystery.

Cancer

Cancer mortality tends to be lower among those from the Indian subcontinent, Caribbean or African commonwealth. Once again the Irish are exceptional with a considerably raised incidence of lung cancer and cancer of the cervix, mouth and pharynx. Breast, cervical and lung cancers are particularly low in those from the Indian subcontinent and from the African commonwealth. High rates of oral cancer are also to be found in South Asian populations and in the African commonwealth. For the former it has been suggested that betel nut chewing may be involved but such an association has not been directly proven and not all South Asian populations chew betel. Data on the incidence of cancer in ethnic minority groups are limited because the cancer registry does not record ethnic origin.

Mental illness

Evidence for the rates of mental illness among the ethnic minority population is derived mainly from hospital admissions but also from community studies. Discussion based upon the rates of admission to hospitals is, of course, subject to difficulty, since not all cases come to hospitals and the routes by which people arrive at mental hospital may vary considerably. The highest rates of hospital admissions are found in Irish migrants, whether from Northern Ireland or Eire. The next highest group are people of the Caribbean-born population and finally South Asians whose rates are lower than the population of UK (in the case of Pakistan and Bangladesh considerably lower). There are also considerable gender differences with higher rates for women in every category except for the Caribbean-born. The all-admissions rate for the ethnic minority population is 9% greater than for the UK population but admissions for schizophrenia and paranoia display a threefold excess for men and a twofold excess for women among the Caribbean-born.

Mental hospital admissions among African-Caribbeans are more likely to have been a result of police activity and to be related to compulsory detention under the 1983 Mental Health Act.

Patients are more likely to be described as violent and detained in locked wards or secure units. They have a greater chance of receiving physical treatments and to be attended by junior staff rather than consultant staff.

Patterns of admission and treatment have been subject to a great deal of controversy. Some writers have argued that psychiatrists are more likely to diagnose schizophrenia in African-Caribbean patients or to exaggerate the importance of minor symptoms. Research in the USA does suggest that there is evidence of misdiagnosis and that cultural misunderstandings on the part of psychiatrists may contribute to this. On the other hand some writers have argued that the stresses associated with migration, racism and disadvantage are responsible for producing a real 'schizophrenia epidemic' among young African-Caribbeans.

Generally speaking, community studies as well as hospital studies show lower rates of psychological symptoms in Indian populations. The relatively low rate of admission to mental hospital displayed by persons of South Asian origin has been explained in three different ways. The first is the 'healthy migrant' effect. The second suggests that there are barriers to seeking help, for example for mental illness, because people think that the help offered is inappropriate. A study of Bangladeshi parents' responses to mental illness among their children showed that they saw such disturbances in some cases as being the province of a spiritual healer or *imam* rather than a psychiatrist (Hillier and Rahman 1996). A third view is that patients of South Asian origin are inclined to express emotional distress by presenting with physical symptoms ('somatization'). There is nothing to suggest that somatization is specifically characteristic of South Asian patients since indigenous British patients also show this behaviour. There is very little recent evidence to show that somatization exists or is a helpful concept.

Haemoglobinopathies (sickle cell disease)

Sickle cell disease (SCD) occurs predominantly in African-Caribbean people. It is an inherited condition. The genetic trait for the disease helps to protect the carrier from malaria, and therefore is most likely to be found in populations where malaria is endemic. According to Ahmad (1993), because the disease is found almost exclusively in a particular minority group it has been marginalized and ignored and relatively little attention has been paid to its care. Britain is well behind the United States in providing screening services.

SCD is clearly an example of a condition where patients can be 'experts'. Their descriptions of pain or factors associated with painful crisis can be seen as a valuable adjunct to clinical care. Ahmad (1995) has drawn attention to research which stresses the social factors involved in SCD (Midence and Elander 1994). These writers emphasize how the 'painful crises' of sickle cell are often neglected or ignored because of stereotyped fears of black people's 'drug seeking'. It has been noted that in Jamaica, where sickle cell patients are regularly monitored on an outpatient basis, they are less likely to require hospitalization for crises.

WHY ARE MORTALITY PATTERNS RAISED FOR ETHNIC GROUPS?

Smaje's (1995) review of evidence considers some of the most common social explanations that are given to account for the differential mortality rates of ethnic groups. He considers a number of explanations for the causes of disease which can be socially located.

Evidence may be an artefact   Numerator data are often derived from cases which may be subject to utilization bias; denominators are based on the census, which has been shown to undernumerate ethnic populations. The health instruments used to measure outcome or morbidity may not be valid for ethnic populations, and confounding factors like social class may have different implications for ethnic minority groups.

Material inequality   Much has been made of the role of material factors in producing inequalities in health in the general population. It is the case that most members of ethnic minority groups are to be found in groups of socioeconomically disadvantaged. Yet simple correlations of material disadvantage (as conventionally used) do not 'fit'. For example, there is higher mortality among social classes I and II for Caribbean-born men. It may be the measures which are at fault, however. They do not capture childhood experiences of disadvantage which might show up in later life. Measures of housing tenure, which is part of the index of socioeconomic status, places owner-occupiership in a advantageous position where health is concerned. Ethnic minorities are likely to possess larger numbers of owner occupiers, but the housing stock itself is often poor, and in the inner city. What is clear is that it is necessary to disentangle these factors to measure their particular influence. It has also been argued that, because of expectations prior to migration, people may perceive material circumstances differently, either positively or negatively, with an unknown impact on mortality and morbidity.

Cultural influences   'Cultural differences' are some times cited as explanations of different patterns of ill health. Unfortunately these differences have sometimes been exaggerated or understood in a shallow or narrow way by researchers or health service providers. They are almost always seen in negative terms, and are not usually based on any in-depth ethnography. Examples include the assumption that rickets resulted from the Muslim tendency to cover the female body; the 'drug seeking' behaviours of those with SCD (quoted above); the attack on consanguinity as being the sole rather than a contested contributory cause of congenital abnormality in Pakistani babies; and the stereotypical 'surgery-haunting' of isolated 'Asian' woman. These prevalent stereotypes suggest that cultural differences in terms of values, beliefs and lifestyles have been inadequately researched up to now.

WHAT ARE ETHNIC MINORITIES' EXPERIENCES OF HEALTH SERVICES?

Relatively few studies of the use that ethnic minorities make of health services have been carried out, but those that have suggest higher than average use of the acute services by the young males and older age groups, and by women of childbearing age. Outpatient attendances are slightly lower. Take-up of preventative services like childhood immunization has been shown to be consistently greater among South Asian and African-Caribbean groups, even controlling for socioeconomic status. In general practice, consultation rates were higher for members of the Indian ethnic group. Overall ethnic group members consulted more for endocrine, nutritional and metabolic disorders, skin and respiratory conditions, circulatory problems and 'signs and symptoms' of ill-defined origin. These higher consultation rates suggest that, where an ethnic minority general practitioner is available, as is often the case for Indian groups, utilization may be easier. However, the number of 'signs and symptoms' which remain unexplained suggest that there are areas of health belief which need to be explored.

Health beliefs which exist in ethnic minority groups may differ from those of orthodox medicine, or may exist alongside them. Comparative studies of white UK populations have also shown a wide range of beliefs about the causes of disease and the best way disease may be remedied. Looked at this way, the beliefs of many white people may also be seen to reflect their ethnicity and values. Some general outlines are shown in Table 10.3.

Health beliefs about specific diseases have also been researched. Morgan (1996) has noted a preference for liquid tonics rather than dry pills among African-Caribbean patients, and examines the nature of compliance and causation in a group with hypertension. Rather than submit themselves to a daily regime people preferred to monitor their own physical state and take pills when they felt a physical change. Pierce and Armstrong (1996) and Lambert and Sevak (1996) have noted the importance attached to diet among diabetic patients from ethnic minorities. However, they do not necessarily follow the medically prescribed diet. Moderation in consumption and fresh foods were thought to be more important than the one-sided avoidance of particular foods, recommended by clinics.

People from different ethnic groups may well have different ways of dealing with illness or keeping healthy. One East London study of the Muslim community stressed the importance of prayer as a way of dealing with behavioural disturbances in children (Hillier and Rahman 1996). The lack of availability of traditional remedies was seen by some African-Caribbean women as contributing to their hypertension (Clarke 1996). Unani and Ayurvedic practitioners continue in practice, and Chinese and British acupuncturists flourish. Members of ethnic minorities may often consult private practitioners for the same reasons that the majority population do – better control, communication and understanding in the consultation. Going to a traditional practitioner or one from the same ethnic group is often explained thus: 'He is the same as us, and understands our situation better'. Creams and oils to keep the skin supple, tonics, close attention to diet and a carefully monitored approach to the 'balance' of the body may be found in any or all ethnic minority groups, where 'health' as a value may have more salience than in the majority population.

TABLE 10.3 General health beliefs by ethnic group.

	White	[Afro-Caribbean	Indian]
Health is	Strength and fitness	ability to do what you have to	
Health has improved because of better health care and higher living standards	Yes	No	No
Good/bad health is	The fault of the individual		A matter of luck
Important cause of disease is	Stress	Alcohol and smoking	

Reproduced with permission of Carfax Publishing Ltd from Howlett et al. (1992).

Although both the majority and minority ethnic populations express general satisfaction with health services, suspicions exist of the policing role of health service workers, particularly in relation to children. The health services can also be a source of distrust and dissatisfaction because they fail to take account of important cultural sensitivities in sexual matters. Failure to provide a female doctor may be causing an underreporting of gynaecological conditions among Pakistani women. The necessity of a female clinician, especially in obstetrics and gynaecology, has been repeatedly stressed, for in the institutional medicalized culture of the hospital negative attitudes which can be perceived as racism occur. Midwives and doctors' behaviour may be experienced as cold and unfeeling. A Pakistani woman recounted her experience of childbirth thus: 'The pain was unbearable . . . they were shouting . . . . why you never took antenatal class . . . you should have, then there wouldn't be that much problem for you and us as well' (Bowes and Domokos 1996).

Bowler's (1993) study showed how midwives viewed South Asian women as attention seeking, demanding and rude. It would have been valuable to find out what the patients thought about their carers. People may not complain at the time, but their silence, their 'muted voices', cannot be taken as evidence that all is well (Bowes and Domokos 1996).

How can the Health of Ethnic Minority Groups be Improved?

The socioeconomic context is an important cause of ill health. Redressing the socioeconomic context in its broadest sense is not within the remit of health services, but it should be regarded as a constraint upon what the health services, committed to free and equal care at the point of need, can provide. There are three main areas where health care improvements may be made:

1. Better communication and translation services and establishment of advocates (those who speak the patient's language and represent the patient) in particular specialities (e.g. antenatal care, coronary care) (Audit Commission 1993). Currently, translation is provided by family members, sometimes children, and in many cases this is unacceptable to patients, breaches confidentiality, and can result in misinformation.
2. Better involvement of ethnic minority members in purchaser and provider activities at local level.
3. Specialist service delivery for particular disorders which have a specific ethnic dimension (e.g. sickle cell disease).

These, together with ethnic monitoring, will provide a constant input into the changing situation of ethnic minority health. It remains uncertain whether the new NHS structures will worsen the situation or whether they will allow greater flexibility for localities to respond to the needs of the ethnic minorities who live there.

References

Ahmad, W.   (1993) *Race and Health in Contemporary Britain*. Buckingham: Open University Press.
Ahmad, W.   (1995) Review article 'race and health' *Sociol. Health Illness*, **17**, 418–29.
Audit Commission   (1993) Communication with non English speaking patients. In: *What seems to be the matter?* London: HMSO, pp. 53–9.

Balarajan, R.   (1991) Ethnic differences in mortality from ischaemic heart disease and cerebrovascular disease in England and Wales. *Br. Med. J.*, **302**, 560–4.

Balarajan, R. & Bulusu, L.   (1990) Mortality among immigrants in England and Wales 1979–1983. In: *Mortality and Geography: a Review of the Mid 1980s*, ed. M. Britton. OPCS Series. DS No 9. London: HMSO, pp. 103–21.

Balarajan, R. & Raleigh, V.S.   (1992) The ethnic populations of England and Wales: the 1991 census. *Health Trends*, **24**, 113–96.

Blakemore, K.   (1982) Health and illness among the elderly of ethnic minority groups. *Health Trends*, **14**, 68–72.

Blakemore K. & Bonham, M.   (1994) *Age, Race and Ethnicity*. Buckingham: Open University Press, pp. 6–7.

Bowes, A.M. & Domokos, T.M.   (1996) Pakistani women and maternity care: raising muted voices. *Sociol. Health Illness*, **18**, 45–6.

Bowler, I.   (1993) 'They're not the same as us' – midwives' stereotypes of South Asian descent maternity patients. *Sociol. Health Illness*, **15**, 157–8.

Clarke, A.   (1996) African Caribbean women's health beliefs in the UK and Trinidad. PhD Thesis, London University.

Department of Employment   (1991) *Employment Gazette*, February 1991, Table 7. London: HMSO.

Department of Health   (1991) *The Patient's Charter*. London: HMSO.

Ebrahim, S., Smith, C. & Giggs, J.   (1991) Elderly immigrants – a disadvantaged group? *Age Ageing*, **16**, 249–55.

Hillier, S. & Rahman, S.   (1996) Childhood development and behavioural and emotional problems as perceived by Bangladeshi patients in East London. In: *Researching Cultural Differences in Health*, ed. D. Kelleher & S. Hillier. London: Routledge, pp. 38–69.

Howlett, B., Ahmad, W. & Murray, R.   (1992) An exploration of White, Asian and Afro Caribbean peoples' concepts of health and illness causation. *New Commun.*, **18**, 281–92.

Lambert, H. and Sevak, L.   (1996) Is cultural difference a useful concept? Perceptions of health and the sources of ill health among Londoners of South Asian origin. In: *Researching Cultural Differences in Health*, ed. D. Kelleher & S. Hillier. London: Routledge, pp. 38–69.

Marmot, M.   (1992) Coronary heart disease: rise and fall of a modern epidemic. In: *Coronary Heart Disease. Epidemiology from Aetiology to Public Health*, ed. M. Marmot & P. Elliot. Oxford: Oxford Medical Publications.

Marmot, M., Adelstein, F. & Bulusu, L.   (1984) *Immigrant Mortality in England and Wales, 1970–78* (OPCS studies on medical and population subjects No 47). London: HMSO.

McKenzie, K. & Cowcroft, N.   (1994) Race, ethnicity culture and science. *Br. Med. J.*, **309**, 286–7.

Midence, K. & Elander, J.   (1994) *Sickle cell Disease, a Psychological Approach*. Oxford: Radcliffe Medical Press.

Morgan, M.   (1996) The meanings of high blood pressure among Afro Caribbean and White patients. In: *Researching Cultural Differences in Health*, ed. D. Kelleher & S. Hillier. London: Routledge, pp. 11–37.

Norman, A.   (1985) *Triple Jeopardy: Growing Old in a Second Homeland*. London: Centre for Policy on Ageing.

Ohri, S. & Faruqi, S.   (1988) Racism, employment and unemployment. In: *Britain's Black Population*, ed. A. Bhat, R. Carr-Hill & S. Ohri. London: Radical Statistics Race Group/Gower, pp. 61–9.

OPCS (Office of Population Censuses and Surveys)   (1991) London: HMSO.

OPCS   (1991) *Ethnic groups by age in Great Britain*. London: HMSO, p. 25.

Parsons, M. et al.   (1993) Pregnancy, birth and maternity care. In: *Race and Health in Contemporary Britain*, ed. W. Ahmad. Buckingham: Open University Press, pp. 51–75.

Pierce, M. & Armstrong, D.   (1996) Afro Caribbean beliefs about diabetes: an exploratory study. In *Researching Cultural Differences in Health*, ed. D. Kelleher & S. Hillier. London: Routledge, pp. 91–103.

Raftery, J., Jones, D. & Rosato, M.   (1990) The mortality of first and second generation migrants to the UK. *Soc. Sci. Med.*, **31**, 577–84.

Smaje, C.   (1995) *'Race' Ethnicity and Health: Making Sense of the Evidence*. London: SHARE/Kings Fund Institute, pp. 35–6.

Teague, A.   (1993) Ethnic group: first results from the 1991 census. *Popul. Trends*, **72**, Summer 1993.

Williams, B.   (1994) Insulin resistance: the shape of things to come. *Lancet*, **344**, 521–24.

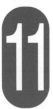

Older People, Health Care and Society

PAUL HIGGS

POPULATION CHANGES

The existence of large numbers of older people in countries such as Britain is a relatively recent feature, characteristic only of the last century and a half. This is not to say that there were no old people in the past. There were many individuals surviving until their 70s and 80s, but there were not enough for them to constitute a significant part of the population. Surviving into old age was an achievement, not an expectation for the majority of the population. In contrast, in modern Britain the vast majority of the population can expect to live beyond the age of retirement. Indeed many will live beyond the age of 80. In 1991, life expectancy at birth in Britain was 73.2 years for men and 78.7 years for women (HMSO 1995) (Table 11.1). In contrast, in 1841 the figures were 40.2 for men and 42.2 for women, and according to Victor (1994) it had taken 400 years for these figures to increase eight years. This process has been described as squaring the rectangle of survival (Fig. 11.1).

That the increase in life expectancy accompanied industrialization is not surprising. The advent of public health measures which substantially controlled infectious diseases had the effect of lowering the infant and maternal mortality rates (see Chapter 1). Consequently, the large majority of deaths in England and Wales occur to those aged over 65, with the rate increasing with age.

Not only has life expectancy increased but the nature of the population has also changed. Over 20% of the population is aged 60 or over and this is projected to increase to around 24% in 2051. This increase is caused in part by the relative balance between the birthrates of different

generations. As those born during the post–war 'baby boom' grow older they affect the composition of the population, because relatively fewer people were born in the decade that followed.
It is for this reason that the proportion of those aged over 80 is not set to rise significantly until
the next century when, by 2051, they will have risen from 4% of the population to just over 9%.

TABLE 11.1 Expectation of life[a]: by gender and age, UK.

	1901	1931	1961	1991	1992	1996	2001	2021
Males								
At birth	45.5	57.7	67.8	73.2	73.6	74.4	75.4	77.6
At age								
1 year	54.6	62.4	69.5	73.8	74.1	74.8	75.7	77.9
10 years	60.4	65.2	69.9	73.9	74.3	75.0	75.9	78.0
20 years	61.7	66.3	70.3	74.2	74.5	75.3	76.1	78.2
40 years	66.1	69.3	71.4	75.1	75.4	76.3	77.2	79.3
60 years	73.3	74.3	74.9	77.7	77.9	78.6	79.5	81.4
80 years	84.9	84.7	85.2	86.4	86.5	86.8	87.2	88.2
Females								
At birth	49.0	61.6	73.6	78.7	79.0	79.7	80.6	82.6
At age								
1 year	56.8	65.3	75.1	79.2	79.5	80.1	80.9	82.8
10 years	62.7	67.9	75.4	79.4	79.6	80.3	81.1	83.0
20 years	64.1	69.0	75.6	79.5	79.8	80.4	81.2	83.1
40 years	68.3	71.9	76.3	80.0	80.2	80.9	81.7	83.5
60 years	74.6	76.1	78.8	81.9	82.1	82.6	83.3	84.9
80 years	85.3	85.4	86.3	88.3	88.5	88.8	89.1	90.0

[a] *Total number of years which a person might expect to live.*
Reproduced with permission of the Controller of HMSO and the Office of National Statistics.

Fig. 11.1 *The increasingly rectangular survival curve. Reproduced with permission from Churchill
Livingstone from Brocklehurst et al. (1992).*

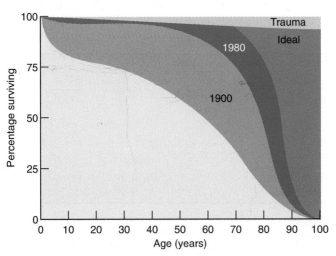

In contrast, the 16–39 age group, which peaked at 36% of the population in 1986, is projected to fall to 28% by the middle of the next century.

These changes are not just happening in Britain. In 1990 just under 20% of the total population of the European Community was aged 60 or over (Walker 1993). In numerical terms this added up to 60 million people. By the year 2020 the corresponding percentage of the population is calculated to be a quarter of all EC citizens. As in Britain, the number of over 80s is also set to increase; by the year 2025 they are projected to rise by up to 115% in Portugal and by nearly an extra million in both Italy and Germany. Life expectancy has also been increasing throughout Europe over the past 30 years, where it has increased by up to 10 years in some countries. In 1989 the average European woman aged 60 could expect to live for another 22 years, and if she had been 80 for another 7.5 years.

HEALTH AND ILLNESS

What kind of life can older people expect to lead when they reach retirement age? One remarkably similar to that experienced by other people in the population. Although there is a connection between old age and physical disability, the extent of it is not as profound and pervasive as popular image would have it. Acute health problems such as colds or accidental injuries increase with age, but even among the very oldest age groups these only affect 20% of males and 25% of females. Chronic health problems such as arthritis do increase with age, with 60% of the over 75 age group reporting a long-standing illness. As Victor (1994) points out, such long-standing illnesses or disabilities do not necessarily impede levels of activity. Almost 50% of those aged over 75 do not have conditions that impair their activity levels.

ACTIVITIES OF DAILY LIVING

Many researchers have looked at the health status of older people from the perspective of their ability to undertake what are called 'activities of daily living' (ADL). There are many different ways of measuring these abilities but most concentrate on a few distinct activities such as bathing, climbing stairs and cutting toenails (Table 11.2). Again, it should be noted that the majority of

TABLE 11.2 Activities of daily living: percentage usually unable to manage on their own.

	Age (years)					
	65–69	70–74	75–79	80–84	85+	90+[a]
Cutting toenails	16	24	34	48	65	78
Bathing self	4	5	10	16	31	35
Brushing hair (women)/ Shaving (men)	1	1	1	3	7	20
Washing face and hands	—	1	1	1	3	12
Feeding self	—	1	—	1	2	4
Negotiating stairs	4	5	10	17	31	34
Getting to the toilet	1	1	2	2	7	15

Reproduced with permission of the Controller of HMSO and of the Office for National Statistics from OPCS General Household Survey 1986, HMSO 1989, Tables 12.14 and 12.31.
[a] Data on 90+ sample derived from Bury and Holme (1990), Table 5.

older people can undertake these activities. Using data from the 1985 General Household Survey, Johnson and Falkingham (1992) point out that even among those aged over 85, 14% of males and 11% of females are described as having no functional disability. However, nearly half of all women in this age group are deemed to have severe disability. Henwood (1992) summarises these data in Table 11.2.

MULTIPLE PATHOLOGY

One important conclusion explicitly acknowledged by those who construct and use ADL scales is the importance of what is known as multiple pathology among older people. What this is referring to is the fact that an older person is likely to have more than one medical condition and these will often be of a disabling nature. But again, although the average number of multiple pathologies increases with age, it should be remembered that nearly two-fifths of older people are not subject to any disabling conditions.

One common belief about old age is that it is inextricably linked with mental decline, so much so that senile, which is the Latin word for old, has become a pejorative term for mental incapacity. The idea of mental decline as an accompaniment of the ageing process is not supported by the evidence. Senile dementia is probably the most well known organic disorder of the brain to affect old people. Its most common symptoms include memory loss and behavioural disturbances, but the prevalence of dementing conditions is in fact less than 10% for older people living in the community. The incidence of dementia does increase with age but not to a point where more than one fifth of the oldest age group are severely affected. Affective disorders such as depression do feature highly among the older population, with around one quarter reporting either a mild or severe clinical affective disorder. Suicide rates seem to increase with age, with people over 65 accounting for 27% of male and 32% of female successful suicides in England and Wales (Victor 1994).

RESIDENTIAL AND INSTITUTIONAL CARE

Another common image of older people is that many of them are residents in some form of institution. This could be an old people's home, a residential or nursing home or a long-stay ward in a geriatric hospital. It is true that nearly 500 000 older people were in some kind of institutional setting by 1990 and that this had grown from 250 000 in 1970 (Henwood 1992). However, such absolute numbers should not be allowed to disguise the fact that these only represent a small fraction of the older population. Even among those aged over 90, nearly three-fifths lived in private households (Bury and Holme 1992). Moreover, the designation of institutional care may be misleading given that nursing care is not provided by old people's homes (sometimes known as part III homes). Many commentators have pointed out that although the numbers of places in institutions has nearly doubled between 1970 and 1990 the real growth has occurred within the private sector; places in private residential homes have increased from 24 000 in 1970 to 156 000 in 1990, and places in private nursing homes have grown from 20 000 in 1970 to 123 000 in 1990. Part of this growth can be accounted for by the absolute growth in the numbers of older people, but this can only explain half of the increase. A more plausible explanation is provided by the massive increase in social security expenditure, which through Income Support paid for older people to stay in private residential and nursing homes rather than funding community-based forms of care (Higgs and Victor, 1993). Expenditure on this part of the welfare budget increased from £10 million in 1979 to nearly £1.5 billion by 1993. Curtailing this increase was one of the objectives of the 1993 Community Care Act, which transferred responsibility for funding this group to local councils (see Chapter 16).

USE OF HEALTH CARE SERVICES

Older patients comprise the largest single group of users of hospital services. This is not just confined to those specialisms with an interest in the conditions of old age such as geriatric medicine but throughout most of the major specialities. The admission rate increases with age, with the 1985 General Household Survey showing 15% of those aged over 75 reporting an in-patient stay in the previous year compared with only 11% of those aged 65–74.

Consulting the general practitioner also increases with age, as does the average number of consultations made. Women tend to consult the doctor more often and they are more likely to receive a home visit. However, Victor (1994) notes that less than 10% of older people in Canada accounted for 35% of all visits to the doctor.

Older people are major users of prescribed medicines, having on average more than two and a half times more items than the rest of the population. When non-prescribed drugs are taken into account, only a small proportion of older people are not taking drugs of any sort. Consequently, one of the notable features of older patients is the existence of what is known as polypharmacy, namely, the taking by one patient of many different medicines. This is a particular problem often associated with the fact that many items are prescribed on repeat prescriptions, leading to a build-up over time. This can also lead to problems in acute hospital care, where doctors may not be sure what medication older patients are on when they are admitted.

AGEING POPULATIONS AND HEALTH POLICY

Ageing may not be synonymous with infirmity and illness but policy makers assume that a population with a high proportion of older people is also one that produces greater demands on its health care services. In Britain the Government calculates what is known as a 'dependency ratio' based on the proportion of the population under 16 and over 65 to those of working age. It is assumed that the former represent a drain on expenditure that the latter will have to pay for. As the percentage of older people in the population increases so the burden on the working population increases. This is not just a British phenomenon. A study by the International Labour Organization suggested that throughout Europe medical expenditure on healthcare for the over 65s will increase from 37% of all health care spending in 1985 to 58% by the year 2015. Individual countries such as Switzerland will find that their expenditure will rise to 70% (Walker, 1993).

Whether or not this rising expenditure is a continually developing scenario is hotly debated. Arguments centre around the prospects for what is known as the 'compression of morbidity' in old age (Fries 1983). This poses the question: Is the level of disability and chronic illness among older people stabilizing or increasing as people live longer, or, are individuals having a longer active life expectancy? One argument presented is that there has been a decrease in morbidity among higher socioeconomic classes. This is seen to relate to the prevention or delayed onset of many non-fatal conditions which increase the age of onset of disability without affecting age of death. This 'squaring of the rectangle of survival' (Fig. 10.1) reduces the proportions of the population dying before they reach their natural lifespan and leads to larger numbers of older people. In this model of 'successful ageing', individual life-style and psychological well-being are seen to be crucial. One implication of this view is that an ageing population would not necessarily be the cause of rising costs. However, in practice all European healthcare systems are preparing for a significant rise in demand. This has led Moody (1995) to argue that modern societies face four possible scenarios. He describes them as follows:

1. *Prolongation of morbidity*: this describes the state whereby an increase in years is not accompanied by an equal increase in quality of life. This prompts demands for the 'right to die' and rationing based on quality-of-life measures.

2. *Compression of morbidity*: as noted above, this describes a situation where the majority of the population experience good health almost up to the end of their lives and are then subject to a 'terminal drop' just before they die. This strategy advocates health promotion and individual responsibility as the way forward in health care.

3. *Lifespan extension*: here the abilities and successes of modern medicine are such that the natural lifespan can be extended upwards, leading to the delaying or abolition of many of the features of 'normal ageing'. The emphasis is put on basic medical research into the ageing process. Problems of who gets access to discoveries and treatments would emerge.

4. *Voluntary acceptance of limits*: this scenario recognizes the problems inherent in the other three positions and argues for a shared 'meaning of old age' that maintains the common good by stressing limits beneficial to coming generations. It is accepted that there must be a point where interventions should be appropriate rather than life extending.

OLDER PEOPLE AND SOCIETY

The only characteristic shared by all older people is chronological age and even this is not consistent between societies. In Britain the state retirement age is often used to designate the onset of old age. This has meant that until recently men became old on their 65th birthday whereas women did so on their 60th birthday. In countries such as Kenya state employees are expected to retire at 40 and live on their pensions in order for younger people to be employed. The arbitrariness of when old age occurs means that all we can safely say about it is that it marks the end of participation in the formal economy. Even this is being eroded by the increase of people taking early retirement in their 50s and not being seen as conventionally old.

It is not the case that older people are either richer than the rest of the population or poorer. There are considerable numbers of relatively well off older people, but it is also the case that some of the poorest people in Britain are old. Although retired households comprised 26% of all households in 1993 only 7% of them were in the wealthiest 20% of the population as opposed to 37% who were in the bottom 20%. The respective figures for non-retired households with two adults were 9% and 36% (HMSO, 1995). It is also the case that among retired households the poorest seem to be single women. This is sometimes described as the 'feminization of poverty'.

It would be a mistake to assume that the poverty of older people is something intrinsic to old age. The poverty of many old people is an effect of the fact that many of them rely upon state benefits as their main source of income; as these are set very low it is not surprising that large numbers are poor. It should be noted that households with children but only one adult are also disproportionately likely to be in poverty. Among those entering retirement now, the growing numbers with an occupational pension, together with other sources of income, has meant that the proportion of total income that they receive from social security payments only amounts to 41% of their income, as opposed to 55% for other pensioners (Fig. 11.2). They also have a relatively higher income at £225 a week against £150 a week.

Fig. 11.2 *Real income of pensioners by source, 1992, in the UK. Other income forms less than 1% of pensioner income and is excluded. Recently retired pensioners are single women aged 60–64, single men aged 65–69 and couples where the husband is aged 65–69. Reproduced by permission of the Controller of HMSO and of the Office for National Statistics.*

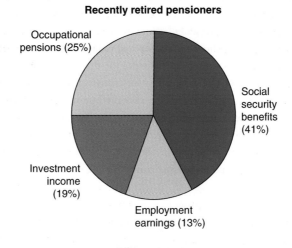

Recently retired pensioners

Occupational pensions (25%)

Social security benefits (41%)

Investment income (19%)

Employment earnings (13%)

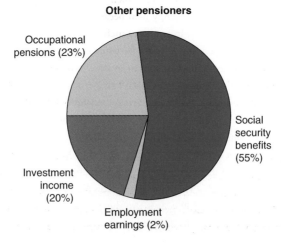

Other pensioners

Occupational pensions (23%)

Social security benefits (55%)

Investment income (20%)

Employment earnings (2%)

DOMESTIC CIRCUMSTANCES

The social circumstances of older people also vary greatly. Family structures are dominated by the cultural norm of the nuclear family, where only two generations of a family live under the same roof. This is different from the extended family, where many different generations live together, which is prevalent in some other cultures. Older people who have been married have tended to live in forms of nuclear family when their children have left home. As older people have aged so the chances of them still living with their spouses decreases. This, combined with the relatively high number of women who have never married, means that a substantial number of older people live alone. Social networks therefore become crucial. Although the vast majority of older people do not live with their children this does not mean that they have little contact. The majority of older people have children and/or a sibling living close to them and contact is frequent. The family does not provide the only source of social contact. Surveys report, unsuprisingly, that friends and neighbours play an important part in maintaining the older person's place in social networks. Age does affect the nature of these contacts in that 'younger' old people tend to visit friends whereas 'older' old people tend to be visited. The percentage of reported contact with both family and friends tends to diminish with age, but only a small minority (2%) of older people are actually seen as totally socially isolated. A slightly larger percentage (5%) report that they are lonely.

Most care for physically frail and mentally confused older people is provided by members of such social networks. There are 6 million carers in Britain and 75% are looking after an elderly person. Family relationships are of extreme importance to this process of informal care, with 80% of carers looking after a relative (Henwood 1992). Women, and especially daughters, are the main carers. However, a third of all carers are men, though they often do different things. Sometimes the caring relationship can continue for so many years that the carers themselves may be elderly people. The effect of caring on carers can be immense both in physical and financial terms. The majority receive no help from formal agencies and what help is offered is often designed to stop the informal caring relationship breaking down rather than alleviating stresses. Community Care policy depends on informal care 'by the community' in order to keep costs down (see Chapter 16).

SOCIOLOGY AND OLDER PEOPLE

The existence of a state of retirement for large numbers of the population is a feature of most industrialized societies. As such it has prompted the interest of many different sociologists who have constructed a number of different theories to account for the position of older people.

Disengagement theory

One of the first generalized accounts to look seriously at old age was an American approach centred on the theme of 'disengagement' (Cumming and Henry 1961). This was a process whereby older people in industrial societies disengaged themselves from the roles that they occupied in the wider society. This was so younger generations would have opportunities to develop and society could continue. Such disengagement not only occurred in relation to work roles but also in relation to families where retired generations became much less central to their children's lives. Seen from this perspective old age presented the individual with many difficulties. In pre-industrial societies the inheritance of skills and property accorded older people a social function. In industrial societies the lack of property or skills that could be handed on meant that older people did not have 'scripts' with which to negotiate their new roles. This led many researchers to stress the importance of finding ways to facilitate 'successful ageing' with the priority being psychological adjustment.

A large amount of research was undertaken in the USA during the 1950s and 1960s to provide evidence for this theory. A longitudinal study in Kansas City (Neugarten et al. 1964) showed that older people did indeed disengage, although women started this process at widowhood whereas men began on retirement. Again the processes were seen as involving difficulties in the roles being played by older people and the answers in psychological adaptation. This approach, which for a long time was the dominant paradigm in social gerontology, saw the way in which old age occurred in modern societies as an inevitable and natural process. Questions about whether older people wanted to 'disengage' or were forced to do so by society were not asked. The emphasis on psychological adjustment also avoided looking at the very real social processes that structured old age.

Structured dependency theory

If the above approach centred on the perspective of the individual older person, then the analysis put forward by the predominantly British 'structured dependency' writers such as Townsend (1981), Walker (1981) and Phillipson (1982) stresses the importance of social policy in creating the circumstances older people find themselves in. For the structured dependency school the most important fact about the ageing process is the existence of the notion of retirement. In most industrial societies the age at which this occurs has been set by the state, and it is from this point that people are entitled to the state retirement pension. Retirement not only marks the withdrawal from the formal labour market but also the shift from making a living to being dependent on the state. In fact, until the 1990s it was a requirement that in order to receive a state pension the recipient was not allowed to do paid work, at the risk of having the money deducted from his or her pension. In this way the state pensioner was treated in the same 'punitive' way as the unemployed person on income support.

As a consequence, decisions made by the government have a dramatic effect on how individuals live their lives. A good example is the decision by the post-war government to set different retirement ages for men and women. Women were to retire at 60 because it was estimated that the average age difference between husband and wife was five years, and if men were to retire at 65 it would be intolerable that their wives would still be working and have access to wages. After all, this might challenge the moral authority of the head of the household. For similar reasons many Governments allowed married women to opt out of paying a full national insurance contribution on the grounds that they could share their husband's pension rather than having one in their own right.

Earlier we saw how a large proportion of older people are in poverty. For the structured dependency school this is not a coincidence. State retirement pensions are kept at a deliberately low level, even falling in relation to average living standards. One study concluded that they were only worth 20% of average earnings and that their value will drop by half by 2020 (Evandrou and Falkingham, 1993). The 'disengaged' nature of many old people is therefore because of low pensions and not any process suddenly brought on by the ageing process. That this can be seen as a continuing feature of modern Britain can be seen by the abolition of the State Earnings Related Pension Scheme (SERPS), which had been set up in the 1970s to create a more generous pension for those not covered by private or occupational schemes.

Structured dependency is not just limited to the economic sphere but rather pervades the whole of society as a consequence of this inferior status. The association of age with infirmity may not be factually true but rather 'represents' the position of older people, as does the exclusion of older people from various forms of social involvement. Often lack of resources may be the main reason for what are taken to be the characteristics of older people. The cultural emphasis on 'youth' is one which sees ageing as only negative and can lead to 'ageism', where it is acceptable to discriminate against older people. This can manifest itself in policies seeking to limit medical or health care resources to older people; in discriminatory employment practices; and in the treatment of physically frail or mentally confused older people.

If the dependency of older people is structured then the obvious response to it is to change those policies that most reinforce the inferior position of older people. Increasing pensions is one obvious answer, but, because a whole raft of policies is needed, many advocates of the structured dependency thesis argue that what needs to be done is to establish the right of older people to be accepted as full citizens in their own countries rather than adopting a position of special pleading. Such citizenship rights would establish the rightful basis for high pensions and full access to health care (Bornat et al. 1985).

Third ageism

However, the validity of this approach has been challenged by writers such as Laslett (1989), who argues that modern societies present opportunities for a fulfilling 'third age' of relative good health and affluence. He argues that the portion of most people's lives spent in retirement is increasing all of the time. The idea of a fixed retirement is increasingly being challenged as many individuals choose early retirement or are made redundant. For many this provides possibilities for undertaking the self-enriching activities that there was not time for when they were preoccupied with the tasks of working or bringing up children. Laslett identifies education as one of the key areas for a successful third age and to this end he has been a proponent of the University of the Third Age.

This theme meshes well with the work of sociologists of culture such as Featherstone and Hepworth (1991), who argue that there has been a blurring of the distinction between 'middle' and 'old' age with the increasing cultivation of life-styles and consumerism by significant numbers of people. Instead, old age is seen as a 'mask' detracting from the person beneath. This has led to a denial of some of the negative effects of ageing in favour of youth orientated activism. As examples of this they point to the growing involvement of older people in entertainment and tourist markets, where they are able to enjoy pleasures previously deemed inappropriate for their age group. Both counter positions to the structured dependency argument can be described as only partial accounts of the position of older people in modern society; however, it is difficult to dismiss them, because they focus on the central issue of ageing in our times, that of change and instability.

CONCLUSION

If the twentieth century is the first epoch to see large numbers of people survive into old age then it is likely that the twenty first century will be one where the implications of this transformation will become apparent. Not only will the priorities of social and health policy have to change but so also will the whole of our understanding of the stages of life. How, or whether, these issues will be resolved is unclear, but it is an inescapable fact that they will become a more and more pressing context for all of us.

REFERENCES

Bornat, J., Philipson, C. and Ward, S.   (1985) *A Manifesto for Old Age*. London: Pluto Press.
Brocklehurst, Tallis and Fillet   (1992) *Textbook of Geriatric Medicine and Gerontology*. Edinburgh: Churchill Livingstone.
Bury, M. & Holme, A.   (1993) *Life after Ninety*. London: Routledge.
Cumming, E. & Henry, W.   (1961) *Growing Old: The Process of Disengagement*. New York: Basic Books.
Evandrou, M. and Falkingham, J.   (1993) Social security and the life course: developing sensitive policy alternative. In: *Ageing, Independence and the Life Course,* ed. S. Arber and M. Evandrou. London: Jessica Kingsley.
Featherstone, M. & Hepworth, M.   (1991) The mask of ageing and the post-modern lifecourse. In: *The Body: Social Process and Cultural Theory*, ed. M. Featherstone, M. Hepworth & B. Turner. London: Sage.
Fries, J. (1983) The Compression of Morbidity. *Milbank Q.*, 397–419.
Henwood, M.   (1992) *Through a Glass Darkly: Community Care and Older People*. London: Kings Fund.
HMSO   (1995) *Social Trends 1995*. London: HMSO.
Higgs, P. & Victor, C.   (1993) Institutional care and the life course. In: *Ageing, Independence and the Life Course*, ed. S. Arber & M. Evandrou. London: Jessica Kingsley.
Johnson, P. & Falkingham, J.   (1992) *Ageing and Economic Welfare*. London: Sage.
Laslett, P.   (1989) *A Fresh Map Of Life*. London: Weidenfield and Nicholson.
Moody, H.   (1995) Ageing, meaning and the allocation of resources. *Ageing Soc.*, **15**, 163–245.
Neugarten, B. et al.   (1964) *Personality in Middle and Late Life*. New York: Atherton.
Phillipson, C.   (1982) *Capitalism and the Construction of Old Age*. London: Methuen.
Townsend, P.   (1981) The structured dependency of the elderly, *Ageing Soc.*, **1,** 5–28.
Victor, C.   (1994) *Old Age in Modern Society*. London: Chapman and Hall.
Walker, A.   (1981) Towards a political economy of old age. *Ageing Soc.*, **1,** 73–94.
Walker, A.   (1993) *European Attitudes to Ageing and Older People*. Brussels: Commission of the European Communities Directorate General V.

THE SOCIAL PROCESS OF
DEFINING DISEASE

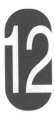

The Limits of Medical Knowledge

PAUL HIGGS

WESTERN MEDICINE

In today's world, the existence of infective agents is seen as such as an obvious truth that it hardly needs stating. In a similar way most people are aware that they risk infection if they allow wounds to be exposed to the environment. Two hundred years ago such precautions were not so obvious. The threat to health posed by micro-organisms was not part of everyday understanding since such organisms had not yet been identified by science.

This did not mean that until the introduction of the theory of sepsis people did not know about the dangers of leaving a wound open to the air; however, their understanding of what was happening was often very different from the idea of infective agents. All societies have had ways of dealing with the problems of illness and disease and these ideas made (and in many cases still do make) perfect sense to the people involved. From our vantage point at the end of the twentieth century the dominant views of earlier centuries or other cultures may seem strange, if not irrational. Modern medicine may seem to be qualitatively different from these other approaches because it is based on the obviously superior rationality of modern science. The evidence to support this view is compelling, given that medical science can diagnose, treat and cure many of the afflictions that have affected human beings for thousands of years. The difficulty with this approach is that it only tells part of the story. Both medicine and science exist in social contexts which can place limits as well as challenges to their activities. This chapter looks at some of the issues involved.

As an example we can return to germ theory. The discovery of germs is only part of the picture given that this particular theory of illness causation can and has been overextended to account for many other processes. Part of the problem lies in the fact that an idea like the 'germ' can catch the public imagination and can become part of popular mythology (Lupton 1994). It has been used both to label certain individuals or groups as potentially dangerous and as a metaphor for social persecution where the undesired group are seen as germs infecting the wider society.

To understand fully the workings of medicine in the modern world we must look at the circumstances in which medical knowledge comes about and how people understand and are influenced by that knowledge. Our starting point must be the inextricable link between modern medicine and the world of science. Again this might seem an unnecessary point to make but the history of medicine need not have culminated in the dominance of what has been described as 'western scientific medicine'. Other highly complex systems of medicine have flourished in other cultures, often for thousands of years.

Conventional accounts of the development of western science stress its emergence out of irrationalism and magic. Although applauding prescientific thinkers for their energy in trying to understand and change the natural world around them, science and the work of scientists starts to come into existence when the metaphysics of explaining things through external media are replaced by approaches which emphasize observation and experiment. Seeking out the regularities of phenomena and explaining why they should be so allows science to be both rational and neutral. Such understanding forms the basis for technological innovation.

Normal science and paradigm shifts

However, as some historians and philosophers of science have pointed out, the idea of a simple distinction between irrational prescience and rational science is not always convincing. In his work *The Structure of Scientific Revolutions* Thomas Kuhn (1970) pointed out that the way in which science operates is often very far from a rigorous objective assessment of evidence. Instead, Kuhn argues, scientific ideas are organized into definable paradigms of ideas which create a state of what he describes as 'normal science'. Such paradigms define the areas of acceptable knowledge and most scientists work within the framework of ideas provided by such approaches. This means that theories that work in accordance with the paradigm are regarded as the commonsense of scientific investigation. Where problems with evidence occur they are treated as anomalies to the paradigmatic understanding. New phenomena can only provide the basis for a new theory when the conceptual understanding necessary for the new theory has been established. When scientific change does occur it is often the result of a crisis in the existing theory which brings about a radical change in ideas which Kuhn calls a 'paradigm shift'. This, rather than the empirical 'falsification' of theories, is what happens in the development of science.

The development of hospital medicine

The idea that scientific knowledge can be understood in terms of successive paradigms, each one replacing the last, has been applied to the development of western medicine where, as Jewson (1976) has noted, there has been a progressive displacement of the patient from the centre of medical interest. The point is made that prescientific medicine can be characterized as 'bedside medicine' because the doctor or physician had to pay particular attention to the complaints of patients who were consulting him (and it was always a man) and it was their payments which provided his living. The nature of the medical knowledge at the time was based on the notion of imbalances in the four basic humours of the sanguine (yellow bile), the choreric (blood), the melancholic (black bile) and the phlegmatic (phlegm). Diagnosis and treatment were in terms of restoring the appropriate balance between the humours whose disequilibrium had brought about the illness. In this system of medicine, illness was the same thing as the symptoms reported and not the outward sign of something else. Hence the focus of medical activity had to be individual patients and their concerns.

This system of medicine had its origins in the works of ancient Greeks and Romans and was still the basis of medical knowledge well into the seventeenth century. However, according to the work of the American sociologist Robert Merton (1970), the impact of the protestant Reformation in sixteenth century Europe provided the impetus for a more experimentally-based theory of how the body worked. Crucially it allowed the anatomical dissection of corpses which had been suppressed under conventional Catholicism. Up to this point the knowledge that most physicians had about anatomy was gleaned from Galen's *On the Conduct of Anatomy* which had been written in the second century AD and was based on the dissection of monkeys and not humans. Consequently the publication of works using direct observation to illustrate a human dissection provided one of the bases for an empirical programme of comparative anatomy where the normal could be distinguished from the pathological.

The need to look at patients in the context of what was normal allowed medicine to move away from bedside medicine and towards what Jewson describes as 'hospital medicine'. The requirement to provide material for scientific investigation resulted in a need for 'cases' to study. Hospitals came to dominate the healthcare scene in the nineteenth century, where the poor would often be allowed access to medical diagnosis if they would offer themselves up for study. Patients' reports of their symptoms became less important than the physical signs their bodies manifested, and both were merely indications of underlying pathological lesions which were the real problem.

Under hospital medicine the patient's physical body became crucially important in aiding the understanding of illness. The way in which medicine was practised also changed with the physical examination being privileged by doctors as a more objective method of investigation than the personal accounts of the patient. As the nineteenth century progressed medical science developed a number of methods for investigating the bodies of patients, such as the stethoscope and the X-ray. The invention of the stethoscope by the French physician Rene Laennec in 1816 was particularly important given that it allowed the patient to be examined rather than just observed. Pathology could be localized, confirmed by autopsy and be compared with the experience of other physicians. In turn, essential bodily activities such as the pulse could be quantified, leading to standardized measures of physical functioning.

To hospital medicine Jewson adds a further development specific to the twentieth century – that of 'laboratory medicine'. Here the importance of the body and the physical examination is undermined by the molecular processes underlying normal physical functioning. By studying these, and by the patient providing specimens, medicine can diagnose difficulties which may not even give rise to symptoms or expressions of illness, and through the use of pharmacology deal with them.

Surveillance medicine

All of this results in the essential 'dualism' of the body and mind in medical practice (Longino and Murphy 1995), where the individual's body is treated as separate from his or her understanding of it. That such approaches have had a negative effect on the practice of medicine is suggested by the popularity of holistic approaches to medical care. Possibly in response to this, Armstrong (1995) suggests a new development in the emergence of what he describes as 'surveillance medicine'. In this development it is not just the ill patient who is the focus of concern but the whole population. Using the results of surveys of the health of the nation, surveillance medicine works from the premise that no-one is really healthy, and that as people go about their everyday lives they exhibit, to varying degrees, many different risk factors, such as diet, weight, behaviour, etc. Instead of localized pathology occurring at specific moments, all symptoms, signs and diseases become 'factors' of constructed 'risks'. Diets rich in saturated fats allied to obesity (measured by the body-mass index) occurring among people who smoke are illustrative of factors increasing the risk of coronary heart disease. Unlike the underlying pathology identified by hospital medicine, which would eventually erupt into illness or 'clinical consciousness', all that risk factors identify are propensities to future outcomes which may in turn be transformed into new risk factors. Consequently the time frame for medicine is the whole lifespan. This has effects on the form of clinical intervention taken by this new form of medicine which must approach healthcare through the medium of population medicine and which seeks to encourage the self-monitoring of risk by individuals.

SOCIAL CONSTRUCTIONISM

Michel Foucault and the clinical gaze

The French philosopher Michel Foucault claims that the development of modern medicine has taken the particular route that it has because it simultaneously constructs its own object of inquiry and comes up with ideas to explain and deal with it. To the prescientific physician the evidence for the existence of humours was as compelling as the modern doctor's acceptance of the evidence provided by X-rays. The medieval anatomists using Galen's account of the body could 'see' what he had told them was there because that was what they were supposed to see. Foucault (1976) argued that with the creation of the hospital came what he describes as the 'clinical gaze', which established the idea that disease was a discrete phenomenon of the human anatomy. For Foucault the gaze is a way of seeing and understanding which becomes identical with the thing itself.

Social constructionism and the sociology of the body

For Foucault there are no fixed meanings or even the possibility of an appeal to an external reality. For this reason he has often been identified with a theoretical approach known as 'social constructionism'. This approach is marked by an interest in how health and illness are created and understood by society and social processes, rather than seeking to find a biological basis for them. The anthropologist Mary Douglas (1970) has written that in many cultures the body has often been seen as an image of society. As a result, our notions about the body will often relate to prevailing ideas about society.

Consequently, for Foucault, it is not only how medical science sees the body that is affected by discourses of knowledge, but also how people themselves view their own bodies. The shift from traditional agricultural forms of society to modern industrial ones, as Shilling (1993) points out, has also been marked by a transition from a concern with the 'fleshy' body to an interest in the 'mindful body'. What this means is that instead of the body being just an object synonymous with the person, the mind is given a central role in directing what the body does and is made responsible for it. We can see in the emphasis given to health promotion an echo of this approach.

The rise of the 'mindful body' itself also changes the nature of health and illness as new 'problems' and new 'solutions' become commonplace in medicine. In the nineteenth century, Foucault (1981) argues a concern developed regarding the nature of sexuality and the problem of the 'hysterical woman' and the 'masturbating child'. The worry arose that if these tendencies were not countered then the health of the nation would be harmed. In a different way, current worries regarding fitness and slimming are seen as ways of being desirable and attractive in a consumer society that puts great store on image.

The work of Michel Foucault has acted as a challenge to many sociologists to look at how what is taken as normal and benign is in fact the product of our own contemporary imagination. In fields as diverse as dentistry and surgery Foucaldian analyses have been put forward to account for what is described as the 'fabrication' of discourses and to locate the operation of 'micro-power'. Ultimately, Foucault was interested in how power permeated every aspect of society to such a degree that everybody was involved in the exercise of it. In his studies of madness (1973) and penal policy (1977) he demonstrated that far from there having been progress to a more humane situation, what resulted from psychiatry and penology was more controlling and more invasive. Ironically one of the dilemmas that has resulted from these pieces of research has been the relativization of the subject under study. It can become impossible to see the benefit in any system of knowledge and, as a consequence, impossible to believe there is any point in changing it. This has been particularly true of some feminist researchers who have been influenced by Foucault.

Erving Goffman and bodily idiom

The work of the American sociologist Erving Goffman provides another way in which the body plays a role in constructing our understanding of health and illness. He argues that fundamental to human interaction and communication is the level of non-verbal language in which the body plays a major part. What is called 'body idiom' indicates to all those who share a culture all sorts of important knowledge. What a person says needs to be backed up with the appropriate clothes, gestures, expressions, etc., if it is to be accepted. Body idiom allows people to classify, label and grade others. It is a process that is continual and ever present in all public interactions. It plays a crucial role in creating individuals' self-identities as well as their social identities.

Control over the body is therefore important for people in social interactions with strangers. People with physical disabilities are at a disadvantage because if they lack control over parts of their bodies this may interfere with the process of communication. Goffman argues that this can lay the basis for the 'stained' identity that forms the basis of 'stigmatization'. It is not at all surprising, therefore, that many disabled people would prefer to 'mask' and 'pass' off their disablement in public rather than be classified in terms of their disability. However, this strategy also has its drawbacks given the continual need for the individual to be wary of 'leaking' their discredited identity to others and then being reclassified. Epilepsy is one condition where this can occur (Scambler 1989).

Goffman's (1968) account of the social construction of disability as stigma is very useful when we look at how the interaction of people in society plays an important role in creating healthcare problems. The existence of stigma leads one part of medicine to become involved in attempting to find ways of countering the visible signs of stigmatizing conditions with techniques such as corrective surgery, while another part attempts to find causes and cures. As a result medicine becomes involved with issues such as erasing face-disfiguring port-wine birthmarks, providing prosthetic limbs and providing growth hormones for children of lower than average height.

MEDICINE, MEDICALIZATION AND SOCIAL CONTROL

The fact that medicine is inextricably wrapped in social processes means that it is continually expected to move into fresh areas and deal with new problems. Part of the reason for this is the very success of medical science and technology. The capacities opened up by drug research, computerization and the new genetics mean that potentially most areas of life can be the focus for medical intervention. Although this is widely welcomed as providing more and more sick people with ways of being made better, it also represents problems on a number of fronts. People may feel that many of their own life experiences are being taken over by a detached biomedical elite. The experience of many women giving birth has been precisely this: that pregnancy was treated like an illness and that the procedures of giving birth to a child were constructed with the doctor in mind rather than the mother. A dispute still rages as to whether high-tech deliveries are less hazardous than ones which perhaps take place in the mother's home and at the mother's pace. However, the very fact that such a debate exists illustrates that there is some unease at the direction taken by modern medicine. This can become even more of a problem if it is combined with what Giddens (1991) has called 'manufactured uncertainty'. Such uncertainty is the result of too much information about risks and no real way of assessing their true impact. The controversy over the safety of eating beef against its potential for causing the devastating dementia of Creutzfeld Jacob disease illustrates this phenomenon. Despite there being no specific evidence linking the two, a fear of the potential risks still pervades.

Iatrogenesis

Another aspect of the increasing involvement of medicine in many different aspects of social life is what the radical Latin American priest Ivan Illich (1975) calls 'iatrogenesis', or self-caused disease. He claims that there are three distinct types of iatrogenesis: clinical, cultural and social.

Clinical iatrogenesis is when medical treatment makes that patient worse or creates new conditions. As the old joke goes, the last place you want to be if you are ill is a hospital because that is where all the other sick people are and you'll catch whatever they have got. Although this may be a gross simplification it is not entirely without foundation. It is also possible that the medical intervention itself may be unnecessary or irrelevant. Social iatrogenesis is the label Illich attaches to the way in which medicine expands into more and more areas, creating an artificial demand for its services. This in turn leads on to cultural iatrogenesis, where the ability to cope with the issues surrounding life and death is progressively eroded by medical accounts. This leads to a reliance on medicine to solve problems and a corresponding decrease in autonomy. Illich believes that as a consequence the scope of modern medicine should be demystified if not curtailed.

Connected to these notions is the fact that medicine can, as we have seen, create its own problems by medicalizing hitherto non-medicalized areas of life. A good example is the case of heroin addiction (Dally 1995). At first sight, this may seem an area of obvious medical action but through most of the nineteenth century it was regarded as a pastime and not a medical concern. This changed when it became a controlled drug in 1906. However, even up to the 1960s a small but significant number of addicts were enabled to maintain their addiction through private prescriptions provided by some general practitioners in private practice. What this meant was that these addicts were not criminalized and were thus enabled to live lives of relative stability. What problems these individuals had were ones of life-style and not necessarily the result of a medical condition. What changed this state of affairs was a number of people abusing the system and the identification of the medical category 'drug dependency' as a field of activity for the speciality of psychiatry. Addiction was to be cured rather than controlled. Gradually there was a change in the approach taken towards addicts; now they were to be actively treated to remove their dependency on heroin. Methadone replacement therapy was offered as an alternative. Unfortunately it did not have a particularly high success rate and many addicts dropped out of the programmes, usually resorting to illegal 'street' heroin. This in turn brought them into conflict with the police and ensured that in order to maintain supplies for their addiction they had to adopt a criminal life-style.

In this manner it could be argued that medicine, in being morally pressurized to do something about a social problem, ends up adding to, rather than dealing with, the real issues of drug addiction. Part of this attitude can be seen in the dilemma about the high rates of HIV infection among intravenous drug users. Do you give out syringes and thereby condone illegal drug use, or do you refuse and let infection rates increase?

Mental illness

A way of understanding these issues is to utilize the concept of social control. All societies need to have some form of generally accepted value system if they are to remain relatively stable. This by definition creates people who refuse to, or cannot, fit in. These people become seen, and are often treated, as deviants. Various groups at different times can be seen to occupy this category. They could be members of youth subcultures, new-age travellers or criminals but they all play the same role in that they enable the majority to define themselves in terms of who they are not.

Medicine can, and has, played a role in defining populations of deviants by finding medical conditions for them. This happened most notoriously in the former Soviet Union, where people opposing the nature of the state were often diagnosed as having severe psychiatric problems necessitating hospitalization. However, similar things happened in Britain up until the early decades of the twentieth century, where pregnancy outside of marriage was regarded as indicative of an absence of morals which could only have a medical cause.

To this end a number of 'rebels' within the psychiatric profession, such as Szasz (1966), have argued that psychiatry's main role is to control deviant populations because of the tremendous legal and categorizing powers capable of being invoked. Often those subject to psychiatric control lose all social and civil rights and are subject to controversial treatments such as electroconvulsive therapy. In addition, those labelled as mentally ill are completely at the mercy of those treating them and can only regain their lives if they agree with them.

In contrast to the ideas of those who have been described as the 'anti-psychiatrists', Hirst and Woolley (1982) have argued that whereas many notions of mental illness are dependent on the observation of the behaviour of the patient rather than any independently existing physiological indicator, it would be wrong to assert that there is no real negative context. They point out that all cultures have categories to express the idea that a person is not functioning properly. These may be seen as episodic occurrences or more long-term difficulties, but they are identified by most people as problems none-the-less. Psychiatry does become involved in controlling some members of society, but this is not sufficient reason to claim that this is its only function.

MEDICINE, SOCIAL STRUCTURE AND SOCIAL POWER

The practice of medicine is not confined to the ideas that determine what is and what is not a medical problem. Modern medicine has come into being at the same time as industrialization and has become an integral feature of it. As countries have become more technologically advanced so has medicine. Since the Second World War breakthroughs with groups of drugs such as antibiotics has meant that many infectious diseases can now be successfully dealt with. Previously deadly diseases such as smallpox have been officially eradicated from the planet. With this success has come a growth in demand for health services throughout the world. Because modern medicine is perceived as being capable of achieving great things with people's health, then more and more people want access to it. This has meant that many developing nations are put in impossible situations trying to provide costly hi-tech medicine in environments where there are few resources.

At this point it is useful to remember the point made by McKeown (1979) that the improvement in the health of the British population during the nineteenth and early twentieth centuries owed more to improvements in diet, sanitation and public health than to the efforts of doctors (see Chapter 1). The impressive strides made by medical knowledge therefore depend crucially on the existence of a wider social infrastructure that can support such advances. In most societies this is formalized into some form of health care system. There are many different types of health care system (Roemer 1989) (see Chapter 19). Some organize health care on free market principles with the state playing a minimal role except to provide a safety net for certain underprivileged groups, whereas others are based on compulsory state insurance as in France. Britain is quite unusual in the way it organizes its health services because it is funded out of general taxation rather than through individual contributions.

However, the differences between healthcare systems do not just reflect national characteristics but are different solutions to the problems of providing access to medical and health services and being able to pay for it. At its most simple this accounts for the disparities in health care provision in some developing countries, where if you have wealth or are an expatriate of a western nation you can use medical facilities as good as those in the industrialized countries, but if you are poor your access to services is minimal and what may be provided rudimentary.

Marxist accounts of welfare

The existence of welfare states in the industrialized countries is a relatively recent phenomenon. Although Britain introduced old age pensions and a limited medical insurance scheme at the beginning of this century, the welfare state of which the National Health Service was a cornerstone did not come into being until the middle of the century. Among the reasons for this delay was the belief that state welfare was a victory for the working class because it shifted responsibility for paying for welfare away from the poorest sections of society. Marxist writers such as Navarro (1994) and Gough (1979) argue that healthcare is a key battlefield in the conflict between labour and employers in all societies. The working class wants to ameliorate as many of the adverse conditions created by capitalism as they can, while the employers want to make as much profit as they can at as little cost. Sometimes, as in post-war Britain, concessions have to be made to allow profitability to continue, but at other times, such as during the 1970s, cuts have to be made to this 'social wage' in order that money can be diverted to profit. This is not to suggest that health care is only an outcome of political struggle. Marxist theorists have also identified that the role of the welfare state is central to the continuation of a profitable capitalism. The welfare state carries out three roles: to ensure the health and education of the existing workforce; to produce the next generation of workers; and to justify the inequalities of capitalism. Of course not all of these things can be done successfully all of the time, and this is why the welfare state is in now in a constant state of crisis.

It is not only Marxists who have noted the close connection between the economy and the welfare state which has resulted in a crisis for the idea of a welfare state. Mishra (1984) noted that if money is to be spent on welfare the first thing that has to be established is economic prosperity. All welfare states seem to be coming to this conclusion, with governments of all persuasions, from New Zealand to Holland, trying to reduce expenditure. This difficulty is sometimes known as the 'fiscal crisis of the state' and results from the tendency for welfare, and particularly health spending, to increase over time. Many policy analysts believe that a limit to spending is essential if health care is to continue to be publicly funded and organized. This has meant that much of the impetus to reform health care systems in Britain and throughout the industrialized world has concentrated on finding ways of controlling costs and making the delivery of health care more effective and efficient. The favoured solution in Britain has been the introduction of what has been known as 'managed competition' or 'quasi markets' (Le Grand and Bartlett 1993). The merits or drawbacks of these reforms are not the concern of this chapter (see Chapter 19), but what is important is the way they represent the reorganization of medicine and healthcare as fundamentally consumer issues. If this is true then the social context in which medicine operates is probably going to be of critical importance in determining its future.

CONCLUSION

This chapter has attempted to cover some of the limits to medicine that exist in the modern world. It has drawn attention to the importance of social and cultural aspects of even the construction of medical knowledge. It has also pointed out that medicine and healthcare can, and have, been involved in the construction and maintenance of forms of social power through the socially sanctioned authority to define what are medical problems. These concerns might seem incidental to the way that modern medicine is practised today with its emphasis on resource allocation and clinical effectiveness. However, to ignore these issues is to neglect in some part the way in which we have reached this point of success. A failure to integrate scientific medicine with its social context, or to face some of the difficult implications of its practice, will in the long run separate medicine from its humanitarian project.

REFERENCES

Armstrong, D. (1995) The rise of surveillance medicine. *Sociol. Health Illness*, **17**, 393–404.

Dally, A. (1995) Anomalies and mysteries in the war on drugs. In: *Drugs and Narcotics in History*, ed. R. Porter & M. Teich. Cambridge: Cambridge University Press.

Douglas, M. (1970) *Natural Symbols: Explorations in Cosmology*. London: Cresset Press.

Foucault, M. (1973) *Madness and Civilisation*. London: Tavistock.

Foucault, M. (1976) *The Birth of the Clinic*. London: Tavistock.

Foucault, M. (1977) *Discipline and Punish*. London: Penguin.

Foucault, M. (1981) *History of Sexuality*, Vol. 1, Harmondsworth: Peregrine.

Giddens, A. (1991) *The Consequences of Modernity*. Cambridge: Polity.

Goffman, E. (1968) *Stigma*. Harmondsworth: Penguin.

Gough, I. (1979) *The Political Economy of the Welfare State*. London: Macmillan.

Hirst, P. & Woolley, P. (1982) *Social Relations and Human Attributes*. London: Tavistock.

Illich, I. (1975) *Medical Nemesis*. London: Calder and Boyars.

Jewson, N. (1976) The disappearance of the sick man from medical cosmology, *Sociology*, **10**, 225–44.

Kuhn, T. (1970) *The Structure of Scientific Revolutions*. Chicago: University of Chicago Press.

Le Grand, J. & Bartlett, W. (1993) *Quasi Markets and Social Policy*. London: Macmillan.

Longino, C. & Murphy, J. (1995) *The Old Age Challenge to the Biomedical Model: Paradigm Strain and Health Policy*. Amityville: Baywood.

Lupton, D. (1994) *Medicine as Culture*. London: Sage.

McKeown, T. (1979) *The Role of Medicine*. Oxford: Oxford University Press.

Merton, R. (1970) *Science, Technology and Society in Seventeenth Century England*. New York: Howard Fertig.

Mishra, R. (1984) *The Crisis of the Welfare State*. Hemel Hempstead: Harvester Wheatsheaf.

Navarro, V. (1994) *The Politics of Health Policy*. London: Blackwell.

Roemer, M. (1989) National Health Services as Market Interventions, *Journal of Public Health Policy* **10**: 62–77.

Scambler, G. (1989) *Epilepsy*. London: Routledge.

Shilling, C. (1993) *The Body and Social Theory*. London: Sage.

Szasz, T. (1966) *The Myth of Mental Illness*. New York: Harper.

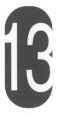

Deviance, Sick Role and Stigma

GRAHAM SCAMBLER

Social norms are definite principles or rules which people are expected to observe in a given culture or milieu. Only a tiny minority of norms are likely to be codified as laws. Deviance can be defined as non-conformity to a norm, or set of norms, which is accepted by a significant proportion of local citizens or inhabitants. Deviant behaviour is behaviour which, once it has become public knowledge, is routinely subject to sanctions – to punishment, correction or treatment. Importantly, behaviour which is acceptable in one culture may be deviant in another. For example, smoking marijuana is deviant in British culture while consuming alcohol is not; the reverse is the case in some Middle Eastern cultures.

ILLNESS, DEVIANCE AND THE SICK ROLE

Few analysts before the 1950s regarded illness as a form of deviance. The term 'deviance' was reserved for behaviour for which individuals could be held responsible; infractions of the law were seen as paradigmatic. A significant change of outlook dates from the work of Parsons (1951), who defined illness as a form of deviance on the grounds that it disrupts the social system by inhibiting people's performance of their customary or normal social roles. If such disruption is to be minimized, then the behaviour associated with illness – which unlike other forms of deviant behaviour cannot be prevented by the threat of sanctions – must be controlled. Control is exercised through the prescription of social roles for the sick and for physicians (see Chapter 4).

According to Parsons, the sick role consists of two rights and two obligations. The rights are that sick people are exempted (1) from performing their normal social roles, and (2) from responsibility for their own state. Sick people are at the same time obligated (3) to want to get well as soon as possible, and (4) to consult and co-operate with medical experts whenever the severity of their condition warrants it. Failure to meet either or both of these obligations may lead to the charge that people are responsible for the continuation of their illness, and ultimately to sanctions, including the withdrawal of the rights of the sick role. Gerhardt (1987) describes Parsons' sick role as a social 'niche' where 'the incapacitated have a chance to recover from their weakness(es), and overcome their urge to withdraw from rather than actively tackle the vicissitudes of the capitalist labour market'. In fact, it can afford its incumbents a legitimate breathing space from a wide range of social demands, and not only from those associated with the labour market.

The sick role is a temporary role into which all people, regardless of their status or position, may be admitted. It is also 'universalistic', in that physicians are held to draw upon general and objective criteria in determining whether or not individuals are sick, how sick, and what kinds of sickness they are suffering from. Its main function is to control illness, and to reduce its disruptive effects on the social system by ensuring that sick people are returned to a healthy state as speedily as possible. Physicians serve as 'gatekeepers', policing access to the sick role by authoritatively determining who is sick and who is healthy. They also spur the urge to leave the sick role (Gerhardt 1987). Unlike some other commentators, Parsons is not at all critical of physicians functioning as agents of social control. Indeed, he sees the sick role, and physicians' policing of it, as important contributions to the stability and health of the social system.

Freidson (1970) is among those who are less sanguine about physicians' social control functions. He acknowledges Parsons' pioneering work in linking illness and deviance, but insists that the argument must be taken a step further:

> *Unlike Parsons, I do not argue merely that medicine has the power to legitimize one's acting sick by conceding that he really is sick . . . I argue that by virtue of being the authority on what illness 'really' is, medicine creates the social possibilities for acting sick. In this sense, medicine's monopoly includes the right to create illness as an official social role.*

Freidson adds that it is in medicine's interests – because it enhances the demand for its practitioners' skills – to pursue actively 'the proliferation of situations that create deviant illness roles'.

It is not necessary to adhere to a thesis of 'medical imperialism' – namely, to claim a conspiracy on the part of physicians to 'medicalize' society – to acknowledge either that a multiplicity of new deviant illness roles have in fact been created this century, perhaps most conspicuously as a product of the growth of psychiatry, or that this has accorded physicians greater powers and responsibilities as agents of social control. Freidson's contribution is to have pointed out that these powers and responsibilities have social – not merely scientific – origins, and require careful analysis and evaluation. After all, to diagnose disease is to define its bearer as in need of correctional 'treatment' of body or mind (even if in practice this often involves little more than recognizing a disease's self-limiting natural history). Contrary to Parsons, Freidson sees physicians' social control functions as extending far beyond the policing of the sick role and as possessing negative as well as positive potential for society.

THE FORCE OF A LABEL

In modern societies professionally trained physicians are generally responsible not only for (collectively) constructing but also for (individually) selecting and applying diagnostic labels. It is now recognized, however, that the application and communication of some diagnoses can have especially serious and unwelcome consequences for patients. This occurs most conspicuously when the conditions being diagnosed are personally or socially stigmatizing. Stigmatizing conditions can be defined as conditions that set their possessors apart from 'normal' people, that mark them as socially unacceptable or inferior beings. Thus, people experiencing deafness, mental illness, severe burns, diabetes, psoriasis, acquired immunodeficiency syndrome (AIDS) and numerous other diseases or symptoms of disease have been in the past and continue to be avoided, rejected or shunned to varying degrees by others.

Another unhappy consequence of being labelled in this way is that people's stigma can come to dominate the perceptions that others have of them and how they treat them. In the vocabulary of sociology, an individual's deviant status becomes a *master status*: whatever else she may be – for example, mother, teacher or school governor – she is regarded primarily as a diabetic, cancer victim, or whatever. In other words, her deviant status comes to dominate and push into the background her other statuses. Even her past may be unsafe and subject to retrospective interpretation. Especially pertinent to this line of reasoning are the concepts of 'cultural stereotyping' and 'secondary deviation'.

Cultural stereotyping

Those afflicted with a stigmatizing condition may be expected to conform to a popular stereotype. An American study, for example, found that blind people are often attributed distinctive personality characteristics that differentiate them from sighted people: 'helplessness', 'dependency', 'melancholy', 'docility', 'gravity of inner thought' and 'aestheticism' (Scott 1969). However far-fetched or misleading such stereotyping may be, the blind person cannot ignore how others expect him or her to behave; to do so might well be to ignore key factors in his or her interaction with them. The author goes on to claim that blind people adapt to cultural stereotyping in five major ways by (1) simply concurring; (2) 'cutting themselves off' to protect their self-conceptions; (3) deliberately adopting a facade of compliance for expediency's sake; (4) making people pay something for a 'performance' (e.g. begging); or (5) actively resisting. It should be mentioned that they may also be obliged to respond to stereotypes of blindness held by physicians and other health professionals.

Secondary deviation

One distinction which has gained currency among those investigating links between crime and deviance is that between 'primary' and 'secondary' deviation (Lemert 1967). Study of the former focuses on how deviant behaviour, for example, stealing, originates. Study of the latter focuses on how people are symbolically assigned to deviant statuses, for example, thief or criminal, and the effective consequences of such assignment for subsequent deviation on their part. The importance of studying secondary deviation has been increasingly acknowledged since the 1960s. It is now accepted, for example, that disapproving cultural and professional reactions to deviant behaviour can often foster rather than inhibit a continuing commitment to deviance.

Similarly, some have claimed that a negative, stereotyped reaction to a stigmatizing illness or handicap can confirm individuals in their deviant status, can constrain them to see themselves as others see them and to behave accordingly. For example, a blind person who is expected to be and is consistently treated as 'helpless' and 'dependent' may actually become so; he or she may find it less exacting to concur with and ultimately adopt the prescribed role than to resist it. Those in institutional or custodial care for long periods are particularly vulnerable in this respect.

Perhaps the area in which 'labelling theory' has had the most controversial impact in relation to medicine has been that of mental illness. In the mid-1960s an American sociologist, Scheff (1966), claimed that labelling is the single most important cause of mental illness. He argued that there exists a residue of odd, eccentric and unusual behaviour for which the culture provides no explicit labels: such forms of behaviour constitute 'residual rule-breaking' or 'residual deviance'. Most psychiatric symptoms can be categorized as instances of residual deviance. There exists also a cultural stereotype of mental illness. When for some reason or other residual deviance becomes a salient or 'public' issue, the cultural stereotype of insanity becomes the guiding imagery for action. In time, contact with a physician is established, a psychiatric diagnosis made and, perhaps, procedures for hospitalization put into effect. Problems of secondary deviation follow with a degree of predictability.

Scheff's theory has been criticized by others, notably Gove (1970). Gove agreed that there is a cultural stereotype of mental illness, but not that people are treated as mentally ill because they inadvertently behave in a way that 'activates' this stereotype. If anything, he argued, 'the gross exaggeration of the degree and type of disorder in the stereotype fosters the denial of mental illness, since the disturbed person's behaviour does not usually correspond to the stereotype'. Scheff is also wrong, according to Gove, in suggesting that, once publicly noticed, the person will be routinely processed as mentally ill and admitted for institutional care; public officials, he argued, 'screen out' a large proportion of those who come before them. Finally, Gove claimed that Scheff overstated the degree to which secondary deviation is associated with hospitalization for mental illness. Although the dispute between Scheff and his critics continues, it seems reasonable to conclude that he fell foul of the temptation to explain too much in terms of a single, if important, insight.

LIVING WITH A STIGMATIZING CONDITION

Stigmatizing conditions vary in terms of their visibility and obtrusiveness and of the extent to which they are recognized. Not surprisingly, there is an equivalent degree of variation in their effects on individuals' lives. People who are 'discredited', to use Goffman's (1963) terminology, are those whose stigma is immediately apparent, such as amputees, or widely known, such as someone whose fellow workers know of his suicide attempt. The discredited will often find they have to cope with situations made awkward by their stigma: their problem will be one of managing tension. Davis (1964) found that the physically handicapped typically pass through three stages when meeting with strangers: the first is one of 'fictional acceptance' – they find they are ascribed some sort of stereotypical identity and accepted on that basis; the second stage is one of 'breaking through' this fictional acceptance – they induce others to regard and interact with them normally; and the third stage is one of 'consolidation' – they have to sustain the definition of themselves as normal over time.

One major criticism of Davis' account is that it overestimates people's strength of will and psychological stamina to engage in what he calls 'deviance disavowal'. It was noted earlier that some blind people regard it as less taxing to defer to than to contest cultural stereotypes of blindness. Higgins (1980) found that deaf people sometimes actually 'avow' their deviance, and even extend it by acting mute, in order to simplify and smooth their relations with the hearing: written messages can minimize misunderstandings and save time and embarrassment.

People who are 'discreditable' are those whose stigma is only occasionally apparent, such as people with epilepsy who suffer infrequent seizures, or little known, such as someone whose status as human immunodeficiency virus (HIV) positive is known only to his or her doctor. The discreditable will usually find they have to take care to manage information; to 'pass as normal' they will have to censor what others know about them. In Goffman's (1963) words, the main quandary is: 'To display or not to display; to tell or not to tell; to lie or not to lie; and in each case, to whom, how, when and where'. People with epilepsy frequently opt to pass as normal, and hence find themselves having to manage information with extreme caution. The following paragraphs illustrate this, and these and the succeeding sections on rectal cancer and HIV/AIDS afford some indication of the types of factors that affect adjustment to stigma.

Epilepsy

The adults with recurring seizures that Scambler and Hopkins (1986) studied clearly felt that, in an important sense, physicians had 'made them into epileptics' by selecting and communicating the diagnosis of epilepsy. It was a diagnostic label that most found unpleasant and threatening and some openly resented and contested, largely, it seems, because they saw the status of 'epileptic' as highly stigmatizing. Those who had been diagnosed in childhood often seemed to have learned to think of their epilepsy in this way as a result of their parents' behaviour: for example, well-intentioned advice never to use the word 'epilepsy', especially outside the home. Schneider and Conrad (1983), reporting the same finding in the USA, graphically refer to such parents as 'stigma coaches'. They add that careless or over-protective physicians can also function as stigma coaches.

Once applied, diagnostic labels tend to be difficult to shake off. Nevertheless, the stigma of people with epilepsy is dormant between seizures; for much of their time, therefore, they are discreditable rather than discredited. Scambler and Hopkins found that, fearing discrimination, people tended to conceal their epilepsy whenever possible. Witnessed seizures were often 'explained away' – for example, as faints – and 'stories' constructed to account for the fact that people could not drive, because of the law, or drink, because of their anticonvulsant medication. Two-thirds of those experiencing epileptic seizures at the time of marriage hid the fact from their partners, at least until after the ceremony. Of those with full-time jobs outside the home, 28% had disclosed their epilepsy to their employers, and only 1 in 20 – all of whom were experiencing seizures daily at the time – had done so before taking the job.

The same authors made a distinction between *felt stigma* and *enacted stigma*. The former refers to the shame associated with 'being epileptic' and, most significantly perhaps, to the fear of being discriminated against solely on the grounds of an imputed cultural unacceptability or inferiority; and the latter refers to actual discrimination of this kind. Scambler (1989) has utilized this distinction to formulate a 'hidden distress model' in relation to epilepsy. This states that the sense of felt stigma is so strong that people with epilepsy typically do their utmost to maintain secrecy about their symptoms and the diagnostic label: they disclose only when it strikes them as prudent or necessary. Non-disclosure, in turn, reduces the likelihood of encountering enacted stigma. Thus felt stigma leads to a policy of concealment which has the effect of reducing the incidence of enacted stigma. Paradoxically, felt stigma was more disruptive of people's lives and well-being than was enacted stigma, which was in fact rarely experienced.

Rectal cancer

If in the nineteenth century tuberculosis stood out as the disease arousing the most dread and repulsion, cancer is its twentieth-century equivalent. Sontag (1977) has argued that it is likely to occupy this role until its aetiology is clarified and its treatments as effective as those of tuberculosis. Rectal cancer accounts for 10% of cancer diagnoses. Two-thirds of those with rectal cancer are left with a permanent colostomy following amputation of the anus and rectum. A colostomy is an incontinent, artificial anus which, with no sphincter to control it, can release faeces and flatus unpredictably, generally into a plastic bag attached to the abdomen. Macdonald (1988) has examined patients' perceptions of what amounts to a family of stigmas: 'the shame, taboos and fears associated with mutilation of the body, with faecal incontinence, with seeing and handling faeces, and with cancer'.

MacDonald found that 49% of her sample reported 'some stigma' and 16% 'severe stigma'; these proportions rose to 54% and 26%, respectively, for those with a colostomy. Most felt as if they had been assaulted and were unclean. Like those with epilepsy, many opted for concealment as a first-choice strategy, felt stigma once more being the motivating factor. They were ashamed by noise and odours from the stoma and filled with self-disgust at the need to handle bags of faeces and to clean faeces from their bodies. They feared exposure because they thought others would be embarrassed or offended and drift away. Some practised 'withdrawal' rather than confront the potential hazards of passing as normal. Many of those in situations where they were discredited rather than discreditable adopted a strategy of 'covering': they took all possible steps to reduce the salience of their stigma for others, to render it unobtrusive (Goffman 1963). A third had never shown the colostomy to their spouses, and more than four-fifths had never shown it to anyone outside the hospital. MacDonald concludes that, although most people in her study learned to accommodate their stomas fairly well, 'a large fraction' suffered impaired quality of life because of their experiences of the stigma of cancer and colostomy.

HIV/AIDS

Since its recognition in 1981 the Human Immunodeficiency Virus (HIV) has aroused strong responses. In the USA, where the HIV epidemic emerged among gay men and intravenous drug users, a persistently negative societal reaction has continued to play a vital role in the experiences of individuals with the virus. Alonzo and Reynolds (1995) suggest that individuals' adjustments to HIV/AIDS must be seen against the background of a 'biophysical disease trajectory'. They note that disease progression varies widely among individuals, but suggest that over a period of 12 or more years they will usually experience a number of stages. These are summarized in Box 13.1.

The authors then go on to identify four phases of an 'HIV stigma trajectory', which is linked to, but can vary independently of, the biophysical disease trajectory. These four phases are outlined in Table 13.1. They again stress individual variation, and also add that stigma can on occasions be 'expansive', pervading all corners of an individual's biography and identity, and on other occasions 'containable, limited and controllable in terms of consequences and, more importantly, personal and social identity'.

BOX 13.1

HIV/AIDS Disease Trajectory

1. A transient flu-like syndrome associated with seroconversion, developing within weeks or months of infection.

2. An asymptomatic period of more than four years average duration.

3. Symptomatic HIV infection of more than five years average duration.

4. AIDS characterized by opportunistic illnesses, HIV wasting syndrome, HIV dementia, lymphomas, and other neoplasms, averaging 9–13 months for treated and untreated individuals combined, and 21 months for those receiving antiviral medical treatments.

Reproduced with kind permission from Elsevier Science Ltd from Alonzo & Reynolds (1995).

TABLE 13.1 *Four phases of the HIV stigma trajectory.*

1. At Risk: pre-stigma and the worried well	This does not correspond to a stage of the disease trajectory. It denotes a time of uncertainty when an individual thinks behaviours might have put him at risk of HIV. He may cope through denial or disassociation. Much depends on the support available. The phase may end with testing for HIV.
2. Diagnosis: confronting an altered identity	An individual may be diagnosed early or late in the disease trajectory. A typical stress response involves disbelief, numbness and denial, followed by anger, acute turmoil, disruptive anxiety and depressive symptoms. Identity and self-esteem may be threatened, stigma becomes salient, and decisions on disclosure have to be negotiated.
3. Latent: living between health and illness	This is when the disease is asymptomatic and perhaps at its least disruptive. Individuals may normalize, conceal and even deny their positivity. They may choose to pass as normal, thereby avoiding enacted stigma, but felt stigma can exact a heavy price.
4. Manifest: passage to social and physical death	There may be no fixed disease course because of widespread individual variation. However, there are fewer symptom-free periods and opportunistic infections accumulate. Stigma tends to be less salient as matters surrounding social and biological death become paramount. Intense felt stigma may nevertheless be associated with isolation and withdrawal as means of concealing 'abominations of the body'. Courtesy stigma may extend to carers who hesitate to reveal cause of death.

Reproduced with kind permission from Elsevier Science Ltd from Alonzo and Reynolds (1995).

AIDS, STIGMA AND HEALTH POLICY AND PRACTICE

The epidemic of HIV/AIDS also raises important issues of health policy and practice. Throughout its brief history, AIDS has been both medicalized as 'disease' and moralized as 'stigma'. Weeks (1989) elaborates on this theme by tracing three distinct phases in social responses to AIDS through the 1980s; these are described below.

The dawning crisis (1981–82)

It was not until the summer of 1981 that the health problems increasingly being experienced in the gay community, and leading to much debate therein, became 'an embryonic public issue' in the USA, with physicians and the press beginning to take note. Exploratory attempts were made to understand the nature of the disease known initially as 'the gay cancer', then GRID (gay-related immune deficiency). (The acronym AIDS was finally accepted in 1982.) Risk categories outside the gay community were soon identified: heroin users, haemophiliacs and, most controversially, Haitians. The Federal Administration, however, remained largely inactive, partly because it was intent on public expenditure cuts at the time, and partly because AIDS seemed to be confined to marginal and, with the possible exception of haemophiliacs, 'politically and morally embarrassing' groups.

Moral panic (1982–85)

From about 1982 a moral panic set in, with a rapid escalation of media and public hysteria. This was the period of the New Right and Moral Majority onslaught in the USA, and of stories of the 'gay plague' in the tabloid press. Around the same time, 1983–84, HIV was identified and named, opening up new opportunities for medical engagement. In addition, the communities most affected, notably the gay community, began to organize for self-help, for example through Gay Men's Health Crisis in New York and the Terrence Higgins Trust in London. The identification of the virus and progress in understanding modes of transmission shifted attention from risk categories to risk activities.

Crisis management (1985–89)

The last phase identified by Weeks commenced in 1985, when it was recognized that AIDS as a disease constituted a global threat, and to heterosexual as well as to gay or socially marginal communities. Governments in the USA and Britain, mobilized by the perceived threat to 'the general population', began to commit resources, especially to prevention. It is ironic that in so doing they drew on the experience and expertise of the gay self-help groups. The self-help groups themselves became more professional as public funds became available to them and as demands on their services increased. An uneasy alliance was formed between the self-help groups and the medical profession.

Weeks' brief history of the first decade of AIDS and current debates highlight a number of important issues concerning the role of physicians. First, not only was AIDS – uniquely combining sex, drugs, death and contagion – itself highly stigmatizing, but it was initially discerned in an already markedly stigmatized population, that of gay men. For several years political and popular homophobia meant that both effective research and health interventions were delayed, and that specialist physicians came under some pressure to sanction or facilitate punitive action against 'guilty' HIV/AIDS carriers – like gay and bisexual men and, later, injecting drug users – if not against 'innocent' carriers – like haemophiliacs and babies of infected mothers. Fortunately such pressure, and the guilty/innocent dichotomy underlying it, has been largely resisted by the British medical profession. The evidence of history is that the punitive medical policing of socially marginalized groups, quite apart from infringing civil rights, is counterproductive in that it leads to further marginalization and losses of contact and capacity to influence through health education or 'user-friendly' services.

There is some indication that, although the great majority of AIDS cases at the end of the 1980s involved gay or bisexual men and injecting drug users, analysis of known cases of HIV infection in Britain suggests increased spread into the heterosexual population. Whether or not this turns out to be true, a second issue is the certain involvement of an increasing number of general, as opposed to specialist, physicians in the care of HIV/AIDS patients. This will constitute a considerable challenge to the primary-care sector. Although general practitioners have become better informed about AIDS, there is evidence of lack of commitment to health education about AIDS and of wide divergences of attitude towards the provision of counselling and treatment and over the issue of confidentiality. In one national study, 70% of general practitioners reported that they found it difficult to discuss the sexual practices of gay men during consultations. Nearly half of the same sample said they would not knowingly accept anybody injecting drugs onto their practice list (Rhodes et al. 1989). It is not surprising, perhaps, that many people with HIV or AIDS are reluctant to consult their general practitioners, either uncertain of the reaction, in fear of a negative one, or anxious about confidentiality (King 1988).

STIGMA AND PHYSICIAN–PATIENT ENCOUNTERS

Whether patients have epilepsy, rectal cancer, HIV/AIDS or any other stigmatizing condition, the quality of the care they receive is a major concern. The enhanced salience of medical audit will be important here. But quality of care encompasses more than biomedical thoroughness, and numerous studies have documented patient unhappiness at physicians' preoccupation with diagnosis and management and apparent lack of interest in psychological and social aspects of care. Scambler (1989) has noted that the accusation that physicians, especially hospital specialists, lack the time, training or motivation to elicit and address patients' own perspectives on their epilepsy is a common one. He goes on to distinguish analytically between three dimensions to patients' perspectives: (1) 'felt stigma' – a sense of shame and apprehension at meeting with discrimination; (2) 'rationalization' – a deep need to make sense of what is happening, to restore cognitive order; and (3) 'action strategy' – a need to develop modes of coping across a diversity of roles and situations. Research suggests that physicians tend to be interested in those aspects of patient rationalization that promise to facilitate diagnosis or management, but not in the process per se. Neither felt stigma nor action strategy tend to be on the medical agenda for consultations, and are typically handled inexpertly and cursorily if raised by patients.

The point has often been made that patients' perspectives need to be respected and explored in their own right. Physicians do not merely need to inform and advise, but also to listen. To do this effectively, particularly in relation to stigmatizing conditions, requires what Schneider and Conrad (1983) have termed 'co-participation in care'. Scambler (1990) has argued that physicians need to provide a competent and up-to-date technical service covering the investigation, diagnosis and management of epilepsy – at optimum cost – and to engage in health education oriented to demythologizing and destigmatizing epilepsy in the community. As far as physician–patient encounters are concerned, he suggests four guiding principles, which are summarized in Box 13.2.

The literature suggests that these prescriptions are pertinent to a wide range of chronic and stigmatizing illnesses, and to surgical procedures such as mastectomy and colostomy which have stigmatizing results.

BOX 13.2

FOUR CRITERIA OF GOOD CARE

1. Acceptance of the principle of *co-participation in care*, which involves coming to terms with 'patient autonomy', or the patient as decision-maker;

2. Acceptance of an *open agenda* in physician–patient encounters;

3. An *holistic* rather than exclusively biomedical orientation to care, with the emphasis on informing, advising and helping 'persons in context' rather than merely managing disease;

4. The development of *counselling skills* to complement technical skills, which presupposes both an awareness of the impact of epilepsy on quality of life and learned expertise in advising on coping strategies.

Reproduced with permission from the Royal Society of Medicine from Scambler (1990).

REFERENCES

Alonzo, A. & Reynolds, N.   (1995) Stigma, HIV and AIDS: an exploration and elaboration of a stigma strategy. *Soc. Sci. Med.*, **41**, 303–15.

Davis, F.   (1964) Deviance disavowal: the management of strained interaction by the visibly handicapped. In: *The Other Side*, ed. H. Becker. Glencoe, IL: Free Press.

Freidson, E.   (1970) *Profession of Medicine*. New York: Dodds, Mead & Co.

Gerhardt, U.   (1987) Parsons, role theory and health interaction. In: *Sociological Theory and Medical Sociology*, ed. G. Scambler. London: Tavistock.

Goffman, E.   (1963) *Stigma: Notes on the Management of Spoiled Identity*. New York: Prentice-Hall.

Gove, W.   (1970) Societal reaction as an explanation of mental illness: an evaluation. *Am. Soc. Rev.*, **35**, 873–84.

Higgins, P.   (1980) *Outsiders in a Hearing World: A Sociology of Deafness*. Beverley Hills, CA: Sage.

King, M.   (1988) AIDS and the general practitioner: views of patients with HIV and AIDS. *Br. Med. J.*, **297**, 182–4.

Lemert, E.   (1967) *Human Deviance, Social Problems and Social Control*. New York: Prentice-Hall.

MacDonald, L. (1988) The experience of stigma: living with rectal cancer. In: *Living with Chronic Illness: the Experience of Patients and their Families*, ed. R. Anderson & M. Bury. London: Allen & Unwin.

Parsons, T.   (1951) *The Social System*. London: Routledge & Kegan Paul.

Rhodes, T., Gallagher, M., Foy, C., Philips, P. & Bond, J.   (1989) Prevention in practice: obstacles and opportunities. *AIDS Care*, **1**, 257–67.

Scambler, G.   (1989) *Epilepsy*. London: Tavistock.

Scambler, G.   (1990) Social factors and quality of life and quality of care in epilepsy. In: *Quality of Life and Quality of Care in Epilepsy*, ed. D. Chadwick. London: Royal Society of Medicine.

Scambler, G. & Hopkins, A.   (1986) Being epileptic: coming to terms with stigma. *Soc. Health Illness*, **8**, 26–43.

Scheff, T.   (1966) *Being Mentally Ill*. Chicago, IL: Aldine.

Schneider, J. & Conrad, P.   (1983) *Having Epilepsy: the Experience and Control of Illness*. Philadelphia: Temple University Press.

Scott, R.   (1969) *The Making of Blind Men*. New York: Russell Sage Foundation.

Sontag, S.   (1977) *Illness as Metaphor*. New York: Allen Lane.

Weeks, J.   (1989) AIDS: the intellectual agenda. In: *AIDS: Social Representations, Social Practices*, ed. P. Aggleton, G. Hart & P. Davies. London: Falmer Press.

ORGANIZATION OF HEALTH SERVICES

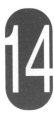

Origins and Development of the National Health Service

Nicholas Mays

There is a wide range of arrangements for the organization and financing of health care in different countries. Each health care system is the product of the social, economic, demographic and technological context and the political philosophy of the country. All exhibit their own balance of advantages and limitations when judged on criteria such as equity, efficiency, accessibility, acceptability and relevance to needs (see Chapter 19). The history of health care in the United Kingdom (UK) in the last 150 years mirrors the trend in all advanced Western countries towards greater government involvement in health care in response to calls for better access to and co-ordination of services (Thane 1982). However, the National Health Service (NHS) which emerged from the interplay and conflict between the medical profession, government, experts, public opinion, employees and insurers was unique to the UK, primarily because it provides services which are predominantly free at the point of use, accessible to all and paid for out of general government taxation. The NHS is perhaps the best known example of a *health service* solution to the financing and allocation of health care in which the vast majority of health care is publicly financed and provided through a publicly managed system. The goal of the NHS is to make health care available to all the population through an arrangement in which there is universal access to a general practitioner (GP) through whom nearly all referrals for specialist and hospital care are made.

Until very recently in the UK, this meant increasing state funding *and* state provision of services. Following the major changes to the NHS introduced in 1991, the role of the state as a direct provider of health care may be reduced for the first time, even though health care continues to be primarily publicly financed.

The purpose of this chapter is to place recent changes in the NHS in a historical context by briefly surveying the evolution of health care in the UK since the nineteenth century and the development of the Service since its inception in 1948, before describing and analysing the Conservative Government's programme of change initiated in 1991.

HEALTH CARE IN THE UK BEFORE THE NATIONAL HEALTH SERVICE

Health care provision in the UK in the nineteenth century and until the mid-twentieth century comprised a number of disparate elements: GP services; the voluntary hospitals; municipal hospitals; and local authority public health measures and related services.

General practitioners

In the nineteenth century, hospitals were primarily used by the poor. They remained dangerous places until the very end of the century when developments in anaesthesia and antiseptic surgery improved the success rate of treatments. For those of the population who could afford it, fee-for-service consultation with a qualified practitioner, either in his surgery or at home, was the main means of obtaining medical care. Gradually, a variety of insurance schemes was also developed, organized by Friendly Societies (non-profit-making, mutual-benefit organizations) and trade unions, which enabled other groups, mainly skilled workers, to use GPs. Increasing numbers of GPs participated in these schemes, particularly in poorer areas where private fees alone did not provide an adequate income. The GP was paid by capitation, receiving an annual sum for each patient enrolled on his list by the insurer. By providing the GP with a modest but reasonably secure income, and protection against competition from unqualified practitioners, the Friendly Societies and trade unions put themselves in a strong position to specify standards of care, such as home visiting, and to limit the clinical freedom of the GP in order to control costs on behalf of their working-class subscribers. Ironically, this degree of lay control forced leaders of the medical profession to conclude that state intervention would be preferable to Friendly Society interference, leading eventually to the National Health Service (Honigsbaum 1989).

By the end of the nineteenth century, only about half the working class was covered by these schemes of contributory insurance. The poor physical condition of recruits for the Boer War (1899–1901), one-third of whom were judged unfit to serve, alarmed military planners in the government at a time of international tension. Industrialists were anxious to see a healthier and, therefore, more productive male work-force. The early twentieth century was also a period of considerable social unrest with working-class uprisings in Germany and an attempted revolution in Russia in 1905. In Britain, the Labour Party, based on the new mass trade unions and the widening of the franchise in 1885, had gained seats in Parliament. Britain's rulers were actively seeking ways of halting the spread of socialist ideas. The German government had already sought to diffuse the revolutionary potential of disaffected sections of the working class by social reforms designed to improve living standards and quality of life. In 1883, for example, Germany's Chancellor, Bismarck, had introduced a system of state-run social insurance covering sickness, accidents at work and old age and invalidity pensions to reduce social unrest. Influenced in part by Germany, Britain introduced old age pensions in 1908 and in 1911, Lloyd George, the Chancellor of the Exchequer, introduced a National Health Insurance (NHI) scheme which the rank-and-file of the medical profession had opposed because the scheme still gave the Friendly Societies a share in its administration. Many members of the profession were equally suspicious of state schemes, fearing control of their work and lower pay. Neither fear was justified in the event.

The scheme, covering manual workers between 16 and 65 years of age whose earnings were below the threshold for payment of income tax, provided funds for sickness, accident and disability benefits in cash, and access to GP services free of charge. Hospital and specialist care were not included. It excluded the self-employed, agricultural workers, many unemployed people and nearly all non-manual workers. Crucially, it excluded all dependants of the insured person, mainly women and children, who had either to pay directly for care or make their own private insurance arrangements. Contributions to the NHI fund were made by the employer, the employee and the Treasury. Entitlement to benefits and GP services was limited to the level of past contributions, so that in cases of chronic illness and unemployment workers could find themselves without cover. Like the earlier Friendly Society schemes, the participating GPs had a list or 'panel' of insured workers and were paid a capitation fee for each, rather than a salary. The NHI scheme was administered in a fragmentary way through the existing Friendly Societies and commercial insurance companies, each of which exercised considerable discretion in deciding the level and entitlement to benefits.

The NHI improved the remuneration of GPs because it provided additional public funds to subsidize the treatment of many more poorer patients while continuing to allow 'panel' doctors to work for other insurers and to continue as fee-for-service private practitioners. This strengthened the financial position of the GPs, which enabled them to resist the Friendly Societies' previous control over their clinical activities. However, it meant that GPs in poorer areas (usually industrial areas and in the north), though better off than before 1911, were paid far less and had far larger lists than those in more affluent areas such as the Home Counties, where private practice was more profitable.

By 1939, approximately 40% of the working population had coverage for GP services through the NHI scheme and about two-thirds of GPs were involved in 'panel' work (Carpenter 1984). Unfortunately, the economic recession of the 1930s had caused high levels of unemployment which had, in turn, led the scheme into financial difficulties. Millions of people failed to keep up with their contributions and there were insufficient funds to meet the needs of the working population.

Hospital services

Hospital care was available from two separate sources: the voluntary hospitals and the municipal or local authority hospitals.

The voluntary hospitals   There were 1100 voluntary hospitals with 90 000 beds in Britain before the Second World War. They were charitable foundations and treated 36% of all hospital patients in 1938 (Abel–Smith 1964). They ranged from GP cottage hospitals, financed by local subscription, to the large, prestigious teaching hospitals which were chartered institutions, established as far back as the Middle Ages in some cases, and supported by extensive endowments. The teaching hospitals concentrated on acute medicine and surgery and undertook most of the training of doctors and nurses. Their consultants offered their services at the hospital without payment so that the hospital could provide free care to patients who could not afford private treatment. In return, they were relatively free to choose to treat the complex and 'interesting' cases. Consultants' incomes were derived from private practice undertaken outside the hospital. GPs, and those doctors who worked for Friendly Societies or the municipal hospitals, were largely prevented from admitting and treating their own patients in the voluntary hospitals. In return, consultants agreed only to accept patients when they were referred to them by GPs.

After the First World War, inflation reduced the real value of the income from bequests and donations to the voluntary hospitals. Medical science and technology were becoming increasingly complex and expensive. As a result, the voluntary hospitals found themselves with mounting financial problems. They responded by trading on their reputations to raise money from the public – as well as by means-testing and charging the growing numbers of more affluent patients who were now using their services – as the effectiveness of hospital care increased. Hospitals set up their own contributory prepayment schemes for those who had some money but could not afford to pay a lump sum when they used services. Another source of income was to undertake work on contract to local authorities, some of which were extending their provision of hospital care in the 1930s. By 1937, at least one-third of the voluntary hospitals were virtually bankrupt (Political and Economic Planning 1937). The government had given them some money in the 1920s to reduce their deficits but had refused to take over responsibility for their finances.

Despite the prepayment schemes, many middle-class people found that acute hospital care between the two World Wars was very expensive since the charges they paid had to finance the care of lower-income patients who were still entitled to free services. However, poor patients brought no income to the voluntary hospital and so there was an increasing incentive for the hospital to neglect them, passing responsibility for their care to the municipal hospitals. Both poor and affluent people became dissatisfied with this state of affairs.

Municipal (local authority) hospitals   The nineteenth-century system known as the Poor Law provided public assistance to the very poorest people and the unemployed. The system distinguished between the 'undeserving poor' whose poverty was presumed to be the result of indolence and fecklessness, and the 'deserving poor' made paupers by old age, mental infirmity or sickness. Provision for the first group was the bare minimum available in the workhouse where conditions were deliberately harsher than those facing the poorest people in work according to the principle of 'less eligibility'. This was to encourage the recipients to find employment and leave. The second group, essentially the sick and elderly poor, were supposed to be treated better in separate infirmaries which were often attached to the workhouses.

In 1929 the Poor Law hospitals were taken over by the local authority health departments headed by the Medical Officer of Health (MOH). They continued to provide mainly chronic, means-tested care for those unable to obtain treatment in the voluntary hospitals or by private means. By 1939 there were 400 000 beds in public hospitals run by the local authorities: 200 000 in 'asylums' serving the mentally ill and mentally handicapped, and 200 000 in a range of tuberculosis sanatoria, isolation hospitals for infectious diseases and former Poor Law infirmaries.

The local authority hospitals tended to be less well equipped than the voluntary hospitals, although standards in the local authority hospitals rose appreciably during the 1930s. They were generally regarded as being of lower status because of the taint of their Poor Law origins. The local authorities paid doctors relatively poorly and attempted to control their work, which antagonized the profession. As a result, by the early 1940s, the medical profession was almost uniformly hostile to the idea of municipal control of health services.

There were big differences in the extent to which local authorities attempted to develop a modern public hospital system in their areas, with some simply perpetuating Poor Law standards, particularly outside London. Indeed, the economic depression of the 1930s meant that many local authorities lacked the money to invest in hospitals. Although the two hospital movements were, in a loose sense, complementary, there was little liaison or co-ordination between them.

Public health and community health services

The earliest and most significant aspect of state involvement to protect the population's health in the nineteenth century had comprised the public health legislation enacted between 1848 and 1875. This had led to major improvements in water supplies and sewerage and, ultimately, the control of infectious diseases, which made a far greater impact on the general standard of health than anything undertaken in the field of curative medicine up to that time (see Chapter 1). By the end of the nineteenth century, each local authority was required by law to have a MOH who was responsible for environmental health, control of infectious diseases, certification of causes of death and a range of preventive services. By the 1930s, the MOH, who was the predecessor of the public health physician in today's NHS, headed a health department in every local authority, with responsibility for services primarily focused on people excluded from the health care available under NHI, such as maternity services, child health and welfare (health visiting in modern terminology), the school medical service and a range of services provided particularly to the elderly in their own homes (e.g. district nursing).

Overview of health care in UK before the Second World War

Despite a reasonably effective pattern of public health and preventive health services, a series of reports between the two World Wars, both official and unofficial, identified major deficiencies in the other health services:

1. financial barriers to the use of health services remained since NHI was not available to more than half the population and did not cover the dependants of the insured worker;

2. NHI did not include hospital care;
3. specialists, GPs and hospital beds were unevenly distributed across the country;
4. there were wide variations in standards in all services;
5. there were mounting financial problems, especially in the voluntary hospitals, and shortages of equipment and skilled staff; and
6. the local authority services, the voluntary hospitals and the GP services were uncoordinated.

ESTABLISHING A NATIONAL HEALTH SERVICE

By the late 1930s there was growing support for the idea that everybody should have the right to good quality health care, but how this should be accomplished was a matter of hot dispute. Decisions would have to be made about, for example, whether services should be funded from general taxation or local taxes or by extending contributory NHI; whether hospitals should be administered by ad hoc bodies or by the existing local authorities; whether doctors should become salaried employees of the state or remain independent contractors; and whether services should be free at the point of use or whether there should be charges and tests of the ability to pay (Webster 1988).

The experience of the Second World War showed how the state could intervene positively in many areas of national life; it also generated demands for a better postwar society. Key factors in relation to the development of health services after the Second World War were the Emergency Medical Service and the Beveridge Report of 1942. The necessity for a national, universally available health care system and the removal of the insurance industry from administering a state scheme was a central plank in Beveridge's famous blueprint for postwar reconstruction, which proposed a 'welfare state' to combat the five 'giants' barring the road to progress: 'want, disease, ignorance, squalor and idleness' (Beveridge Report 1942). Beveridge's report was supported by the Trades Union Congress which joined forces with the medical profession to resist the influence of the insurance companies and Friendly Societies over health policy (Honigsbaum 1989).

BOX 14.1

AIMS OF A COMPREHENSIVE HEALTH SERVICE WITH FREE TREATMENT PAID FOR FROM TAXES

'To ensure that everybody in the country – irrespective of means, age, sex and occupation – shall have equal opportunity to benefit from the best and most up-to-date medical and allied services available. To provide, therefore, for all who want it, a comprehensive service covering every branch of medical and allied activity.

'To divorce the case of health from questions of personal means or other factors irrelevant to it; to provide the service free of charge (apart from certain possible charges in respect of appliances) and to encourage a new attitude to health – the easier obtaining of advice early, the promotion of good health rather than only the treatment of bad.'

Source: Ministry of Health (1944 : 47).

Box 14.1 sets out the ambitious aims of a comprehensive health service from the 1944 Government White Paper. In 1939, a state-run centrally organized Emergency Medical Service (EMS), funded by the Treasury, was set up to deal with the large numbers of civilian casualties which were expected. It was free; it took over two-thirds of the hospitals; it established a national blood-transfusion service and co-ordinated ambulance services; and it showed that a NHS of some sort was feasible. Working in the EMS, leading members of the medical profession also saw for themselves the weaknesses in the existing services, particularly the poor conditions outside the prestigious teaching hospitals.

It was not possible to establish a NHS without securing the co-operation of the medical profession. Although the British Medical Association (BMA) had published its own report in 1942 calling for a comprehensive health service, covering all but the 10% of people with the highest incomes, it was at loggerheads with the civil servants in the Ministry of Health over the means of implementation, particularly the Ministry's support for a municipal health service. Between 1942 and 1948 there was continuous negotiation about almost every aspect of the finance, organization and control of a new unified service between the government and key interest groups, particularly the representatives of the medical profession (Eckstein 1958). The GPs resisted a salaried service to preserve professional autonomy. The hospital specialists refused the proposal for local authority control. Both groups were hostile to anything which hinted at the two nineteenth century systems of lay control – the Friendly Societies and the Poor Law. The system which finally emerged was the product of skilful compromises by Aneurin Bevan, the Labour Minister of Health after 1945, and reflected these concerns to a considerable degree, although it was never formally agreed to by the BMA.

The main concessions to the profession in the 1946 NHS Act were as follows:

1. GPs remained independent contractors but most were made better off by the NHS;
2. Hospital consultants were paid for the hospital work they had previously done for nothing;
3. Consultants were allowed to work part-time in the NHS on good salaries and keep their private practices;
4. Beds for private patients ('pay beds') were permitted in NHS hospitals;
5. A system of distinction (merit) awards controlled by the profession was established for hospital consultants but not GPs;
6. Doctors were to play a major role in deciding policy at all levels; and
7. Hospitals were not to be controlled by local authorities, but 'nationalized' under the control of local appointed bodies.

From the outset, therefore, despite its apparent radicalism, the NHS represented a compromise between principles of traditional medical authority and rational public administration (Klein 1995a). The original Labour intention of placing all services under about 60 local authorities had been abandoned (Webster 1988).

THE NHS IN 1948

The new NHS was open to the whole population solely on the basis of health care need, free at the point of use and mainly funded from the general tax revenues of central government. The aim was to secure equality of access throughout the country and provide a comprehensive range of modern services accessible by referral from a GP except in emergencies.

The NHS which began in 1948 nationalized the existing pattern of services. Thus the NHS inherited many of the strengths and weaknesses of the previous arrangements, including the historical divisions between general practice, local authority health services and the teaching hospitals and inequalities in the geographical distribution of hospital beds, staff and equipment.

The structure in England and Wales was tripartite (Fig. 14.1) since the administration was

Fig. 14.1 *The structure of the NHS in England and Wales, 1948–74. Reproduced with permission from Robinson (1989).*

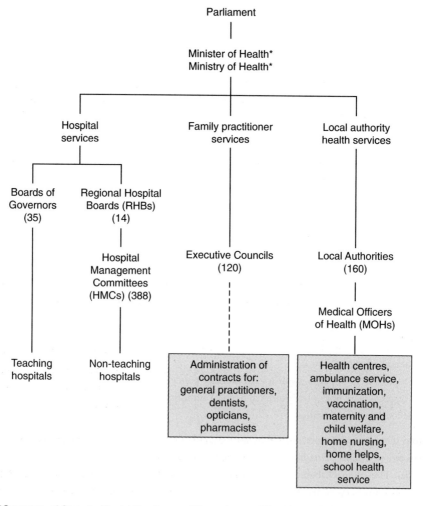

*Secretary of State for Social Services and Department of Health and Social Security (DHSS), respectively, from 1968

——— Direct managerial authority
– – – Administrative responsibility

shared between three statutory authorities (Box 14.2). The teaching hospitals continued to have elite status. Their Boards of Governors were outside the Regional Hospital Board (RHB) structure and had direct access to the Ministry of Health. Thus, the administration of the NHS fell far short of the ideal of full integration. Similar but separate structures existed in Scotland and Northern Ireland. In terms of overall control, finance and access, the system had changed markedly. The assumption was that a 'free' NHS would particularly benefit the working class. In practice, because many working-class people had had access to subsidized or free health care before the Second World War, the NHS, paradoxically, did as much to remove the financial barriers facing middle-class patients as those facing working-class patients.

BOX 14.2

TRIPARTITE ADMINISTRATION IN THE NHS AFTER 1948

1. 14 Regional Hospital Boards (RHBs), appointed by the Minister of Health, were responsible for the Hospital Management Committees (HMCs) which ran the former local authority hospitals.

2. Local authorities ran preventive and community health services under the MOH.

3. Executive Councils dealt with the GPs, dentists, opticians and pharmacists who were independent contractors to the NHS.

THE NHS, 1948–74

The NHS was immediately very popular with the public and rapidly proved financially attractive to the vast majority of medical practitioners. However, two main sources of discontent marked the first 25 years: the level of expenditure and the organization of the service.

The level of expenditure

The original expenditure estimates drawn up by the civil servants in the Ministry of Health were relatively modest and assumed that spending would rapidly stabilize, although Aneurin Bevan was in no doubt that the NHS would be expensive due to previous underfunding and a backlog of untreated illhealth. The planners had reckoned without the popularity of the NHS, rising public expectations, inflation and postwar developments in technology and drugs; all of these drove up the cost of the Service. Charges for spectacles, dentures and, eventually, prescriptions were introduced and have remained ever since. By 1953, expenditure had reached such an unexpectedly high level that the Minister of Health ordered an enquiry into the cost of the NHS (Ministry of Health 1956). Instead of profligacy, the Guillebaud committee could find no evidence of inappropriate treatment and noted that health care spending had actually declined as a percentage of the national income. Most of the increase in spending was due to price inflation and necessary pay awards. The committee recommended an increase in spending to remedy the chronic lack of investment in NHS buildings. In a belated response, the government announced a Hospital Plan for England and Wales in 1962 with the objective of ensuring that a modern district general hospital (DGH) was made available for each population of approximately 250 000 people (Ministry of Health 1962). The priority was to increase the number of consultant specialists in the acute hospital sector and provide the infrastructure to support them.

The demand for health care continued to rise in the 1960s fed by professional and public aspirations and supported by economic growth. The period 1960–74 was marked by a steady expansion in spending in real terms and in the volume of services provided through the NHS. Spending rose from 3.8% to 5.7% of gross national product. By the mid-1970s, when the growth in resources began to slow down, the NHS was having to face up to the dilemmas imposed by the requirement, which faces all health systems, to reconcile seemingly infinite demand for care with inevitably finite resources (see Chapter 19). One possible solution was to get more from the existing level of resources through a more efficient organization.

Towards an integrated service

By the 1960s it had become apparent that the NHS had not only a curative role, but also growing numbers of chronically ill and disabled people to care for who could be looked after best outside hospitals. This emphasis on developing 'community care' (see Chapter 16) highlighted the importance of an integrated pattern of acute (curative), caring and rehabilitative services for client groups (such as elderly people) whose needs crossed administrative divisions. The difficulties encountered in providing continuity of service for such groups highlighted the lack of linkage between the three arms of the NHS (Fig. 14.1 and Box 14.2). By the late 1960s, there was consensus on the need to reform the structure of the NHS to provide better co-ordination and a more efficient, planned allocation of resources. The acute sector catering for short-stay patients had been developed at the expense of all other parts of the service, including primary care.

REFORM BY REORGANIZATION, 1974–82

The NHS reorganization of 1974

After lengthy consultation and analysis, the NHS was reorganized in 1974 (Fig. 14.2). The NHS remained accountable to Parliament through a cabinet minister (the Secretary of State for Social Services). Below the Department of Health and Social Security (DHSS), established in 1968, were 14 Regional Health Authorities (RHAs) in England. Their main function was to allocate finance, plan major projects and monitor the activities of 90 Area Health Authorities (AHAs). The new AHAs had responsibility for both the hospitals and the community health services formerly managed by the local authorities. An AHA could be divided into between one and five operational districts depending on population size. A similar reorganization took place in Wales, Scotland and Northern Ireland.

At each level of administration, management was undertaken by a multidisciplinary team comprising an administrator, an accountant, a senior nurse, a public health physician (now employed by the health authority), a consultant and a GP. Decisions could only be taken when there was a consensus in favour among the members of the team ('consensus management'). This system was deliberately devised to incorporate the main professional groups in the decision-

Fig. 14.2 *The structure of the NHS in England, 1974–82. Reproduced with permission from Robinson (1989).*

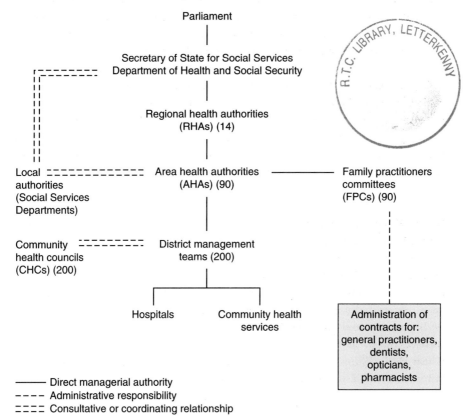

Parliament

Secretary of State for Social Services
Department of Health and Social Security

Regional health authorities
(RHAs) (14)

Local authorities (Social Services Departments)

Area health authorities
(AHAs) (90)

Family practitioners committees
(FPCs) (90)

Community health councils
(CHCs) (200)

District management teams (200)

Hospitals   Community health services

Administration of contracts for: general practitioners, dentists, opticians, pharmacists

——— Direct managerial authority
– – – – Administrative responsibility
= = = = Consultative or coordinating relationship

making process. In each district, there was a Community Health Council (CHC), independent of the health authority, to act as the public's 'watch-dog' and to represent the views of patients and the public to the professionals. The CHC was given rights of access to information from district managers and to premises and had to be consulted on major service developments. The GPs remained independent contractors outside the new structure. The Executive Councils were replaced by Family Practitioner Committees (FPCs) which administered the contracts of family practitioners in much the same way as before. Neither the AHAs nor the FPCs had any significant influence over how the GPs behaved.

The reorganization was designed to facilitate the implementation of an ambitious cyclical process of short- and long-term rational planning and priority setting by region, area and district which began in 1976. This was accompanied by the introduction of the Resource Allocation Working Party (RAWP) formula, the aim of which was to redistribute finance fairly between different parts of the country on the basis of the size and needs of the population. The effects of this redistribution were particularly painful because they were applied to a now near-static NHS budget.

The 1974 reorganization went some way to unifying the NHS and to improving the opportunities for co-ordination with local authority social services. It failed, however, to solve the problem of how to reconcile effectively the role of central government in setting policy, overseeing expenditure and monitoring performance, with the requirement for local, delegated authority and freedom to implement policy at area and district levels. The new structure was criticized for having too many tiers of administration, an overelaborate planning system and too many consultative committees of doctors, nurses and other health workers. Consensus management was said to lead to slow and ineffective decision-making.

MANAGERIAL REFORM, 1982–87

From 1979 to 1983 the Conservative government under Margaret Thatcher had encouraged those at local level in the NHS to take decisions in the light of local circumstances. However, this posed the problem of how to ensure that local managers were using resources efficiently and in line with central policy. There was also a pressing need from the government's perspective to find ways of preventing health authorities overspending their budgets.

Where previous enquiries had concentrated on the structure of the NHS, a small team of private-sector managers, led by Roy Griffiths of Sainsburys, was asked in 1983 to undertake an inquiry into its management practices. Griffiths found a lack of individual responsibility and accountability for the attainment of objectives among the senior officers in the consensus teams. He concluded that the NHS needed a stronger, clearer management system (DHSS 1983). At every level in the NHS the consensus teams were replaced by a single general manager with the power to take executive decisions over the resources under his control. Within the DHSS, two bodies were created: a Health Services Supervisory Board to make strategic decisions about objectives, and an NHS Management Board to direct operations in the NHS.

By establishing a hierarchy of general managers on fixed-term contracts and paid according to their performance, the Griffiths reforms enabled the centre to exercise greater control over activity at all levels, increased the powers of managers and reduced the influence of health authority members, particularly those from local authorities. Full-time managers began gradually to introduce more controls over the way traditionally autonomous clinicians used the resources available to them. For example, clinicians are now increasingly responsible and accountable for delivering an agreed workload efficiently within a set budget through systems of 'resource management' (Packwood et al. 1991).

Overall, far greater emphasis was placed on considerations of efficiency and obtaining greater 'value for money' than ever before. The traditional, professional viewpoint that medical services could and should not be susceptible to measurement, external evaluation and control was increasingly challenged (see Chapter 18 for more on this). For example, the NHS Management Board instituted annual RHA reviews of each of the new District Health Authorities (DHAs) which had replaced the AHAs to ensure that resources had been spent effectively and in line with objectives; set up a system of quantitative performance indicators (PIs) to measure and compare the activity and costs of each district and unit; established a limited list of drugs of proven effectiveness which GPs were allowed to prescribe on the NHS; instituted competitive tendering for support services (e.g. catering, cleaning, portering and security) involving the private sector; implemented new cost–benefit methods for assessing building schemes; and brought in strict DHA cash limits linked to compulsory 'cost improvement programmes' to generate savings for new services.

THE NHS REVIEW, 1988

Why a review?

Despite the emphasis on greater efficiency in the later 1980s, the NHS continued to face the, by now familiar, problem of reconciling increasing demand for its services, generated by an ageing population and new technology, with the available funds. From 1982, health authorities were allocated a sum of cash at the beginning of each year for hospital services with no allowance for unforeseen price increases during the year (for example, in wages or consumables such as drugs). Yet the budgets for the family practitioner services remained largely demand-led. As a result, hospital purchasing power was reducing as a proportion of total NHS expenditure. Despite the fact that more than ever was being spent in total in real terms, and more patients were being treated, by the autumn of 1987 the NHS, and especially its acute hospitals, had entered one of its periodic, but particularly severe financial crises. Many DHAs were having to use their cash reserves, delaying payment of bills, closing wards and cancelling non-emergency admissions to stay within budget while meeting the extra costs of national pay awards. Waiting lists, which had always been a cause of public concern, shot into the headlines. Professional and public pressure for more money for the NHS grew. The RAWP formula was moving money away from inner city areas, particularly in London with its concentration of teaching hospitals. The medical profession was growing increasingly reluctant to manage strictly limited resources on behalf of the Government. In January 1988, the Prime Minister, Margaret Thatcher, unexpectedly announced a wide-ranging, confidential review of the NHS, the results of which were to be published within a year.

An avalanche of analysis and blueprints for reform was submitted to the review team which included the Prime Minister, the Chancellor of the Exchequer and other senior ministers. The review team was forcibly reminded that the advantages of the existing arrangements included the ability to control the level of expenditure (the lack of such control was a problem in most Western countries) and the system of GPs, which allowed many health problems to be dealt with inexpensively without recourse to costly hospital care. These led to a comparatively low level of spending by international standards (6.5% of the gross domestic product (GDP) for most of the 1980s, which was primarily a consequence of relatively poorer economic performance in the UK), for which the whole population was given equitable access to a comprehensive range of high-quality services, regardless of the ability to pay, and with low administrative costs. Although this situation was the envy of many countries:

> the very success of the government in controlling expenditure . . . had turned the NHS into a source of political aggravation. Ministers were being constantly (and successfully) pilloried by the medical profession and the political opposition for their failure to fund the NHS adequately (Klein, 1995b: 803).

The NHS was thus perceived to have weaknesses, often relating directly to its strengths. Evidence was brought forward to show that the NHS was chronically underfunded and that this was reflected in the lack of repair of buildings, waiting lists for elective procedures, the poor quality of care for people such as those with learning difficulties and the low pay of its staff. The most influential economic critique was that the NHS was badly flawed because there were no incentives for health care providers to be efficient (Enthoven 1985). Studies which demonstrated big variations in patterns of clinical activity (e.g. referral rates to hospital (Andersen and Mooney 1990)) were said to prove that resources were not being used as well as they could be (see Chapter 18). Much of the clinical care in the NHS (and in other systems) appeared to be of unknown effectiveness. Furthermore, there was no incentive for hard-working staff in a hospital to become more productive and treat more patients, since the hospital budget would remain the same or could even by reduced in order to produce 'efficiency savings'. This was the so-called 'efficiency trap'.

There was also criticism of the limited extent of patient choice and the insensitivity of managers and clinicians to consumer views in the NHS. These were blamed on the near-monopoly position of the NHS in the health care market, which had allowed a paternalistic, professionally dominated and inflexible system to develop. The NHS was also criticized for perpetuating the divisions between primary care, community care and hospital care, which hampered the effective delivery of services.

Options for reform

The options for reform fell essentially into two categories: options concerned with finance and options concerned with the organization or delivery of health care. The main alternative to finance from general taxation was some form of social insurance (see Chapter 19) or, alternatively, an ear-marked 'health tax'. The idea behind an explicit 'health tax' was that taxpayers would know where their money was going and might be prepared to be taxed at a higher rate than through general taxation. A free-market option was to introduce a basic system of public health care for the poor with private health insurance for the remainder of the population as in the USA. There was, however, little support for this type of radical change in the financing of the NHS towards some system of US-style private health insurance. General taxation was judged to be the cheapest and fairest way to raise money. General taxation for health services normally redistributes resources away from the healthy and wealthy towards those in poor health and the less well off. It is broadly progressive in that those on higher incomes usually contribute a higher proportion of their income. It also redistributes resources over the life cycle since children and elderly people are the main users of health services and most tax revenue comes from people of working age.

The debate about organizational change reflected the influence of American ideas, especially economist Alain Enthoven's proposal in 1985 for an 'internal market' within the NHS as a remedy for the lack of explicit incentives to efficiency in the seemingly monolithic NHS (Enthoven 1985). The basic idea behind the 'internal market' was that it was desirable to separate the role of districts as purchasers of health care from their role as providers (Box 14.3 gives a summary of the basic features of 'internal' or 'quasi-markets'). Under this arrangement, the DHAs would

---

BOX 14.3

KEY FEATURES OF AN 'INTERNAL' OR QUASI-MARKET IN WELFARE
PROVISION

- Somewhere on a continuum between the extremes of a fully private, free market and
  a bureaucratic 'command economy' (fully planned hierarchy)

- Some separation of the demand (purchasing) and supply (providing) functions within
  a service which is still largely publicly funded

- Creation of a network of buyers and sellers linked by more or less binding contracts
  or service agreements specifying the nature of the service to be provided, to whom,
  the volume and the timescale

- Purchasers tend not to be individuals (e.g. patients) but agencies acting on behalf of
  groups (e.g. health authorities)

- Usually some competition between providers or at least the potential for competition if a provider does not perform well

- Variants were developed in 1980s in UK in state education, public housing, community care and the NHS

---

concentrate on planning and purchasing services for their resident populations but would be free
to obtain these services from any NHS unit. Units (e.g. individual hospitals) would concentrate
on providing the best quality of care at the least cost, and in competition with other units. It was
argued that competition within a tax-funded NHS would improve efficiency. A number of variations on this proposal were put forward during the review (Butler and Pirie 1988; Goldsmith
and Willetts 1988), including the idea of using the GP practice as the key purchaser and abolish-
ing DHAs (Maynard et al. 1986). All the proposals for change were accompanied by measures to
strengthen the accountability of doctors to health authorities and steps to manage clinical activity more effectively.

THE CONSERVATIVE GOVERNMENT WHITE PAPER *WORKING FOR PATIENTS*, 1989

For a review initiated by a radical Conservative administration and in response to a perceived
funding crisis, the NHS White Paper of 1989 (Secretaries of State 1989) was notable, firstly, for
the things which it did not change and, secondly, for the fact that the main changes concerned
the means of delivery of health care and not the sources or level of finance (Klein 1995a). It also
said nothing about the balance of priorities in the NHS (e.g. the level of spending on prevention
and public health relative to curative services).

The NHS was to continue to be financed mainly from taxation, to be available to all regardless of income, and to be predominantly free at the point of use. The level of funding would
remain a political decision by the government of the day. The only innovation on finance was

the introduction of tax relief on private health insurance premiums for the over-60s, which was included at the insistence of Margaret Thatcher.

There were four main sets of proposals brought forward in *Working for Patients* (Secretaries of State 1989) and also in a new contract for GPs, which was introduced in 1990. They covered the internal or quasi-market; professional accountability; the management hierarchy; and the development of general practice. The first three are dealt with in Box 14.4.

The internal market: the main proposal for change was the introduction of what is now referred to as an 'internal market' in the NHS, based on the separation of the roles of purchaser and provider along the lines suggested by Enthoven (1985). DHAs would be financed according to the needs of their residents by a variant of the former RAWP formula. They would be free to purchase services from public-, private- or voluntary-sector providers, including their own directly managed units, or from new 'NHS trusts'. Major acute hospitals and other units were encouraged to apply for NHS trust status which would given them freedom from DHA control. Providers such as hospitals would be funded on their ability to win contracts to undertake an agreed amount of work for a DHA. The theoretical incentive for providers, therefore, was to minimize costs and maximize quality in order to stay in business. At the same time, GP practices with more than 11 000 patients were encouraged to become 'GP fund holders' and to take control of their own budgets for the non-emergency hospital care of the patients on their lists. The idea was that the fund-holding practice would act as an informed agent on behalf of its patients and place contracts for services such as routine diagnostic investigations and elective surgery with those providers who were offering a good standard of service at a reasonable price in line with patients' wishes. It was also believed that fundholders would be more likely to challenge providers to produce better services than staff in health authorities.

Fig. 14.3 sets out schematically the main elements in the 'internal market' intended to create conditions for 'managed competition' in the NHS. The aim was to bring the supposed benefits of competition between suppliers, together with business management, to the NHS without jeopardizing its basic principles.

Professional accountability: a second group of proposals aimed to make doctors more accountable to managers for their performance. Medical audit (that is, the systematic analysis of the quality of clinical care) was to be compulsory in hospitals and general practice. Hospital consultants were to have job descriptions which explicitly set out their clinical time commitments in the NHS. General managers were to be involved in the appointment of new consultants and in the allocation of merit awards.

Management hierarchy: a third group of proposals extended the Griffiths' management reforms by removing the remaining local authority and professional representatives from health authorities. The authorities were slimmed down to 10 members and were to become managerial bodies akin to the boards of directors of private companies. Senior managers became members of the new health authorities in their own right. The central NHS Supervisory Board and the NHS Management Board were transformed into a NHS Policy Board, chaired by the Secretary of State for Health, to set overall objectives, and a NHS Management Executive in England (now known simply as the NHS Executive) with a Chief Executive, to run the NHS, including family practitioner services. Fig. 14.4 gives the structure of the Service some years

BOX 14.4

MAIN ELEMENTS IN THE *WORKING FOR PATIENTS* REFORMS
IMPLEMENTED FROM 1991

The internal market

- Health authorities became primarily purchasers not providers, buying hospital and community health services for their populations from providers in public, private or voluntary sectors

- Health authorities' budgets set on the basis of 'weighted capitation' (ie population size and age structure 'weighted' for differences in morbidity between areas)

- GP practices with more than 11 000 patients encouraged to become GP fundholders

- GP fundholders permitted to buy diagnostic, outpatient and selected, non-emergency surgical procedures from providers, including the private sector

- Hospitals and other directly managed units encouraged to apply for 'trust' status in which they remain in the NHS, accountable directly to the Secretary of State for Health, but have greater managerial discretion (eg to buy and sell assets, build up surpluses, establish their own management arrangements, set their own pay and conditions)

- Trusts' income is based on their ability to market their services to purchasers (health authorities, GP fundholders and private insurers)

- Contracts or service agreements devised to link purchasers (health authorities and GP fundholders) and providers (trusts and the private sector) so that funding would follow the patients

Professional accountability

- Compulsory, professionally-led audit of medical practice to ensure quality and efficient use of resources

- Job descriptions for consultants

- Managerial involvement in consultant appointments and allocation of merit awards

Management hierarchy

- Smaller managerial bodies reformed on 'business lines' (ie professional and local authority representatives removed)

- Regions to focus on monitoring performance of district purchasers

- Family Practitioner Committees (FPCs) phased out to be replaced by Family Health Services Authorities (FHSAs) with greater responsibility for monitoring GP prescribing and quality of care and influencing the development of general practice in their areas

Fig. 14.3 *The internal market for NHS services from April 1991. Reproduced with permission from Robinson (1989).*

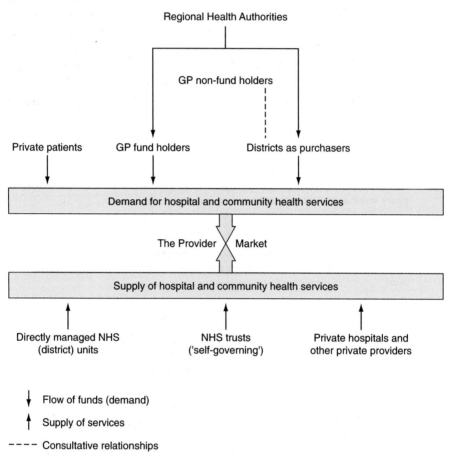

later. Chief executives were also appointed to run the NHS in Wales, Scotland and Northern Ireland through separate management structures.

General practice: the final main set of proposals concerned the new NHS general practitioner contract which was introduced in 1990. The contract aimed to encourage more preventive activities such as screening by GPs, more patient choice between GPs, a degree of competition between practices for patients and greater cost-effectiveness of services delivered in primary care. GPs were required to provide more information to prospective patients about the services which they offered and it was made easier for patients to change their GPs. GPs were allowed to advertise their services. A higher proportion of GP remuneration was to come from capitation (from 46% to 60% on average) in order to encourage GPs to be more responsive to patients' needs. Other elements in the pay of GPs were now linked to the attainment of activity targets set by the government (e.g. achieving specified rates of take-up for child immunization and vaccination and cervical cytology). Subsidies to GPs to employ additional staff in their practices, such as practice nurses to carry out screening and health promotion work, were greatly increased. It was also made easier for patients to change GP. All GPs were given an official indication of the amount they should be spending on drugs to exert downward pressure on their expenditure. High prescribing GPs are now given advice on how to reduce costs without denying patients the drugs they need. Family Practitioner Committees (FPCs) were retitled Family Health Services Authorities (FHSAs) and were given greater powers to audit and monitor the work and spending of family practitioners. FHSAs were merged with the DHAs in April 1996 to produce integrated health authorities (see Fig. 14.4 for the structure of the NHS after April 1996).

Fig. 14.4 *Structure of the NHS in England from April 1996. Reproduced with permission from Robinson (1989).*

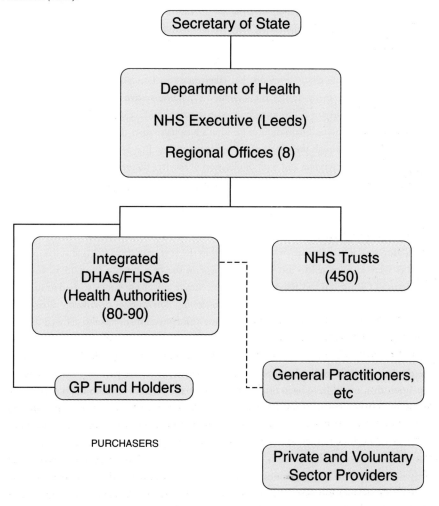

Despite a concerted campaign of opposition from the BMA and the other NHS trade unions, the main elements in *Working for Patients* (Secretaries for State 1989) became law in the NHS and Community Care Act 1990 and were rapidly put in place. The 'internal market' officially began operation in April 1991, although there was a deliberate policy in the first year ahead of a General Election of maintaining a 'steady state' in which district purchasers were discouraged from making major changes to the location or type of services which they bought.

DEVELOPING AND MANAGING THE NHS INTERNAL MARKET

Working for Patients (Secretaries of State 1989) and the NHS and Community Care Act 1990 only provided sketches towards a new system. The true nature of the changes only became apparent in the course of their implementation as Ministers and the Service attempted to decide the extent to which competition should be allowed to shape the future or the degree to which the market should be managed to avoid destabilizing hospitals and harming patients (Ham 1994). Gradually the language used started to change and the phrase 'managed competition' came more frequently into use to signify a more measured approach in which some degree of old-style planning persisted. The most notable example of this has taken place in London, where the government slowed down the implementation of the weighted capitation system of funding so that health authority budgets would not fall too much in relative terms, and set up the Tomlinson enquiry in an attempt to plan the rationalization of London's hospitals rather than see them scaled down in piecemeal fashion through the effects of market competition. London hospitals faced relatively high costs in providing services and with duplication of services there was a noticeable degree of competition. It is perhaps an irony that in London and other big cities, where, in many respects, conditions are best suited to the development of an efficient internal market (e.g. many suppliers in proximity to one another), the government has intervened because of political pressures and the market has been curtailed.

In addition to the 'steady state' which prevailed in the first year, 1991/92 (see above), health authorities were encouraged to use 'block contracts' in the first instance (Box 14.5), based on past patterns of GP referral and activity, and to concentrate any changes they wished to make on the quality criteria built into contracts rather than driving down prices or radically altering the pattern of providers which their patients were to use. The government has also allowed the self-governing trusts less freedom than *Working for Patients* implied. For example, their ability to raise money for capital projects by borrowing commercially has been severely restricted.

Despite developing a more centralized, regulated system at a slower pace and with far less free competition than might have been originally expected, the changes on both the purchaser and provider sides of the 'internal market' have been substantial. In 1991/92, 57 former directly managed units (mainly large acute hospitals) were granted NHS trust status. A further 99 became trusts in 1992/93 and a further 137 in 1993/94. In 1995, over 95% of hospital and community health services were operated by trusts. By 1996/97, only a handful of NHS providers were still directly managed by health authorities. Table 14.1 charts the slower take-up of the GP fund-holding scheme, which remains voluntary. Despite this, by 1996 half the population in England was served by GPs involved in fundholding.

As part of a wider government initiative, not directly related to the 'internal market' changes,

---

BOX 14.5

DIFFERENT TYPES OF CONTRACT USED IN THE NHS INTERNAL MARKET

- **Block**

  The provider receives a sum of money for a specified range of services to a defined population over a fixed period of time. The numbers and types of cases to be treated are not specified in advance. These contracts tend to be based on past patterns of activity and cost, but if demand is unusually high, the provider still has to find a way of paying for the service to be provided.

- **Cost and volume**

  The provider receives a fixed amount for a specified level of service and extra payments for treating additional patients beyond this level, usually up to a pre-set ceiling, with deductions or additions in proportion to volume. This gives an incentive for the provider to increase throughput.

- **Cost per case**

  The provider receives a negotiated price for each case treated based on the expected cost of treating the particular type of case. This is often used for relatively rare treatments and has been particularly popular with GP fundholders.

- **Nature of these contracts**

  NHS contracts are not legally binding but are really 'service agreements' between parts of the larger NHS. Disputes are resolved by regions.

  Initially, contracts tended to be for a year only but longer-term relationships have been developed.

  GPs are allowed to refer outside contracts (Extra–Contractual Referrals) and health authorities have to decide whether to pay for these ECRs.

TABLE 14.1 The expansion of GP fundholding in England and Wales.

Year	Funds	Practices (% of practices)	GPs (% of GPs)	% of population covered	Budget (£bn)[a]	% of hospital and community health services budget
1991/92	303	303		7	0.4	
1992/93	590	590	≅ 3000	13	0.8	
1993/94	1248	1249		24	1.8	
1994/95	1836	2066	8800	34	2.8	
1995/96	2221	2603 (28)	10 410 (39)	41		7
1996/97				50		15

Reproduced with permission from Audit Commission (1995, 1996).
[a] *A typical fundholder is responsible for an annual budget of about £1.7 million or approximately £160 for each patient on the practice list (1995/96 prices).*

the *Patient's Charter* was published in October 1991 to ensure that providers in competition with one another did not overlook issues of patient information, convenience and access to care when required. It sets out the standards which patients can expect from the NHS, covering areas such as waiting times for a first outpatient appointment and for admission for a planned treatment (Box 14.6). The *Patient's Charter* has been criticized for not including rights and standards valued by patients, such as good communication between doctor and patient, information in advance on the risks and benefits of treatments and access to effective pain relief (Consumers' Association 1995), for distracting managers' efforts towards meeting targets which may be irrelevant to standards of *clinical* care, and for ignoring the issue of the resources required to meet its standards. Nonetheless, along with *Working for Patients*, it represents part of a package of changes which are gradually altering the *culture* or taken-for-granted ways of thinking and acting in the NHS. Rather than accepting the views of the provider professionals without question and allowing

---

BOX 14.6

THE PATIENT'S CHARTER

1991 Version

- 10 'rights', 7 of which existed previously (e.g. the right to be registered with a GP and to treatment on the basis of need, not ability to pay), but 3 new rights included:

  no patient to be on a waiting list for treatment for more than 2 years;

  detailed information should be available on local health services, including quality standards and maximum waiting times;

  all complaints to be investigated followed by a full, prompt reply in writing from the trust chief executive.

1995 Update

- New 'guaranteed rights' include:

  an *18-month* maximum waiting time for all admissions;

  advance notice if any patient has been assigned to a mixed-sex ward, except in emergencies.

- New standards which can be expected, but not guaranteed:

  a first outpatient appointment within 26 weeks of referral and 9 out of 10 people to be seen within 13 weeks;

  treatment within one year for coronary bypass and related heart surgery;

  requests for single sex accommodation to be respected, if possible;

  a choice of hospital meals according to dietary needs and preferences;

  children to be cared for in a children's ward.

them to provide what they want, managers and GP fundholders and, to far less a degree, patients are increasingly put in a position through the operating of economic incentives where the appropriateness, effectiveness and costs of care are matters for legitimate discussion. The culture of the NHS is perhaps less trusting and some commentators fear that the new, post-1991 NHS has undermined the traditional values which have motivated NHS staff in the past, such as a sense of vocation and satisfaction in a job well done (McLachlan 1990).

ASSESSING THE EFFECTS OF THE NHS CHANGES FOLLOWING *WORKING FOR PATIENTS*

The changes in *Working for Patients* were complex and had multiple aims which could potentially be in conflict (e.g. greater efficiency in service provision could work against giving patients greater choice of where to go for treatment). Like most governments, the Conservative government did not clearly state the criteria which should be used to judge whether their 'reforms' had been successful or not. The government also refused to support independent evaluation of the changes for fear that research would be used, particularly by the medical profession, as an excuse for delay in implementation. Furthermore, the original changes were constantly modified during the period after 1991/92 as they came into operation in response to political and practical considerations. As a result, evaluation of the effects of the changes is not straightforward. It is difficult to produce unequivocal conclusions (Box 14.7).

Nonetheless, it is possible to make a number of interim observations about the effects of the changes. In each case, however, it is important to be cautious about attributing all the responsibility for what is observed to the internal market as against other policy changes and ongoing initiatives. First, the 'nuts and bolts' of the radical market-style changes were put in place across the country with considerable speed, but without any major disruption of services to patients. In

---

BOX 14.7

DIFFICULTIES IN EVALUATING THE EFFECTS OF THE 1991 NHS CHANGES

- The changes were complex with multiple aims, not always clearly stated

- The changes were constantly modified during their implementation

- Likely to be several years before major effects become apparent

- Effects of changes were influenced by prior changes (e.g. introduction of general management) and parallel policy developments (e.g. initiatives to reduce waiting lists)

- Government's refusal to support independent evaluation of important changes (e.g. GP fundholding) and to undertake formal experiments

- Early waves of fundholders and NHS trusts were self-selected and atypical (selection bias)

most cases, patients were not aware of the upheaval behind the scenes. As Rudolf Klein, a leading health policy analyst, commented:

> *The NHS . . . went on much as before, defying both the government's predictions of radical transformation and the opposition's prophecies of imminent disaster* (Klein 1995b: 804).

In part this was because health authorities as purchasers were actively discouraged, particularly in the first two years of the internal market, from risking destabilizing the finances of their local providers by making significant shifts in their pattern of services purchased. Fundholders were given more freedom and, as a result, were more entrepreneurial, extracting improvements in service from trusts and moving their 'business' between providers, including the private sector. Paradoxically, in those places where the potential for competition between providers was most apparent, such as the conurbations, and particularly London, the risk that inner London hospitals might lose business to less costly providers elsewhere provoked government intervention in the shape of the Tomlinson enquiry (see above) and, in effect, the reintroduction of a planned approach.

Another reason for the relative stability of the service was the fact that additional resources were made available to the NHS in the first two years after 1991 both to support the managerial costs of implementation and for extra patient care. This period also coincided with a general election when governments tend to increase NHS expenditure in order to have good news to tell the electorate.

Secondly, whatever else the changes may or may not have achieved, they have been associated with a change in the operating culture of the NHS and in the balance of power both between managers and health care professionals and between hospital providers and GPs. Providers now have to be far more aware than in the past of the quality and cost of what they provide. Purchasers, after a slow start, are increasingly questioning inherited ways of providing services and encouraging providers to think of new forms of service more relevant to the needs of patients (e.g. development in specialist 'outreach' services in the community, early discharge schemes, shared care between hospital and general practice, use of skilled nurse practitioners rather than medical staff and so on). Managers in trusts have greater influence over the pattern of clinical work than before 1991, although this shift in power should not be exaggerated. Most managers are reluctant to confront clinicians head-on over matters of clinical judgement. GP fundholding on the other hand has significantly increased the ability of GPs with budgets to influence the way in which hospital specialists provide care to their patients. It has also increased the degree of communication between primary and secondary care (Glennerster et al. 1994). Table 14.2 attempts to summarize the benefits and drawbacks of fundholding hitherto. None of these changes appears fundamentally to have increased the power of patients to influence their treatment.

Thirdly, the changes have exposed long-standing issues, but in new and more noticeable ways (Klein 1995a). For example, the purchaser–provider separation and the requirement to contract for specific groups of services has increasingly drawn attention to the fact that purchasers are faced with a finite budget and an ever lengthening list of demands for resources. At the same time, the greater cost consciousness required by an internal market has led trusts and health

TABLE 14.2 *Summary balance sheet of evidence about the benefits and drawbacks following the introduction of GP fundholding.*

Benefits identified (mainly efficiency based)	Drawbacks identified (mainly equity based)	Areas with little or no hard evidence
Shift in balance of power in favour of GPs	Not all fundholders able to make good use of their budgetary power	
Providers more responsive (e.g. shorter waiting times, more information, higher quality standards in contracts)	Preferential treatment of fundholders' patients compared with those of other GPs (two-tier service)	Effect on quality and appropriateness of clinical care purchased (e.g. from hospitals)
More practice-based services,more accessible to patients	Not clear that all practice-based services are cost-effective	'Cream-skimming' (i.e. whether fundholders actively remove expensive patients from their lists to protect their budgets)
Able to make 'savings' from budgets to plough back into patient care	Not all 'savings' have been spent	
Rate of increase in prescribing costs slower in fundholding than non-fundholding practices (but difference small and not sustained)	Administrative costs likely to be higher than health authority purchasing	Level of funding compared to non-fundholding population
No differences in referrals rates between fundholding and non-fundholding practices	Fundholders may fragment pattern of services locally and are less clearly accountable for their use of public funds	

authority purchasers to question where the responsibilities of the NHS for continuing care should end and those of the local authority social services should begin (see Chapter 16). The issue of priority setting (or 'rationing') in health care and the problem of defining the limits of a comprehensive health care system have both existed for many years, but were largely hidden from view under the previous system.

Fourthly, the effects of the changes on the quality of clinical care and on health outcomes (see Chapter 18) have been very little studied. The data which are routinely generated within the NHS tend to cover activity indicators such as trends in the numbers of patients treated and in waiting lists and waiting time, all of which are at best partial measures of improvements in the services received by patients. Such statistics are also open to a variety of interpretations. For example, a vigorous debate broke out between the government and the Radical Statistics Health Group (RSHG) about whether the NHS showed greater improvements in productivity before or after the 'reforms'. Data on numbers of patients treated suggest that the long–term increase over the last 30 years has continued with relatively little sign of an acceleration after 1991

(Radical Statistics Health Group 1995). On waiting, the evidence suggests that although the numbers on waiting lists have changed relatively little, the numbers waiting for over 18 months have fallen substantially (NHS Executive 1995).

Finally, it is increasingly apparent that any improvements in quality or efficiency of services have been achieved at a considerable administrative cost. As critics of the Conservative government's changes predicted, setting up and running a managed internal market generates a requirement to undertake a range of tasks which did not previously exist. For example, trusts have to cost their services, market them, negotiate contracts with purchasers, ensure that contract terms are honoured, raise invoices to ensure payment, collect data on the quality of their services (e.g. wound infection rates after surgery) to report to purchasers and so on. With hundreds of GP fundholders purchasing part of their services, these 'transactions' costs have multiplied. Not surprisingly, the number of posts labelled as 'managerial' rose from 4610 in 1989 to 12 340 in 1991, although part of this increase was brought about by a change in the definition of a 'manager'. For example, numbers of clinical staff such as senior nurses are inevitably and appropriately involved in managing resources and activity with a direct bearing on good patient care. Although the statistics may exaggerate the increase in managerial costs, there has been an undoubted increase which may or may not be judged worthwhile compared with the achievements of the Service since 1991.

CONCLUSIONS

Despite the free market radicalism of some of the proponents of reform in the late 1980s, the NHS of the later 1990s remains a relatively centralized, tax-funded service still pledged to trying to provide a comprehensive range of health services equally accessible to the whole population on the basis of need and largely free at the point of use. The NHS is still accountable for its performance ultimately to Parliament through the Secretary of State for Health. The one planned breach of the equitable basis of the NHS was the introduction in 1991 of tax relief on private health insurance for elderly people. Charges for NHS dental, ophthalmic and pharmaceutical services in the community have also risen substantially during the 1980s and 1990s, further undermining, in practice, the notion of a Service free at the point of use. Nonetheless, this trend has not affected the hospital and other community health services, such as district nursing.

It has been suggested that as long as the bulk of finance comes from public sources and secures access to health care for all, the question of who owns and runs the health care facilities is strictly secondary (Ham et al. 1990). Seen in this light, the 1991 changes were no more than the logical extension of the earlier policy of compelling health authorities to put their support services out to competitive tender (see above). Although the *Working for Patients* changes were accompanied by the rhetoric of market freedoms and competition, they have demonstrated the near-inevitable tendency of governments to intervene in health care in order to produce an acceptable balance between potentially conflicting objectives such as equity and efficiency; responsiveness to patient demand and expenditure control; and between lay and expert definitions of need.

The policy challenge for the future in UK and other Western countries is how best to combine elements of market-style and bureaucratic planned solutions to the universal problems of health care provision (see Chapter 19). Future UK governments with a different ideological slant from the Conservatives of the first half of the 1990s will arrive at a different judgement about the optimum combination of these elements, but will be unlikely to sweep away all the changes made in the NHS since the Conservatives came to power in 1979. Two elements stand out as likely to endure: the formal separation between purchasers and providers; and the growing involvement of GPs and possibly other primary care professionals in shaping the balance and nature of health care to be purchased.

REFERENCES

Abel-Smith, B. (1964) *The Hospitals 1800–1948*. London: Heinemann.
Andersen, T.F. & Mooney, G. (eds) (1990) *The Challenge of Medical Practice Variations*. London: Macmillan.
Audit Commission (1995) *Briefing on GP fundholding*. London: Audit Commission.
Audit Commission (1996), *What the doctor ordered: a study of GP fundholders in England and Wales*. London: Audit Commission.
Beveridge Report (1942) *Inter-departmental Committee on Social Insurance and Allied Services*, Cmnd. 6404. London: HMSO.
Butler, E. & Pirie, M. (1988) *Health Management Units*. London: Adam Smith Institute.
Carpenter, G. (1984) National Health Insurance: a case study in the use of private non-profit making organisations in the provision of welfare benefits. *Publ. Admin.*, **62**, 71–89.
Consumers' Association. (1995) The NHS: what's the verdict? *Which? Way to Health* June, 80–3.
Department of Health and Social Security (1983) *NHS Management Inquiry: Report* (Chairman: Mr R. Griffiths). London: DHSS.
Eckstein, H. (1958) *The English Health Service*. Cambridge, MA: Harvard University Press.
Enthoven, A.C. (1985) *Reflections on the Management of the National Health Service*. London: Nuffield Provincial Hospitals Trust.
Glennerster, H., Matsaganis, M. & Owens, P. with Hancock, S. (1994) *Implementing GP Fundholding*. Buckingham: Open University Press.
Goldsmith, M. & Willetts, D. (1988) *Managed Health Care: a New System for a Better Health Service*. London: Centre for Policy Studies.
Ham, C. (1994) *Management and Competition in the new NHS*. Oxford: Radcliffe Medical Press.
Ham, C., Robinson, R. & Benzeval, M. (1990) *Health Check: Health Care Reforms in an International Context*. London: King's Fund Institute.
Honigsbaum, F. (1989) *Health, Happiness and Security: the Creation of the National Health Service*. London: Routledge.
King's Fund Institute (1989) *Managed Competition: a New Approach to Health Care in Britain*. Briefing Paper No. 9. London: King's Fund Institute.
Klein, R. (1995a) *The New Politics of the National Health Service*, 3rd edn. London: Longman.
Klein, R. (1995b) Review of Ray Robinson and Julian Le Grand (eds) *Evaluating the NHS Reforms*. *J. Health Politics, Policy Law*, **20**, 802–7.
Le Grand, J. (1990) *Quasi-markets and Social Policy*. Studies in Decentralisation and Quasi-markets No. 1. Bristol: School for Advanced Urban Studies.
Maynard, A., Marinker, M. & Gray, D.P. (1986) The doctor, the patient and their contract. III. Alternative contracts: are they viable? *Br. Med. J.*, **292**, 1438–40.
McLachlan, G. (1990) *What Price Quality? The NHS in Review*. London: Nuffield Provincial Hospitals Trust.
Ministry of Health (1994) *A National Health Service*. Cmnd 6502. London: HMSO.
Ministry of Health (1956) *Report of the Committee of Enquiry into the Cost of the National Health Service* (Chairman: Mr C. Guillebaud), Cmnd. 9962. London: HMSO.
Ministry of Health (1962) *A Hospital Plan for England and Wales*, Cmnd 1604. London: HMSO.
NHS Executive (1995) *Annual Report, 1994/95*. Leeds: NHS Executive.
Packwood, T., Keen, J. and Buxton, M. (1991) *Hospitals in Transition: the Resource Management Experiment*. Milton Keynes: Open University Press.
Political and Economic Planning (1937) *Report on the British Health Services*. London: PEP.
Radical Statistics Health Group (1995) NHS 'indicators of success': what do they tell us? *Br. Med. J.* **310**, 1045–50.
Robinson, R. (1989) New health care market. *Br. Med. J.*, **298**, 437–9.
Secretaries of State for Health, Wales, Northern Ireland and Scotland (1989) *Working for Patients*, Cmnd 555. London: HMSO.
Thane, P. (1982) *The Foundations of the Welfare State*. London: Longman.
Webster, C. (1988) *The Health Services Since the War*. Volume 1: *Problems of Health Care, The National Health Service Before 1957*. London: HMSO.

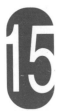

Health Professions

DAVID BLANE

Medical care in contemporary Britain is provided by a work-force which is largely organized into professions. Hospital doctors work alongside nurses, physiotherapists, radiographers, speech therapists and medical laboratory scientific officers. General practitioners integrate their work with pharmacists, midwives, health visitors, community nurses and social workers. Relations between these professions are sometimes strained by a lack of mutual understanding and respect. Given the large number of professions which work within health care, there is considerable potential for such interprofessional conflict.

Better relations between professions can hopefully be fostered by an understanding of the nature of professions and the history of their development. At first sight the far from exhaustive list of professions which have already been mentioned share a commitment to the welfare of their patients or clients and a prohibition against exploiting their dependency. This professional attitude to those in their care is part of each profession's ethics, but a code of ethics is only one of the characteristics of a profession. The general characteristics of a profession as a form of occupational organization are considered in this chapter. The chapter then continues by examining the medical and nursing and other health professions in more detail and ends by considering some of the effects on health care of a professionalized work-force.

PROFESSIONS

Although medical care contains many professions, it does not have a monopoly of them. Lawyers, accountants, teachers, priests, surveyors and civil engineers are examples of non-medical professions (Carr-Saunders and Wilson 1933). Attempts to identify what all these professions have in common, and what distinguishes them from other occupations, have produced a list of core features or defining characteristics (Freidson 1970) (Box 15.1). First, professions tend to be found in the highly skilled sector of the labour market. They possess a body of *specialized knowledge* to which they add by research. This specialized knowledge is passed on to trainees in institutions controlled by the profession, usually in a university setting. Second, professions have a *monopoly* of their field of work which depends on state registration. The state rarely makes unqualified practice illegal, so a profession's monopoly also depends on agreement by the state and other large employers to employ only those who are duly registered. Third, professions have considerable *autonomy* or freedom to organize, define the nature of, and develop their work. This freedom from outside control is defended on the grounds that only a member of the same profession has the specialized knowledge to assess a professional's work. Fourth, professions espouse a *code of ethics* which prohibits the exploitation of clients and regulates intra-professional relations. A further characteristic, namely status, could be added to this list. Professions are middle-class occupations whose members are assigned to social classes I or II on the Registrar General's classification.

BOX 15.1

CHARACTERISTICS OF A PROFESSION

- Specialized knowledge
- Monopoly
- Autonomy
- Code of ethics

Professional socialization

The above characteristics ensure that professions are among the more privileged occupations in the labour market. The nature of their work involves intellectual challenge and interest, their monopoly ensures a measure of job security, their autonomy gives relative freedom from supervision, their code of ethics encourages the satisfaction of aiding others, and their status provides respect and, in some cases, relative affluence. Not surprisingly, therefore, there are many applicants for professional training and professions can be selective about the trainees they choose to admit. This selection is the first stage of professional socialization, which is the process by which members of the lay population are turned into members of a particular profession. Professional socialization involves more than the acquisition of relevant knowledge. It also involves the transfer of what are considered appropriate attitudes and behaviour towards clients, colleagues and fellow workers, although it tends to be only the knowledge which is formally examined. Professional training is, by definition, lengthy and takes place in institutions which are controlled by the profession and somewhat isolated from the rest of higher education. This setting promotes effective socialization and gives considerable power to the senior members of a profession to mould new members in their own image. Professions are, therefore, slow to change and tend to be the focus of their members' self-identity and loyalty.

The process of professional socialization can be illustrated by studies of medical and nursing education. One study of a medical school, which relied heavily on interviews with the staff, stressed the distinction between the formal and the informal curriculum. The formal curriculum consisted of the knowledge considered necessary for a doctor, whereas the informal curriculum involved the attitudes, beliefs and behaviour considered appropriate. A student's success in the former was monitored through regular examinations, whereas their performance in the latter respect was noted, rather than being formally examined, and used to make decisions whenever there was sufficient room for such discretion (Merton et al. 1957). Another study of medical education, which relied on participant observation among the students, drew attention to some of the unintended consequences of this process. Students as they went through medical school increasingly substituted means (passing examinations) for ends (helping sick people) and learned to divide patients into 'good examination material' and 'crocks' (Becker et al. 1961). In other words, the students' initial idealism about the practice of medicine was replaced by a concern with the day-to-day details of getting through medical school, even when this led them to behave in ways which their earlier idealism would have condemned. Whether this was intended or not, the students were being taught to see the disease rather than the patient and to put medical interests before patients' needs.

A study of nursing education found a similar process at work when students were interviewed during both ward and formal academic segments of their training. The student nurses tended to divide their ward work into 'real nursing' and 'just basic nursing care'. The latter, which was the less highly prized, involved serving the basic needs of helpless patients. 'Real nursing' in contrast was more technical, involving drips and drugs, and responsible in the sense that a mistake could harm a patient. 'Real nursing' was emphasized in the formal academic part of their training and to some extent overlapped with the work of doctors. 'Just basic nursing care' received little formal attention and was often performed interchangably with untrained nursing auxiliaries (Melia 1987). Such studies illustrate the ability of a profession to instil into trainees its values and assumptions about what is desirable in its work (e.g. 'good examination material' and 'real nursing') and what can be downgraded (e.g. 'crocks' and 'just basic nursing care'). Professionalization refers to the process by which an occupation achieves such powers.

PROFESSIONALIZATION

The comparative approach which has been used so far in this chapter is useful because it identifies those characteristics which professions share and which distinguish them from other occupations. One limitation of this approach, however, is its inability to inform us about the origins of these characteristics and the order in which they were obtained. The comparative approach might suggest, for example, that society gave medical practitioners their status and power in recognition of their proven ability to save lives and promote health. In order to test such ideas an historical approach is used in the next section which deals firstly with the medical profession and then with the nursing profession.

The historical approach quickly dispenses with the idea that medical practitioners were the passive recipients of their professional powers. These powers were not given by a grateful society; rather they were achieved piecemeal by doctors applying pressure to a series of social institutions. The Voluntary Hospitals of the early nineteenth century, for example, were financed by local subscribers who received in exchange the right to nominate patients to a certain number of hospital beds. The honorary physicians and surgeons who gave their services to these hospitals, which were the only hospitals at the time, had no control over which patients were admitted. The subscribers tended to use their right to admit patients as a way of caring for their elderly relatives and dependants. The physicians and surgeons, however, were interested in patients whom they could use as teaching material, an activity from which they did derive income, and during the course of the nineteenth century they slowly wrested control of admissions policy from the lay subscribers. This measure of professional autonomy was first achieved by persuading the subscribers on humanitarian grounds that accidents and, later, emergencies could be admitted by medical staff without a subscriber's authority. The physicians and surgeons also obtained the subscribers' agreement to a policy of excluding certain categories of patients. The number of excluded categories increased as the century progressed and came to include all infectious diseases, terminal illnesses, pregnancy, children, all psychiatric conditions, mental handicap, epilepsy and the elderly. As a result of a prolonged diplomatic campaign, therefore, the physicians and surgeons obtained sufficient control over admissions policy to ensure that the patients in the voluntary hospitals reflected their interests rather than those of the subscribers (Abel-Smith 1964).

The campaign which achieved professional monopoly was almost as prolonged as that which gained autonomy in relation to hospital admissions policy. By the early nineteenth century a third type of medical practitioner, the apothecary-surgeon or 'general practitioner', was rising in importance to join the physicians and the surgeons. These three types of medical practitioners were united into a single occupational group, called doctors, by the 1858 Medical Act, which established the General Medical Council. This reform of the professional licensing system was neither forced on medical practitioners nor easily conceded to them. The 1858 Act was preceded by 16 unsuccessful Parliamentary bills which failed to become law, partly because of disagreements among their medical supporters but also because Parliament was sceptical about whether medical practitioners could be trusted with this professional monopoly (Peterson 1978). The legislation which was finally enacted did not give medical practitioners the legal monopoly for which they had long campaigned; the General Medical Council was empowered to keep a register of suitably trained practitioners, but unqualified practice was not made illegal. Nevertheless, registration became the basis of the profession's monopoly because an increasing number of employment opportunities were limited to those who were registered. In particular, Poor Law and Friendly Society appointments (of which more later) were restricted to General Medical Council registrants, who also increasingly became the chosen medical practitioners of the growing middle class. The profession's monopoly, therefore, was neither given nor was it complete; rather a sustained campaign by medical practitioners partially succeeded in enlisting the support of the state, and this was subsequently reinforced by the employment practices of local government, voluntary institutions and those private consumers who could afford their services.

Qualified medical practice before 1858 had always been vulnerable to competition from the unqualified who charged lower fees. This was inhibited by the 1858 Act, which thus strength-ened the doctors' market position, a development which was further enhanced when the output of qualified practitioners lagged behind the growth in the proportion of the population able to afford professional care (Waddington 1984). This relative shortage of doctors enabled them to press for further professional powers. The British Army, for example, had refused to grant full officer status to its doctors, who resented the automatic precedence of all combatant officers over them and such slights to their officer status as not being saluted by barrack sentries, having to be dismounted on parade and having to make private arrangements for the grooming of their horses. In 1896 the British Medical Association responded to these longstanding grievances by securing the agreement of medical school deans to actively discourage their students from apply-ing for army posts. As a result of this boycott the army quickly resolved these grievances to the doctors' satisfaction (Cantlie 1973).

At the same time as the doctors were organizing to raise their status within the British Army, they were also engaged in 'the battle of the clubs' for increased autonomy over their working-class patients. These 'clubs', Friendly Societies and, later, some trade union branches, were orga-nizations of, predominantly, working men which offered insurance protection against sickness and death. In order to prevent abuse of the sickness benefit, they hired doctors to certify inca-pacity for work (see Chapter 13) and these duties were gradually extended to include the full range of general practitioner care. By the end of the nineteenth century, Friendly Societies cov-ered more than 4 million members of the working class and employed at least 50% of general practitioners on a full- or part-time basis. Each 'club' tended to employ only one doctor who was responsible to the club's committee and whom all the club's members had to consult. The doc-tors generally disliked supervision by their collective patients, in the form of the club's elected committee, and they particularly disliked the right of dissatisfied patients to complain to the committee, thus risking their employment and the loss of all their patients, not just the aggrieved party. They organized a boycott similar to the one which had recently been successful against the British Army, but lack of solidarity in their ranks frustrated this attempt to increase their auton-omy. The balance of power between the doctors and the 'clubs' of their working-class patients was only altered in the doctors' favour by the 1911 National Health Insurance Act. This act 'nationalized' many of the functions of the Friendly Societies and placed their administration in the hands of local health committees which contained strong medical representation. This degree of medical control was only conceded to doctors in response to persuasive lobbying and the British Medical Association's threat of non-co-operation with the new scheme; the original bill had left control of medical benefit with the Friendly Societies (Honigsbaum 1979). The 1911 Act thus freed general practitioners from any immediate control by these patients, an extension of their autonomy which was not given to doctors but was achieved by them through influenc-ing the state (see Chapter 14).

Two additional points need to be made about these four episodes in the professionalization of medicine. First, success in each case was accompanied by an increase in income. Achieving con-trol of hospital admissions policy allowed physicians and surgeons to select cases for teaching their fee-paying students and for investigating the type of diseases most likely to be seen in fee-paying patients. Achieving registration in 1858 removed much low priced competition and gave relative scarcity value to qualified practitioners. The achievement of full officer status in the British Army in 1898 was accompanied by increased remuneration; and the increase in autonomy which resulted from the 1911 Act was accompanied by a 75% increase in the capitation fee and full reimbursement of the cost of all medicines and drugs. Second, and more importantly perhaps, the acquisition of these professional powers occurred before doctors had the means to alter the course of most diseases to any significant extent (see Chapter 1). Doctors, of course, already had a body of specialized knowledge, but it rarely achieved great success when applied. The development of more effective knowledge came later; it was produced by a health care system over which doctors had already achieved considerable professional control, and it involved an increasingly elaborate division of labour within, particularly, the hospital sector of this system.

Nursing and paramedical staff

Until recently, most general practitioners worked on their own, often with their wives acting as receptionist, chaperone and filing clerk. Only since the mid-1960s has a form of primary care developed in which general practitioners are supported by practice nurses and clerical staff and integrate their work with health visitors, midwives and specialist community nurses (Jefferys and Sachs 1983). The development of a similarly complex division of labour started at a much earlier date in hospitals. In the early voluntary hospitals, medical practitioners, most often apothecary-surgeons, performed much of the skilled care of patients, for example distributing medicines, dressing wounds and monitoring the patient's state. Their only assistants were domestic servants who received no more training than other domestic servants and who performed normal domestic duties in exchange for little more than their own subsistance (Davies 1980). From the middle of the nineteenth century this division of labour began to change under the influence of reformers such as Fry and Nightingale who established a grade of trained nurses and schools of nursing in which to train them. These trained nurses were inserted into the division of labour between the doctors and the nurse–domestics, and they increasingly undertook much of the work at the ward level which had formerly been performed by the apothecary-surgeons. The combination of training and skilled work formed the basis of the professionalization of nursing, a process which continued with the formation of a national professional body, the College of Nursing, in 1916 and state registration in 1918 (Abel-Smith 1960). The new occupation of trained nursing thus adopted a similar form of organization to that which was proving advantageous to medical practitioners.

In contrast to the experience of doctors, however, the professionalization of nursing achieved relatively small increases in autonomy and remuneration. Low pay remains endemic and, although the chain of command lies within the profession, the content of nurses' work is still largely determined from outside (i.e. by doctors). The professionalization of nursing, therefore, demonstrates that those characteristics of a profession which were listed earlier do not necessarily go together, and that the advantages of professionalization do not inevitably follow the adoption of its organizational form (Dingwall et al. 1988). Several explanations have been offered for this comparative failure. One stresses nursing's lack of a distinctive body of specialized knowledge and its dependence on medicine in this respect. Another points to the relatively weak monopoly which has been achieved, which allows the shortage of registered nurses to be met by the recruitment of less qualified enrolled nurses and nursing auxiliaries rather than by an improvement in the position of the fully qualified. Finally, it has been suggested that the professionalization of medicine succeeded because it was the first profession to develop within the nineteenth century's rapidly expanding health-care sector, and that the subsequent professionalization of other occupations within this sector was limited by medicine's already established dominance. The former two types of explanation underlie the efforts, particularly of those who are based in the schools of nursing, to encourage research and university degree courses, and hence the development of a distinctive body of knowledge. The latter type of explanation fits better with the behaviour of those who value their profession as a source of training and qualifications, but who turn to trade unions in order to achieve the benefits which professionalization promised but seems unable to deliver. Both strategies, however, are likely to face similar problems. As a largely female work-force confronting a predominantly male medical profession and administrative civil service, nurses may be met by assumptions of superiority and the belief that women do not need to be paid a 'family wage'. In addition, nursing staff are the largest group employed within medical care (Table 15.1). For the employers, conceding to nurses the salary levels which are normal in most other professions would have far greater cost implications than those which were involved in the professionalization of doctors.

TABLE 15.1 *NHS staff in post by main staff group (WTEs) 1981–89.*

Main group of staff	1981	1985	1987	1989	% change 1981–91
Nursing and midwifery	47.5	49.3	50.6	50.9	3.5
Medical and dental	5.0	5.3	5.4	5.8	12.7
All professional and technical	7.9	9.1	9.9	10.2	24.4
Maintenance and works	3.3	3.2	3.0	2.7	−22.1
Ancillary	20.9	17.1	14.4	12.9	−40.5
Admin. and clerical	13.2	13.7	14.3	15.2	11.6
Ambulance	2.2	2.2	2.4	2.4	3.5
Total	824 400	812 900	799 300	796 000	−3.4
%	100	100	100	100	

Reprinted by permission of Addison Wesley Longman Ltd from Allsop (1995).

Since the mid-nineteenth century, many other occupations within the health-care sector have shared nursing's experience of professionalization. Ophthalmic opticians, health visitors, midwives, medical laboratory scientific officers, pharmacists, physiotherapists, radiographers and chiropodists have all sought to develop their knowledge base, extend control over their work situation and obtain state registration. These developments, however, have been negotiated within a division of labour already dominated by the medical profession and, although they have redrawn the boundaries between these occupations, they have not equalized all the parties involved. It seems relevant to distinguish between those professions which develop within an already established division of labour and those which are agents of the division of labour itself. Occupations such as social work and clinical psychology are exceptions to this general rule, in the sense that they possess a knowledge base which owes little to medicine and which is distinctively their own. They work alongside medicine but are not part of its division of labour, and they can thus claim professional equality with it. In practice, however, the medical profession has proved resistant to this claim. Social workers have obtained an employment base in the local authorities, rather than the health-care sector, in order to maintain their professional autonomy in relation to doctors (Stacey 1988).

The four episodes in the professionalization of medicine, together with the brief consideration of this process within other health-care occupations, suggest certain generalizations. First, the professional characteristics which have been identified by means of the comparative approach are not obtained en bloc by an occupation; rather they are obtained piecemeal in a variety of specific historical situations. Second, these characteristics are not given to an occupation; they are fought for and won by its members, often only after a protracted struggle. Third, knowledge plays a complex role in this process. The claim to a body of specialized knowledge and the establishment of training institutions to pass on this knowledge would seem to be preconditions for professionalization. It does not appear to be necessary, however, for this knowledge to be effective and, in the case of medicine at least, therapeutic effectiveness was a consequence rather than a precondition of professionalization. Fourth, the acquisition of status and income which accompanies professionalization means that it involves a form of occupational upward social mobility which is in contrast to the more usual movement of individuals between social classes. Finally, professional powers are achieved by an occupation through negotiations with the relevant powers-that-be. In the case of medicine these were the state and institutional employers, whereas in the case of the other professional occupations within health care the powers-that-be included the already established medical profession. In the latter case there was less room for occupational improvement through professionalization and trade unionism has subsequently developed as part of a combined occupational strategy.

EFFECTS OF PROFESSIONS

The nature and effects of professions have recently become issues within the policy debate about the provision of health care. The dynamic nature of professionalization implies that an occupation's professional status is not guaranteed for all time and that the level of its professional powers can change. The rising cost of medical care has raised a fear among those who finance this sector that these costs will grow exponentially. The growing involvement of large industrial and financial corporations in hospital construction, instrument manufacture, pharmaceutical production and medical insurance introduces powerful new vested interests into the provision of medical care. Lastly, rising rates of litigation against doctors and protests, such as that by the women's movement against high rates of induced labour, suggest that patients are becoming less deferential. It is thus possible to see the medical profession's autonomy increasingly limited by managerial attempts to control costs, by capital's attempts to ensure profitability and by patients' attempts to shape their own medical care. These changes can be clearly seen in the USA (Light and Levine 1988), where managerial attempts to control costs seem to be having the most immediate impact. Similar developments are discernible in Britain. Many members of the medical profession believe that the health care reforms of the 1990s (see Chapters 14 and 19) have increased management's powers at their expense. In this context, it is useful to attempt a balance sheet of the effects of professionalization.

From the point of view of consumers of health services, professions have the great advantage of guaranteeing the qualifications, and thereby hopefully the knowledge, of those who are registered. The General Medical Council register was established because 'it is expedient that persons requiring medical aid should be enabled to distinguish qualified from unqualified practitioners' (General Medical Council 1980). The ability to make this distinction is equally useful to both individual patients and employers such as health authorities. Similarly advantageous is a profession's code of ethics, which constrains exploitative behaviour on the part of the professional and provides some redress if this nevertheless occurs. Any assessment of professions, however, needs to balance these advantages against other less desirable effects.

Team work

Modern health care involves the work of many different occupations, among whom doctors form a small minority and nurses are the largest group (Table 15.1). The way in which their work is integrated is of considerable importance to patient care. Two models of integration can be seen. One type involves a decision-maker who gives instructions that are carried out by the other participants. This model is appropriate in emergency situations such as a cardiac arrest. In other situations this hierarchical model can be counterproductive because it inhibits the upward flow of information and ideas about patients whose health is changing more slowly. In these situations the model of a team is more appropriate. Although the team may include a final decision-maker, team decisions are made only after an open and equal discussion between its members. The earlier sections of this chapter have indicated that the professionalization of health care has tended to lock integration into the hierarchical model. This historical legacy is in conflict with the growing predominance of chronic diseases for whose care the team model is more appropriate. The logic of many doctors' work therefore drives them to try to create a team approach in a situation where each participant's primary loyalty is to their own profession and relations between these participants reflect the established interprofessional hierarchy. Success in this endeavour tends to depend more on the personal characteristics of those involved than on institutional arrangements, and such teams are always vulnerable to disintegration, with their members drawing back into their traditional professional roles and interprofessional relationships (Beales 1978). Although this problem affects most parts of health care, it is particularly important in relation to the community-care programme which depends on co-ordination of health services and the personal social services provided by local authorities (see Chapter 16). As has already been mentioned, social workers have maintained their professional autonomy in relation to doctors by obtaining separate employment in local authorities rather than the health service. The success of the community care programme, therefore, depends in part on doctors and social workers reconciling their different approaches and establishing a modus vivendi which respects the autonomy of both professions.

Communication with patients

A second unfortunate consequence of health care's professionalized work-force is the power imbalance it creates between the professionals and their patients (see Chapter 4). A number of elements contribute to this imbalance. Professionals usually possess greater medical knowledge than their patients. Second, there is a difference in control over resources, with the doctor being the patient's sole point of access to desired goods such as prescribed medication, sickness benefit and medical care. Finally, there is often a difference in social class and gender, with most doctors being middle-class men and the largest group of patients being working-class women. These differences come from, respectively, the profession's specialized knowledge, state monopoly and status. In some situations these differences may be small, for example, where the patient possesses considerable medical knowledge. In general, however, they combine to produce a marked inequality in power between doctor and patient, which is likely to interfere with effective communication between them.

Sometimes this inequality can be justified clinically in terms of facilitating prompt emergency treatment, although even in these cases the patient's informed consent is usually necessary, which requires effective communication. In general, however, patients prefer a consultation style which has been described as 'mutual participation', in which the doctor listens to the patient, encourages the patient's questions and answers them comprehensibly. This more equal relationship between doctor and patient is necessary in many clinical situations, particularly those which involve the management of chronic diseases. Good clinical practice often requires doctors to learn subtle communication skills to overcome barriers to effective communication which themselves are derived from doctors' own collective efforts towards professionalization.

Medical priorities

Control over priorities within health care is a third aspect of professionalization which needs to be considered. It is widely acknowledged that the so-called 'Cinderella services' provide relatively poor care to certain categories of patients – in particular, those who are mentally or physically handicapped, terminally ill, elderly infirm or suffering from chronic psychiatric conditions. This relative neglect is often explained in terms of the values of the wider social system and its impact on health care. This explanation, however, ignores the history of the professionalization of medicine which has already been described. The eventually successful struggle by physicians and surgeons to control hospital-admissions policy resulted in the exclusion of precisely those categories of patients which are now confined to the Cinderella services. There would appear to be a coincidence of interests between the economic system, which values productive workers, and the medical profession which values acute diseases offering the prospect of successful treatment. The profession's interest in acute diseases is based on their traditional employment as curers of the sick, but their professional autonomy over health care allows this interest to shape the whole of the health-care system. A second example of this power can be seen in the health-care system's emphasis on the diagnosis and treatment of disease, rather than the study of its causes and prevention.

Alternative medicine

A final questionable aspect of professionalization concerns its monopoly and consequent power to marginalize rival forms of therapeutic practice. As has been described, the 1858 Medical Act effectively discriminated against unqualified practitioners; some of these were undoubtedly opportunistic quacks, but among their number were also practitioners of other therapeutic traditions. These alternative forms of medical treatment continue to be denigrated by most members of the established medical profession, and treatment by their practitioners has been excluded from the state-financed health-care system. Psychoanalysis and osteopathy are examples of such excluded forms of therapy, as are Vedic and Chinese medicine, to which many recent immigrants from these cultures remain committed. Homeopathy is one partial exception to this general rule. Possibly because of the Royal Family's support for this form of therapy, the National Health Service contains one homeopathic hospital. The professionalization of medicine thus allowed its practitioners' hostility towards alternative therapies to be translated into the marginalization and exclusion of their rivals. In some instances the counterproductive nature of this reflex is, in retrospect, accepted even by the medical profession; for example, the profession's slow acceptance of the germ theory of disease was probably due to Pasteur's position outside the profession as an agricultural biochemist.

Challenges to Medicine

Writers in the 1990s have sometimes maintained that medicine's traditional dominance in the health-care field is increasingly under threat. There are signs, for example, that professional strategies to marginalize and exclude practitioners of alternative medicine are giving way to strategies of 'cooptation' as members of the public consult them in greater numbers. This willingness on people's part to turn to alternative therapists is said to be but one indication of a general decline in the status and authority of medicine and of doctors. Some have characterized this process of decline in terms of a 'proletarianization' or 'de-professionalization' of medicine.

The proletarianization thesis proferred by some Marxists, notably in the USA, contends that doctors are being progressively incorporated into a factory-like system of production and are in consequence experiencing a loss of autonomy and skills. More specifically, they are surrendering control over (1) criteria for recruitment, (2) content of training, (3) terms and content of work, (4) objects of labour (e.g. clients served), (5) tools of labour (e.g. equipment and drugs), (6) means of labour (e.g. premises), and (7) amount and rate of remuneration. Fundamental to this contention is the view that medicine is becoming subordinated to the more general requirements of production under advanced capitalism. One general criticism of this controversial thesis is that its acceptance seems to presuppose the growing proletarianization of virtually the whole labour force in contemporary capitalist societies. Moreover it is sometimes unclear precisely what is meant by 'proletarianization' (Elston 1991).

The de-professionalization thesis too has its origins in the USA. Whereas the proletarianization thesis emphasizes the changing work conditions of doctors, the deprofessionalization thesis stresses changes in the relations between doctors and patients. Its advocates argue that the increased 'rationalization' of medical knowledge and practice – for example through computerization – and enhanced lay knowledge about health have undermined the cultural authority of medicine and weakened its monopoly over health-related knowledge. The public, it is claimed, are more critical than hitherto of the paternalism of professional experts. Although more limited in scope and ambition than the proletarianization thesis, the de-professionalization thesis arguably shares some of its deficiencies: clear definitions are sometimes lacking, it is pitched at a very general level, and it appears as yet to have little unambiguous empirical support (Elston 1991).

Alaszewski (1996) offers an early assessment of the impact of the newly introduced internal market in the NHS on both the medical and nursing professions. The medical profession, he suggests, has attempted to secure some of the benefits of its market position while protecting itself from the competitive aspects of the market. He argues that doctors now face a clear choice: they either become 'players' in an internal market, or they accept 'managerial protection' at the expense of some autonomy. As far as nursing is concerned, he maintains that the authority and status of ward nurses is being enhanced, especially with the development of the new technology of nursing and of the ward manager role. Although the dependence of ward nurses on senior nurse managers and doctors is declining, it is however being replaced with increased control and scrutiny by general managers.

Johnson (1996) has recently developed a quite different approach to the health professions. Drawing on the work of Foucault (see Chapter 12), he rejects the clear distinction between the state on the one hand, and the professions on the other. He argues that modern professions like medicine developed in association with the process of what Foucault calls 'governmentality', in other words, as part of the apparatus of the state. 'The success of medical professionals in constructing a social reality with universal validity', he writes, 'is a consequence of their official recognition as experts. The point at which technical autonomy is established is the very same point at which professional practice is indistinguishable from the state; part and parcel of governmentality'. It follows from this analysis that professions become what Johnson terms 'socio-technical devices' through which the means, and perhaps the ends, of government are expressed. It is in this context that the recent health reforms, together with their impacts on the health professions, must be understood. Further time and research will show the advantages and disadvantages of this distinctive theoretical approach.

CONCLUSIONS

The health care available to patients has been profoundly influenced by the struggles of its providers to increase their authority, status and income. The success of medical practitioners in this respect encouraged other occupations within health care to emulate their strategy, producing a highly professionalized work-force. Patients have benefited from this process in terms of the competence and ethical behaviour of those who care for them, but they may suffer as the result of other effects such as poor team-work, poor communication between themselves and professionals, priorities which reflect professional interests rather than their needs and limitations on the range of treatments available to them.

These disadvantages of professionalization may also handicap conscientious professionals in the performance of their work; for example, when they struggle to integrate the work of a multi-professional team in order to provide effective care, when they coax patients to overcome their diffidence in order to obtain a full account of what is wrong with them, or when they attempt to deal with the financial problems consequent on a patient's need for psychoanalysis. Such problems are endemic in the present organization of health care and individual professionals have little choice but to learn new skills in order to overcome them. In the longer term, however, individual solutions rarely form a satisfactory response to structural problems. The earlier sections of this chapter described how the contemporary structure of health care has its roots in the nineteenth century when its development was part of, and took place in the context of, rapid and profound change in the wider society. On this basis it can be suggested that any major change in health care will depend on a similar period of wider social change.

REFERENCES

Abel-Smith, B. (1960) *A History of the Nursing Profession*. London: Heinemann.

Abel-Smith, B. (1964) *The Hospitals 1800–1948*. London: Heinemann.

Alaszewski, A. (1996) Restructuring health and welfare professions in the United Kingdom: the impact of internal markets on the medical, nursing and social work professions. In: *Health Professions and the State in Europe*, ed. T. Johnson, G. Larkin & M. Saks. London: Routledge.

Allsop, J. (1995) *Health Policy and the NHS*, 2nd edn. London: Longman.

Beales, J. (1978) *Sick Health Centres and How to Make Them Better*. Tunbridge Wells: Pitman Medical.

Becker, H., Greer, B., Hughes, E. & Strauss, A. (1961) *Boys in White*. Chicago, IL: University of Chicago Press.

Cantlie, N. (1973) *A History of the Army Medical Department*, Vol. 2. London: Churchill Livingstone.

Carr-Saunders, A.M. & Wilson, P.A. (1933) *The Professions*. Oxford: Clarendon Press.

Davies, C. (1980) *Rewriting Nursing History*. London: Croom Helm.

Department of Health (1989) *Health and Personal Social Services Statistics for England*. London: HMSO.

Dingwall, R., Rafferty, A.M. & Webster, C. (1988) *An Introduction to the Social History of Nursing*. London: Routledge.

Elston, M.A. (1991) The politics of professional power: medicine in a changing health service. In: *The Sociology of the Health Service*, ed. J. Gabe, M. Calnan & M. Bury. London: Routledge.

Freidson, E. (1970) *Profession of Medicine*. New York: Dodds, Mead & Co.

General Medical Council (1980) *Constitution and Functions*. London: GMC.

Honigsbaum, F. (1979) *The Division in British Medicine*. London: Kegan Page.

Jefferys, M. & Sachs, H. (1983) *Rethinking General Practice*. London: Tavistock.

Johnson, T (1996) Governmentality and the institutionalization of expertise. In: *Health Professions and the State in Europe*, ed. T. Johnson, G. Larkin & M. Saks. London: Routledge.

Light, D. & Levine, S. (1988) The changing character of the medical profession: a theoretical overview. *Millbank Q.*, **6**, 10–32.

Melia, K. (1987) *Learning and Working*. London: Tavistock.

Merton, R.K., Reader, K. & Kendall, P.L. (1957) *The Student-Physician*. Cambridge, MA: Harvard University Press.

Peterson, M.J. (1978) *The Medical Profession in Mid-Victorian London*. San Francisco: University of California Press.

Stacey, M. (1988) *The Sociology of Health and Healing*. London: Unwin Hyman.

Waddington, I. (1984) *The Medical Profession in the Industrial Revolution*. London: Gill and McMillan.

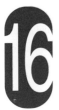

Community and Continuing Care Outside Hospitals

NICHOLAS MAYS

Community care has been the goal of government policy in the UK since the late 1950s for the care of the elderly, the chronically ill, people with learning difficulties and other dependent groups. The aspiration of a series of governments has been to alter the emphasis of care for these people from institutional to community-based or home-based (domiciliary) settings. Although it has been acknowledged that there will always be a core of people who require long-term institutional care because of their frailty or social circumstances (DHSS 1981a), for the vast majority community care has been seen as a solution to the many problems associated with long-term care in institutions (Hunter, 1993) (see Chapter 5). An important element in the durability of the policy and in its appeal to successive governments lies in the fact that it appears self-evidently good and humane. Yet, on closer inspection, the meaning and objectives of a policy of community care are surrounded by considerable confusion and ambiguity.

In a very broad sense, the term community care is attractive because it sums up our aspirations towards a society in which close-knit, supportive social relations exist to support dependent people, but, as Jones and colleagues have pointed out, in practice community care can mean very different things to different people:

To the politician it is a useful piece of rhetoric; to the sociologist it is a stick to beat institutional care with; to the civil servant it is a cheap alternative to institutional care which can be passed to the local authorities for action or inaction; to the visionary it is a dream of the new society in which people really do care; to social services departments it is a nightmare of heightened public expectations and inadequate resources to meet them. We are only just beginning to find out what it means to the old, the chronic sick and the handicapped (Jones et al. 1978).

WHAT IS COMMUNITY CARE?

It is helpful to start by attempting to define what is meant by community care. Unfortunately, as the above quotation from Jones et al. (1978) makes plain, there is no single definition of the term. For some people community care is no more than residential care outside a major institution. For others it includes enabling dependent people to participate as fully as possible in normal life. There is an important distinction between the use of the term as a prescription for how people should meet the health and social needs of dependent people, and as a description of a set of services which are currently provided. As a description of services, the term community care is generally used today to refer to those health and social services which provide professional and quasi-professional help as an alternative to large-scale residential or institutional care including hospitals. However, when used prescriptively, the emphasis in official statements of community care policy has altered over time. In the 1950s, 1960s and early 1970s, government policy statements implied that community care consisted mainly of formal domiciliary services provided primarily by staff employed by local authorities. By the mid-1970s the term had expanded, confusingly, to include other services such as day hospitals, hostels and even residential homes. Whatever the precise definition, the emphasis in this period was on formal care in the community. After 1979, when the Conservative Party was elected to office, public services were still discussed, but there was a far greater emphasis in policy documents on an ideal of care by the community; that is, care by family, relatives, neighbours and friends and by voluntary organizations (DHSS 1981b).

THE JUSTIFICATION FOR COMMUNITY CARE

The policy of community care and the desire to reduce the use of institutions and enable vulnerable groups to live an ordinary life has been sustained since the 1950s, firstly, by a belief that community care (however defined) is better than the alternative. This view was prompted and underpinned by a number of influential research studies carried out in the UK and the USA in the 1950s and 1960s, which showed the failure of a variety of institutional settings to meet the emotional, social or physical needs of their inmates and, in some cases, actively to worsen residents' disabilities. In Britain, Townsend (1962) concluded that residential homes for the elderly should be replaced by a different form of help and support which would enable residents to maintain their dignity and independence. In the USA, Goffman (1961) argued that long-stay hospitals for the mentally ill bore many of the characteristics of 'total institutions', in which inmates were separated from the rest of society and managed according to depersonalizing 'batch processes' which, over time, led to a reorganized conception of self subordinate to the requirements of the institution. This debilitating process has been referred to as 'institutionalization', sometimes resulting in 'institutional neurosis' (Barton 1959), and was regarded as incompatible with any possibility of rehabilitation and return to ordinary life (see Chapter 5).

Secondly, the critique of institutional care was stimulated in the UK in the late 1960s and early 1970s by a series of scandals in which cruelty and negligence by staff, together with poor living conditions and unstimulating care regimes, were revealed at a number of long-stay hospitals. A third factor, favouring a policy of community care specifically for the mentally ill, was the development of new psychotropic drugs which could help control some of the more severe symptoms of mental illness and which facilitated the care of patients outside custodial settings. However, this cannot be the clinching explanation since the first bed reductions in UK asylums *preceded* the introduction of these drugs and the effectiveness of psychotropic drugs for community living tends to have been overstated (Busfield 1986). Prior (1991) argues that the shift in mental health care owed more to a change in psychiatric thinking. His argument is that during the 1950s psychiatrists began to focus more on the *behaviour* of their patients and less on their *illnesses*. The best place to observe and produce normal behaviour was in normal settings outside the institution.

From the point of view of the government, community care offered additional attractions since the long-stay hospitals periodically suffered difficulties in recruiting nursing staff and were mainly Victorian institutions which were beginning to require major programmes of maintenance and modernization. The belief that community care might be not only better but also cheaper than institutional care, although far from proven, has attracted successive governments anxious to limit public expenditure.

THE DEVELOPMENT OF COMMUNITY CARE POLICY

The policy of achieving care within community settings began with mentally ill people during the 1950s. The 1959 Mental Health Act set course towards a comprehensive community care service for people with mental illness, with hospital care reserved for acute episodes and a small number of severe cases which, in essence, has remained the line ever since. The 1962 Hospital Plan proposed a massive programme of closures of Victorian psychiatric hospitals with the aim of halving the number of beds by 1975 and locating acute psychiatric care away from the long-stay institutions (Ministry of Health 1962).

During the 1960s, community care principles were gradually extended to other dependent groups. In the 1970s, a series of official policy documents stressed the development of local community-based alternatives to institutional care, better domiciliary services and the importance of joint planning between the local authority and the local health services to meet the needs of elderly, physically handicapped, mentally ill and mentally handicapped people. Specific targets were set by central government, for example, to reduce the number of hospital beds, to build up small-scale hostels and to train staff in the community and increase domiciliary services. However, the needs and problems faced by each client group varied.

Progress towards community care

How successful were the succession of official documents and plans in shifting the balance of care from large-scale, institutional provision towards the range of provision labelled 'community care?'

In 1986, the Audit Commission, an independent body set up by an Act of Parliament to assess the efficiency and effectiveness of local authority and NHS services, investigated the extent to which there had been a change in the balance of care, and, most notably, replacement of institutional care by community care in the previous 15 years. The Commission concluded that progress had been limited (Audit Commission 1986). For example, domiciliary services for the elderly were struggling to keep up with the increasing proportion of the very elderly. There had been a decrease in reliance on long-stay hospital care for the elderly, but this had been more than offset by a rapid increase in private residential care funded out of social security board-and-lodging payments for which elderly people with low income were eligible. There had been much more progress in ensuring that mentally handicapped people were cared for in 'normal' settings outside hospital, most often under the care of the local social services. This was possibly because of a perception that the risks of community care for this group were lower and because of a higher level of public acceptability. There had been very limited progress towards the targets of provision outside hospital for mentally ill people and of day care for mentally handicapped people (now generally known as 'people with learning difficulties'):

> The result is poor value for money. Too many people are cared for in settings costing over £200 a week when they would receive a more appropriate care in the community at a total cost to public funds of £100–£130 a week. Conversely, people in the community may not be getting the support they need (Audit Commission 1986).

The Commission argued that more flexible, cost-effective alternatives to institutional provision were underdeveloped. There was some research evidence from experiments to support this view, showing, for example, that even very frail elderly people could be maintained at home with carefully organized domiciliary support at lower cost than for residential care (Challis and Davies 1986).

The continued dominance of institutional care in the spectrum of formal, professionally provided services for dependent people, despite 30 years of community care policies, was vividly shown in a study of six districts in England in the late 1980s. When spending on acute health services and general practice was excluded from the calculation, as much as 73% of the remaining health and social services expenditure by the Health Service and the local authorities was still devoted to institutional care of one kind or another (Gray et al. 1988). There was also considerable variation between the districts in how much was spent on community care, which appeared to be unrelated to the needs of the locality. Furthermore, there was no evidence that areas which spent little on institutional care spent more on community care or vice versa (Hudson 1987).

PROBLEMS IN IMPLEMENTING COMMUNITY CARE

How can we explain the gap between policy statements and the reality of what has been provided? There have been two main types of obstacle to community care implementation: a lack of resources; and managerial difficulties. The Audit Commission (1986) identified the following problems in more detail:

1. a mismatch between the resources made available and the aims of policy;

2. a lack of 'bridging' finance to enable a simultaneous run-down of institutions and development of community care;
3. the perverse incentive towards institutional care created by the availability without limit of social security board-and-lodging payments, while local authority domiciliary care was strictly cash-limited;
4. organizational fragmentation and confusion between the National Health Service (NHS), the local authority social services and housing departments and the social security system in their responsibility for community care; and
5. inadequate arrangements for training staff to work in community care settings.

The policy of attempting to close old, long-stay, mental illness hospitals exemplified many of these financial and managerial problems. It proved very difficult to close hospitals and transfer resources and personnel into community care without additional finance in the form of 'bridging' loans. This was because resources could not be released, except in a small way, from hospitals until all the patients had been transferred to alternative care; and, in turn, the discharge of patients could not occur until resources were available for community care. However, in the later 1980 and 1990s the process of closing long-stay psychiatric hospitals accelerated and whole NHS hospitals were closed.

The intention was that many of the consequences of closing long-stay institutions in the NHS would be met by the local authorities, which were expected to provide community care alternatives to hospitalization. This required close co-operation between the local authority and the local health authority in the form of joint planning and, ultimately, a substantial transfer of resources from the NHS to the local authorities. In practice, health authorities have proved reluctant to pass funds to the local authorities. This reluctance has been exacerbated by differences in working style, priorities, organization and systems of accountability between doctors, nurses, social workers, occupational therapists, housing managers, home-help organizers and all the other staff involved in caring for dependent groups in the NHS and in local authorities.

In the case of closing mental illness hospitals as opposed to mental handicap hospitals, there has also been powerful resistance from sections of the medical and nursing professions to government policy for a variety of reasons: least laudably, out of professional self-interest and an unwillingness to surrender power to local authority staff; and more appropriately, perhaps, from a genuine belief in the continuing need for places of 'asylum' or refuge for chronically ill people and a fear that adequate community care support would not be forthcoming, leaving vulnerable people to fend for themselves in a harsh environment. More and more of the prison population and of the homeless on the streets of the big cities are former patients of long-stay hospitals. The anxieties of psychiatrists are reinforced by evidence that society as a whole is at best ambivalent, and at worst hostile, to the idea of the mentally ill living outside hospitals. There have been a series of cases in which the fear and stigma attached to mental illness have united the community in campaigns to exclude former mental patients from participation in ordinary patterns of living (see below for further instances of problems with community care for people with mental health problems). These obstacles appear to have been far less prevalent in the case of people with learning difficulties living in the community.

INFORMAL CARE

The preoccupation of public policy towards dependent groups with getting people out of hospitals risks obscuring the fact that the vast majority have always lived outside institutions, cared for informally at home, usually by family, relatives or friends (see Chapter 11).

The scale of informal care

The 1990 General Household Survey revealed that 17% of women and 13% of men said they were looking after, or providing some regular service for, someone who was sick, elderly or handicapped. When applied to the population of Britain, this suggests a total of about 6.8 million carers, of whom about 1.7 million were heavily involved in care, providing at least 20 hours care per week either to someone living with them or in another household (Social Policy Research Unit 1994). It was estimated that this volume of unpaid care would have cost between £35 billion and £40 billion a year in 1993 if it had been provided by the state (Nuttall et al. 1993). This dwarfs the £10 billion contribution to community care from formal health and social services.

About 80% of informal carers help with tasks such as cooking, shopping and gardening; 45% provide nursing care and physical help; and about 20% offer help with personal care such as washing and toileting. Women carers are more likely to be involved with intimate tasks and physical help than are male carers (see Chapter 9).

Who provides informal care?

> 'Care is socially divided between the state and the family and between family members. In practice "community care" is overwhelmingly care by kin, and especially female kin, not the community' (Walker 1982: 23).

Care by the community tends to be based primarily on kinship obligations between the immediate family (e.g. daughters caring for fathers and mothers), with a limited contribution from 'moral communities' such as churches and ethnic groups (Abrams 1980). Care from neighbours is relatively rare. The chances of being a carer are not only increased for women, they also increase with age. It is not uncommon for an elderly person to be responsible for the care of someone far older than themselves.

The relationship between formal and informal care

Only a relatively small amount of help is received by informal carers from the statutory agencies, although it can be crucial in assisting a carer to cope. For example, the General Household Survey (Green 1988) shows that two-thirds of carers who look after a dependent person in the same household receive no regular visits from any formal services. State policies for allocating formal services tend to hinge on the assumption that it is natural for family members, which means in practice women, to provide care for others. The notion of 'natural' family care assumes that the dependent person lives with or near their family and that the family is itself stable and has an able-bodied woman at home supported financially by a husband at work. This applies to only about 15% of contemporary families. State interference in 'natural' caring has thus been regarded as potentially harmful and, as a result, providing support for carers has not been a priority of policy. Indeed, services are frequently withheld on the grounds that a dependent person has help from relatives. For example, an elderly person living alone or living with a spouse is much more likely to receive the services of a home help or meals-on-wheels regardless of the degree of dependency than if they live with other family members (Parker 1990). This approach to rationing formal care is liable to penalize women who take on primary responsibility for unpaid caring rather than complementing what informal carers can offer.

The costs of caring

Official community care policy has tended to ignore the financial and social costs to families of caring. As a consequence, informal care can appear very cheap. However, it has become apparent that the true costs are disproportionately borne by informal carers themselves. For example, combining paid employment with informal caring responsibilities in the absence of financial or practical recognition by the state of the costs of caring, can impose great financial, physical and psychological strains on carers and also on their immediate families (Table 16.1). About 42% of lay carers who care for at least 20 hours per week also have a paid job (Henwood 1990). The relatively private, and therefore invisible, daily grind of physical and emotional caring has now been vividly documented in a number of studies (e.g. Nissel and Bonnerjea 1982; Finch and Groves 1983; Parker 1990). Although respite care is now accepted as an integral part of support to informal carers in the community, it is frequently in short supply.

Financial support from the state to informal carers in the UK is also very restricted and low in comparison with other European countries (Glendinning and McLaughlin 1993). The Invalid Care Allowance (ICA) dominates. It is available to low earning people who spend at least 35 hours a week caring for a person who receives the Disability Living Allowance. In 1995, the ICA was set at £34.50 per week. Since it is not possible to live on this level of income (about 10% of average earnings), carers have to rely on other forms of support.

TABLE 16.1 *Effect on the immediate family of caring for a mentally ill adult at home.*

Aspect of family life	% of families	
	Some disturbance	Severe disturbance
Health of closest relatives		
Mental	40	20
Physical	28	—
Bringing up children	24	10
Domestic routine	13	16
Income	14	9
Employment (other than the mentally ill person)	17	6

Source: Sainsbury and Grad de Alarcon (1974).

Trends in informal care

In the future, there will be larger numbers of people living in the community who need care and support, but there may well be fewer people available to provide it. A combination of smaller families, a decline in the proportion of single women, who comprised the traditional recruits to care giving in the population, increased female participation in the labour market and greater geographical mobility, will all limit the extent to which families can care for their dependent members without formal help from outside. The tensions between paid work and unpaid caring, for women particularly, are likely to intensify because of a reduction in the number of younger entrants to the labour market and a rising demand for women's labour. Hence recent concerns about paying for long-term care (see below).

ATTEMPTING TO MAKE A REALITY OF CARE IN THE COMMUNITY

The analysis of the Audit Commission (1986) had shown that community care policy, particularly for the elderly, had been seriously knocked off course during the 1980s by the perverse incentives generated by the open-ended availability of public funds from the social security system to help poorer elderly people in meeting fees in private residential and nursing home care. No such incentives existed to develop provision to support dependent people living in their own homes or in the public sector. As a result, it was likely that residential care was being used inappropriately in many cases. The cost to the taxpayer was mounting rapidly as places were filled (Fig. 16.1). Furthermore, in all areas of community care, there was uncertainty at local level as to where the responsibility for funding and organizing care lay between the Health Service and the local authority social services.

The Audit Commission's critical investigation of community care proposed a strategic review of the available options for the finance and organization of community care services. Ideally, according to the Commission, there should be a single budget for the care of each dependent client group managed by a single agency.

Fig. 16.1 *Nursing and residential care places for elderly, chronically ill and physically disabled people by sector, England, April 1967–95. The discontinuity in the number of long-stay NHS geriatric hospitals is due to changes in definition. ESMI, elderly severly mentally infirm; YPH, younger physically handicapped. Reproduced with permission of Laing and Buisson (1996).*

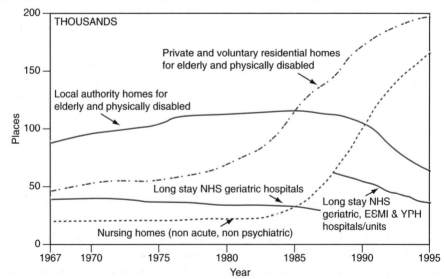

The Griffiths review of community care (1987–88)

In 1987, the government appointed Sir Roy Griffiths, the Deputy Chairman of the Sainsbury supermarket chain and, at that time, the government's chief adviser on health service management, to report on ways of making more effective use of the public funds available for community care of elderly people and people with mental health problems. Griffiths concluded that the respective roles of health authorities and local authority social services departments had to be clarified to avoid confusion and overlap and each should be made accountable for particular care groups and services (Griffiths 1988). Access to private residential homes should be controlled by the local authority on the basis of need to avoid unnecessary or inappropriate placement subsidized by social security payments. Overall, the Griffiths proposals meant a transfer of funds from central to local government and from health and social security to social services.

Caring for People (1989)

In response to the Griffiths report, the Conservative Government's plans called Caring for People defined the tasks of community care as 'providing the right level of intervention and support to enable people to achieve maximum independence and control over their own lives' (Secretaries of State for Health, Social Security, Wales and Scotland 1989). There were three main elements in the proposals:

1. The care element in the social security board-and-lodging payments to residents of private residential homes was to be transferred from social security to the local authorities, where it would form part of an overall budget to meet the costs of care in relation to need, irrespective of whether an individual was living at home or in a residential setting.
2. The local authorities were to become the lead agency in community care and appoint 'case managers' whose job was to assess the needs of individual clients, design appropriate packages of care for them, ensure that services were delivered and monitor their quality. Local authorities were to make the maximum use possible of the voluntary and commercial (private) sectors of care by contracting out provision to produce a cost-effective 'mixed market' or 'mixed economy' of services.
3. A specific grant was to be paid to NHS Regions, subject to central approval of a care plan, to enable the NHS to discharge mental patients to new community care facilities run by local authorities. There were to be no similar ear-marked community care grants for other client groups.

An assessment of Caring for People and the 1993 community care changes

The proposals in Caring for People (Secretaries of State 1989) formed part of the 1990 NHS and Community Care Act which also introduced an internal or quasi-market based on the separation of purchasers from providers in health care (see Chapter 14 for discussion of the so-called NHS reforms). The community care changes, which were not implemented in full until April 1993, aimed to develop a similar publicly financed quasi-market in community care. Unfortunately, as can be seen below, the two sets of market changes were introduced without sufficient recognition of the interdependence of the health and social care systems. The emphasis in *Caring for People* was on developing a 'mixed economy of care' with a diversity of private, voluntary sector and public providers whose services were to be purchased by local authority social services departments and health authorities in collaboration in order to create 'packages of care' available in, or close to, where people lived and appropriate to their needs to 'enable people affected by ageing or disability to live as independently as possible' (Secretaries of State 1989). Local authorities were to become 'enablers' or 'facilitators' putting together 'packages' of care provided by others rather than being primarily *providers* of services. The care or case manager who is normally a social worker but on occasions a community nurse, has the pivotal role of selecting and co-ordinating a range of services in response to individual needs provided and funded by a range of health and social services agencies to support dependent or vulnerable clients outside institutions. These changes have met with varying degrees of success (Box 16.1).

Whereas the Griffiths proposals had envisaged the local authority taking the lead for *all* client

---

BOX 16.1

CHANGES IN COMMUNITY CARE SINCE 1993

Unresolved general problems

- Co-ordination of resources and 'care packages' across the boundaries between health and social services

- Defining the responsibilities of the NHS and the local authority social services for continuing care of dependent people

- Allocating fixed budgets in relation to needs when demand for health and social care in the community is rising

- How best to support informal carers to maintain dependent people in the community

Specific examples of problems

- Difficulties faced by NHS Trusts in getting elderly people discharged to supportive environments outside hospital funded by social services

- Co-ordination and adequacy of resources for care of the seriously mentally ill in the community

Achievements

- Greater use of appropriate non-institutional forms of care

- A wider range of providers of community care

- A greater range of types of services and support

- Greater flexibility in the intensity of support and in its availability round-the-clock to enable people to live in their own homes groups and holding a unified budget for all the elements of community care (i.e. care outside hospital), the April 1993 arrangements maintained separation of budgets for health, social services and housing. For example, much of community care (the home or hostel elements) is financed by housing benefit and related payments and not from health or social services budgets. For mental health services, the social services departments have to agree care packages with the local health authorities before the social or non-NHS care element can be funded. The degree of understanding between the NHS and the local authority social services thus remains crucial in mental health and also, similarly, in the care of elderly people and those with learning difficulties. As the length of stay in acute hospitals for medicine and surgery continues to fall, patients are returned to their own homes in ever-increasing numbers requiring professional support, much of which presumes a major contribution from the local social services (e.g. in the form of home helps).

A series of now notorious cases in the early 1990s drew attention to the difficulties of implementing care in the community for people with mental health problems and revealed the 'precarious consensus' (Walker 1989) in favour of the principle in this area. In one case, a severely schizophrenic young man entered the lions' enclosure at London Zoo and was mauled to death. In another case which generated enormous public anxiety, Christopher Clunis, a schizophrenic with a history of violence, stabbed Jonathon Zito to death in a London tube station. The official enquiry into the Clunis case identified major failings in the co-ordination of his care in the community. A large number of agencies and different professionals had been aware of his condition, but none had taken decisive action to protect the public. New guidelines followed in 1994 on co-operation between health, social services, housing and other agencies which encouraged them to focus their efforts preferentially on people who are severely mentally ill, who are unable to care for themselves, or who are a significant risk to themselves and others. Such patients are now put on a supervision or 'at risk' register in the hope that this will allow them to be more closely monitored in the community. However, client mobility and lower levels of compliance with treatment in the community may work against this.

Caring for People and the April 1993 changes have not altered long-term policy aspiration to shift care for all sorts of dependent people from institutional to community-based or home-based (domiciliary) settings. However, they do represent a very important shift in the *funding* of care for poorer elderly people from the open-ended system of subsidy to residential and nursing home provision in the independent sector to a budget-capped system of grants to local authorities (Hudson 1994). Health authorities have had strictly cash-limited budgets since the 1970s. Through income support, elderly people in the 1980s had enjoyed, in effect, a *right* to a residential care subsidy, albeit for inappropriate care in many cases. Now, both health and social services have the difficult task of balancing their obligation formally to assess the care needs of people with their awareness of how many people of which types they can afford to care for in the community and how much can be spent on each.

FINANCING LONG-TERM CARE OUTSIDE HOSPITAL

The removal of the open-ended subsidy derived from income support to independent residential and nursing home provision has also starkly exposed a problematic feature of the British welfare state present since its beginning in the late 1940s, but largely ignored: namely, the fact that local authority social services such as residential care, home helps, day centres and so on are generally *means-tested* (for example, clients admitted to residential homes normally pay varying levels of fees, depending on the local authority, in proportion to their savings above a very modest level), whereas services purchased by health authorities, such as continuing care beds, are free to all patients irrespective of means at the point of use. Historically, there had been considerable overlap between the sorts of dependent people cared for in NHS continuing care beds and those looked after by the local authority. Two consequences of this arrangement have increasingly become apparent in the 1990s. First, it has been possible to find examples of similar elderly people in adjacent rooms in the same private nursing home, one of whom was having to deplete his/her savings in order to contribute to the cost of care arranged through the local authority, and the other who was receiving free care from the NHS. Secondly, the NHS involvement in long-term care has been progressively reduced through the 1980s and 1990s. This was made possible by the subsidy provided by the social security system but which has now been withdrawn.

Continuing care beds for the elderly and long-stay hospitals for people with chronic mental health problems and learning difficulties have been closed. In the case of the provision of continuing care for older people this was on the implicit grounds that most of them did not need medical and/or nursing care and, therefore, it was inappropriate for them to be in NHS facilities. In the case of long-term care for those with chronic mental health problems and people with learning difficulties, this was part of the explicit strategy of closing large Victorian asylums and reproviding care in the community. In the case of mental health services, there have been disputes between health and social services about the transfer of resources between the NHS and the local authorities and *within* the NHS concerns about the adequacy of the community support put in place before institutions close (House of Commons Social Services Select Committee 1990). In the case of the continuing care of dependent or frail elderly people, NHS acute hospital trusts came under increasing pressure from Government to reduce waiting times for elective surgery and to increase their throughput of patients and, as a result, many reduced their continuing care work despite instructions from the NHS Executive not to do so. Between 1989/90 and 1993/94, the number of NHS geriatric beds fell by 22%, since the main performance targets in the NHS related to the acute sector (Wistow 1995). Box 16.2 describes a notable case which brought this problem to public attention and compelled Government to issue central guidance.

Cases like the Leeds one have intensified discussion of how long-term care, particularly in old age, should be paid for and made available to those who need it. There is a fear that, in future, taxpayers will be unwilling to pay more to support the care needs of very elderly people. Box 16.3 and Table 16.2 highlight the main reasons why the issue has come to prominence in the 1990s (Laing 1993).

The debate has generated some alarmist commentary on future costs which has tended to overlook the fact that only a very small proportion of people are likely to require very expensive care (e.g. nursing home care can cost £20 000 per year and be needed over a number of years). Also, the UK is fortunate in facing a far smaller increase in the proportion of over 85s than many other Western industrialized countries such as Germany and the USA (see Chapter 11). It is

---

BOX 16.2

WHAT ARE THE LIMITS OF NHS RESPONSIBILITY?

The Leeds case

- In Leeds in 1993, a 55-year-old man who was profoundly brain-damaged and totally unable to look after himself was discharged from a NHS hospital to a private nursing home on the grounds that the hospital could no longer improve his condition and, therefore, he was no longer a NHS responsibility

- His wife complained to the Health Service Commissioner (the Health Ombudsman who investigates complaints relating to non-clinical aspects of Health Service care) on the grounds that she had been obliged to pay for nursing care which should have been provided free of charge by the NHS

- The Ombudsman ruled that the health authority owed the man a continuing duty of care and that he should have remained the financial responsibility of the NHS

Government guidance on responsibility for long-term care following the Leeds case (HSG (95)8, February 1995)

- The NHS is responsible for funding and/or providing free continuing care for those with incurable/chronic conditions only if complex or intensive medical and nursing care requiring supervision by specialists such as a consultant or a specialist nurse is needed

- The same criteria are to apply to patients who are likely to die in the very near future and to those with rapidly degenerating conditions

- The social services have responsibility for the rest of continuing care, which is means-tested

- It is up to local authorities and GP fundholders to define precise eligibility for NHS continuing care in light of local resources and after consultation with the social services

Continuing concerns

- Differences in financial regime between NHS and social services remain

- The financial consequences for the small proportion of people who require long periods of professional care or receiving either NHS or social services care are vastly different

- The boundary between health and social care remains unclear

---

apparent that the scale of future cost increases is very uncertain. However, the issue has begun to raise fundamental social questions concerning the balance between state, family and individual responsibilities to provide for care in the event of either mental infirmity, illness or old age. Paying for care in old age also threatens the ability of individuals to keep their assets intact to pass onto their children, as against having to use them to pay for their own care. It can be argued that the current 'system' of means-tested care creates a 'savings trap' which either penalises the thrifty or compels them to transfer their wealth to their children before they become old. It is also said

---

BOX 16.3

WHY IS LONG-TERM CARE IN OLD AGE SUCH A PROMINENT POLICY
ISSUE?

- People over 85 years and those living alone are those most likely to need long-term supervised care not provided by NHS

- Both groups are increasing as a proportion of the elderly

- Estimates of the number of over 85s in UK in 1991, 2001 and 2051 are 897 000, 1.3 million and over 3 million, respectively

- Long-term care can cost £15 000–£20 000 per year in residential settings, but it is very difficult to predict who is going to require such care in old age

- The supply of informal care is likely to diminish as the proportion of very elderly rises

- NHS is increasingly focused on specialist medical and nursing care and facing rising pressure to fund new acute treatments

- Removal of social security open-ended subsidy to independent residential and nursing home care in 1993, but no private insurance alternative

- Increasingly stringent means testing of other care through social services

- Lack of state support to heavily involved informal carers

- Majority public belief that the state should provide free care

- Perception that better off elderly people could fund their own long-term care

---

TABLE 16.2 *Cost to society and to individuals and their families of long term care.*

	Cost of care including informal care at 1991 prices (£bn)	% Gross National Product	Cost per adult of working age (£)
1991	42	7.3	1345
2001	44	7.7	1365
2011	49	8.5	1485
2021	55	9.6	1689
2031	62	10.8	2014

Reproduced with permission of the Institute of Actuaries from Nuttall et al. (1993).

to create a disincentive for people to save, which could harm the economy by reducing the resources available for investment.

Box 16.4 summarizes the main policy options discussed for financing long-term care outside the NHS in the next century, regardless of whether it is in the form of rehabilitation, respite care, residential care, or intensive care in people's own homes. The options fall into three main groups:

BOX 16.4

POLICY OPTIONS FOR FUNDING LONG-TERM CARE OUTSIDE THE
NHS

- Public finance (not-for-profit)

  General taxes (as in current NHS)

  Social insurance (compulsory 'earmarked' tax)

- Private finance

  Personal savings

  Personal assets (i.e. including houses owned)

  Private insurance (usually for profit)

- Mixed finance

  For example:

  Guaranteed minimum, publicly funded and available to all (universal system)
  Guaranteed minimum, publicly funded, but means-tested (selective)
  Separation of hotel costs (paid for privately) and care costs (paid for publicly)

- Informal care – essential to underpin all schemes

- those based on forms of *taxation* in which today's taxpayers pay for today's users of care;
- those based on some form of *private finance*, mainly insurance;
- *mixed schemes* incorporating taxation and private finance.

Responses based purely on private insurance principles are likely to face major practical problems, most notably the near-impossibility of estimating the likelihood of specific individuals requiring different forms of care up to 65 years in the future and of predicting the cost of such care, together with the need to guard against insurers trying to offload high risk people (e.g. by using genetic testing) onto the state. Premiums would be very costly. It seems likely that some form of mixed arrangement based on an 'earmarked' tax to provide a minimum level of continuing and community care together with a facility to 'top-up' care through private insurance will be adopted. Another option under consideration is for the state to organise some form of insurance enabling people to pay a premium on retirement in order to protect their assets (primarily their homes) should they later require means-tested long-term residential care. However, a solution based on using *general* tax revenues, as in the NHS currently, also has considerable public appeal. It would be simple to implement, would spread the costs of care as widely as possible across society and, in the case of old age care, would express solidarity between the generations as younger people provided resources for older people.

Whichever scheme is eventually taken up, three things stand out:

1. The question of how much society can afford to spend on long-term care of all kinds is the same, irrespective of who pays and how (public, private or mixed finance).

2. Any scheme will have to include a means of paying for the long-term care of those who live outside institutional (nursing home or residential home) settings since they represent the vast majority of people with such needs who are often poorly supported currently by domiciliary services.

3. Any scheme will have to be built on a recognition that informal care by close kin will remain central to the provision of continuing care for the foreseeable future. Such care will have to be sustained in the face of adverse socioeconomic trends by a range of cash payments to recompense informal carers (Glendinning and McLaughlin 1993).

CONCLUSIONS

The partially reformed formal care system in Britain continues to be dominated in financial terms by institutional provision, but the nature of these institutions has changed since the 1950s. Their average size has dropped and there has been a multiplication of mini-institutions away from hospital sites 'in the community'. However, these settings continue to provide care for the minority of dependent people. The assumption remains that the bulk of caring for vulnerable people will continue to be provided mainly by female kin with little help from the state. Domiciliary and day care for dependent people remain relatively weak. Rather than acting to share care between formal and informal carers in order to avoid putting an excessive burden on informal carers, the formal system is still largely funded and organized, with the exception of small amounts of respite care, to intervene only when informal caring relationships have broken down. It is becoming increasingly doubtful whether this approach can be sustained in the future. Demographic trends and women's increasing participation in the paid economy are combining to increase the need for care, while reducing the supply of informal carers. This is likely to lead to growing pressures on lay people to care, but there is also a greater awareness of the financial and emotional costs to carers. In this situation the state will have to find ways of 'caring for the carers', particularly to ensure that they do not suffer financially or in their employment, as well as enabling people to pay for long-term care in new ways. To do this, formal care will need to be far more closely dovetailed with the pattern of informal care, rather than operating as an entirely separate system. One possibility for the future which might be attractive to some carers would be to categorize caring for a frail or disabled relative as a proper job attracting a full or part-time salary from the state paid for out of some form of 'earmarked tax' (or social insurance) scheme.

REFERENCES

Abrams, P.   (1980) Social change, social networks and neighbourhood care. *Soc. Work Serv.*, **22**, 12–23.
Audit Commission   (1986) *Making a Reality of Community Care*. London: HMSO.
Barton, R.   (1959) *Institutional Neurosis*. Bristol: Wright.
Busfield, J.   (1986) *Managing Madness: Changing Ideas and Practice*. London: Unwin Hyman.
Challis, L. & Davies, B.   (1986) *Case Management in Community Care*. Aldershot: Gower.
Department of Health and Social Security   (1981a) *Care in Action: a Handbook of Priorities for the Health and Personal Social Services in England*. London: HMSO.
Department of Health and Social Security   (1981b) *Growing Older*. London: HMSO.
Finch, J. & Groves, D. (eds)   (1983) *A Labour of Love: Women, Work and Caring*. London: Routledge & Kegan Paul.
Glendinning, C. & McLaughlin, E.   (1993) *Paying for Care: Lessons from Europe*. Social Security Advisory Committee, Research Paper 5. London: HMSO.
Goffman, E.   (1961) *Asylums*. New York: Anchor Books.

Gray, A., Whelan, A. & Normand, C.   (1988) *Care in the Community: a Study of Services and Costs in Six Districts*. York: Centre for Health Economics, University of York.

Green, H.   (1988) *General Household Survey 1985: Informal Carers*. London: HMSO.

Griffiths, R.   (1988) *Community Care: Agenda for Action*. A report to the Secretary of State for Social Services. London: HMSO.

Henwood, M.   (1990) *Community Care and Elderly People: Policy, Practice and Research Review*. London: Family Policy Studies Centre.

House of Commons Social Services Select Committee   (1990) *Community Care: Services for People with Mental Handicap and Mental Illness*, Eleventh Report Session 1989–90. London: HMSO.

Hudson, B.   (1987) Steering a course through the myths of community care. *Health Serv. J.*, 28 May (Suppl.).

Hudson, B.   (1994) Community care one year on: an implementation deficit? In: *Health Care UK, 1993/94*, ed. A. Harrison, pp. 57–62. London: King's Fund Institute.

Hunter, D.   (1993) Care in the community: rhetoric or reality? In: *Dilemmas in Health Care*, ed. B. Davey & J. Popay, pp. 121–42. Buckingham: Open University Press.

Jones, K., Brown, J. & Bradshaw, J.   (1978) *Issues in Social Policy*. London: Routledge & Kegan Paul.

Laing, W.   (1993) *Financing Long Term Care: the Crucial Debate*. London: Age Concern/Ace Books.

Laing & Buisson   (1996) *Care of Elderly People: Market Survey 1995/96*. London: Laing and Buisson.

Ministry of Health   (1962) *A Hospital Plan for England and Wales*. Cmnd. 1604. London: HMSO.

Nissel, M. & Bonnerjea, L.   (1982) *Family Care of the Handicapped Elderly: Who Pays*? London: Policy Studies Institute.

Nuttall, S.R., Blackwood, R.J.L., Bussell, B.M.H., Cliff, J.P., Cornall, M.J., Cowley, A, Gatenby, P.L. & Webber, J.M.   (1993) *Financing Long Term Care in Great Britain*. London: Institute of Actuaries.

Parker, G.   (1990) *With Due Care and Attention: a Review of Research on Informal Care*. Occasional Paper No. 2, 2nd edn. London: Family Policy Studies Centre.

Prior, L.   (1991) Community versus hospital care: the crisis in psychiatric provision. *Soc. Sci. Med.*, **32**, 483–9.

Sainsbury, P. & Grad de Alarcon, J.   (1974) The cost of community care and the burden on the family of treating the mentally ill at home. In: *Impairment, Disability and Handicap*, ed. D. Lees & S. Shaw. London: Heinemann.

Secretaries of State for Health, Social Security, Wales and Scotland   (1989) *Caring for People: Community Care in the Next Decade and Beyond*. Cmnd 849. London: HMSO.

Social Policy Research Unit   (1994) *Different Types of Care: Different Types of Carer*. London: HMSO.

Townsend, P.   (1962) *The Last Refuge*. London: Routledge & Kegan Paul.

Walker, A.   (1982) The meaning and social division of community care. In: *Community Care: the Family, the State and Social Policy*, ed. A. Walker, pp. 13–39. Oxford: Basil Blackwell/Martin Robertson.

Walker, A.   (1989) Community care. In: *The New Politics of Welfare: an Agenda for the 1990s*?, ed. M. McCarthy, pp. 203–24. London: Macmillan.

Wistow, G.   (1995) Long term care: who is responsible? In: *Health Care UK, 1994/95*, ed. A. Harrison, pp. 80–7. London: King's Fund Institute.

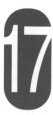

Prevention and Health Promotion

DAVID LOCKER

THREE ERAS IN CONTEMPORARY HEALTH CARE

Resource development and redistribution

By the middle of the twentieth century, health-care systems had become major institutions within industrialized nations. The scientific discoveries and therapeutic successes of modern medicine, which began in the 1930s and accelerated in the following decades, were accompanied by a significant expansion in health-care facilities and a massive increase in the number of health professionals and other workers responsible for the delivery of health care.

Government policies at this time were concerned with increasing the provision of health services and ensuring that the population had access to them. Even within the largely private system of the US, government legislation encouraged development of the health sector in the form of biomedical knowledge, personnel and facilities and, through Medicaid and Medicare programmes, made health services more readily available to the old and the poor. Green and Kreuter (1990) have referred to this period as one of **resource development and redistribution**.

Cost containment

The belief underlying initiatives such as the National Health Service (NHS) in Britain, and universal public health insurance in Canada, was that better access to health care led to better health. When the NHS was founded it was anticipated that health-care costs would rise initially but then fall as the population became healthier and less in need of medical care. This did not happen: the post-Second World War period has been one in which health-care costs have risen systematically, both in absolute terms and as a proportion of gross national product (see Chapter 19).

This belief in the effectiveness of health services was subsequently tempered by a growing scepticism and awareness that increases in spending on health care were having only a limited impact on the health of the population. Increased inputs in the form of financial and other resources were no longer matched by increased outputs such as improvements in life expectancy. Consequently, as the costs of medical care continued to rise, governments began to turn their attention to **cost–containment**, finding ways of stabilizing costs while continuing to secure improvements in health. In the US, for example, emphasis came to be placed on health education in promoting self-care and reducing the utilization of medical services, and on new forms of medical practice such as Health Maintenance Organizations, in which the prevention of disease was encouraged through the way in which health professionals were paid.

From prevention to health promotion

At the same time, it was recognized that the major health problems of modern populations were and continue to be chronic degenerative disorders such as cancer, heart disease and cerebrovascular disease which cannot be cured and are expensive to manage since they frequently entail many years of living with disabilities. However, many of the disorders characteristic of modern populations can be prevented by modifying behaviours and life-styles. This better understanding of the causes of ill-health and mortality reinforced the interest of governments in health education and disease prevention (Green and Kreuter 1990).

Two other influences which encouraged the development of a new approach to the population's health were the historical research of McKeown (1979) (see Chapter 1) and changes in the way in which we think about health. McKeown clearly demonstrated that the improvements in health during the nineteenth and early twentieth centuries were due to social, economic and environmental factors and not to the rise of high technology medicine with its focus on curing disease. This research, along with a broadening of the way in which we define health, provided the basis for a new era in health care, that of **health promotion**.

DEFINING HEALTH

Over the past 40 years, our conception of health and what it means to be healthy has changed considerably. A useful starting point for a discussion of this change and its implications is the definition of health offered by the World Health Organization in 1948 (Box 17.1). In spite of its obvious limitations, this definition of health is a useful one in that it recognizes the essential distinction between disease and health and sees health as being multidimensional, with important social and psychological components.

BOX 17.1

DEFINITIONS OF HEALTH

WHO, 1948:

> A complete state of physical, mental and social well-being and not merely the absence of disease and infirmity.

WHO, 1984:

> Health is the extent to which an individual or group is able, on the one hand, to realise aspirations and satisfy needs; and on the other hand, to change or cope with the environment. Health is, therefore, seen as a resource for everyday life, not the object of living; it is a positive concept emphasising social and personal resources, as well as physical capacities.

From this point of view, disease is a relatively narrow concept and refers to pathological processes and the way in which they compromise the body and its anatomical and physiological systems. Health is a much broader concept and refers to an individual's subjective experience of functional, social and psychological well-being and its consequences for the conduct of everyday life. Whereas disease belongs to the realm of biology and pathology, health belongs to the realm of sociology and psychology, including as it does feelings, behaviours and the quality of life.

The breadth of what we currently mean by health is clearly illustrated by the definition formulated by the World Health Organization in 1984 which clarified and extended the 1948 definition. Here, health is a resource because it maximizes freedom of choice and the opportunities we have for gaining satisfaction from living. It means the capacity to manage everyday life and the ability to pursue our own goals. Based on this definition, Labonte (1993) identified six components of good health (Box 17.2). These components identify some of the aims of health promotion, and indicate what we should take into account when assessing the health of individuals or communities.

BOX 17.2

COMPONENTS OF GOOD HEALTH

- Feeling vital, full of energy
- Having good social relationships
- Experiencing a sense of control over one's life and living conditions
- Being able to do things one enjoys
- Having a sense of purpose in life
- Experiencing being part of a community

Reproduced with permission of the University of Toronto from Labonte (1993).

These definitions lead us to the conclusion that disease and health are separate and discrete events; though they may be related, they often occur and are experienced separately. This is readily illustrated by the simple model presented in Fig. 17.1.

This model suggests the following, much of it credible in terms of our everyday experience. Sector A respresents a situation in which we may have a disease of some kind which does not impinge on our health or sense of well-being. This is not always confined to conditions which are relatively trivial in medical terms. Many people with severe and potentially life-threatening diseases, for example, describe themselves as feeling well and healthy. Sector B represents a situation in which disease imposes a burden on our body systems so that our sense of health and well-being are compromised. Finally sector C suggests that, just as we may feel healthy even in the presence of what may be severe disease, it is also the case that we may experience negative changes to our well-being in the absence of a disease process. What this means is that disease is only one of the factors that threaten good health.

To the extent that diseases of various kinds do impinge on health, the prevention of disease is part of health promotion. However, health promotion goes beyond this to address the other factors which compromise health.

Fig. 17.1 *Model to illustrate the relationship between disease and health.*

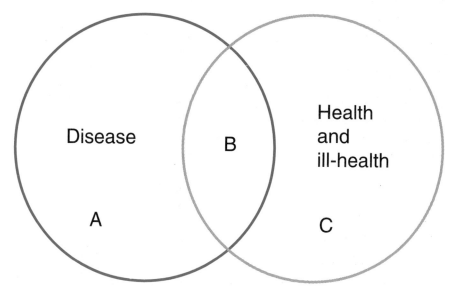

ISSUES IN PREVENTION

The scope for prevention

Some impression of the potential impact of prevention can be gained from a brief overview of the major causes of mortality and morbidity in modern populations. As mentioned previously, these are cardiovascular disease, cancer, motor-vehicle accidents, alcohol-related problems, suicide, respiratory disorders, congenital and genetic disorders and sexually transmitted disease, including acquired immunodeficiency syndrome (AIDS). The majority of these are associated with one or more risk factors which can be modified to prevent disease, disability and death.

Cardiovascular disease (CVD) has been in decline since the 1970s but still ranks as the leading cause of death in most industrialized societies. Its underlying cause is atherosclerosis and contributory factors include: smoking, high blood pressure, obesity, lack of physical exercise, high levels of dietary fat, blood cholesterol levels and genetic factors (see Chapter 2). Many of these factors are amenable to change through preventive health practices. Although controversy surrounds some of the preventive approaches related to CVD, there is no doubt that its incidence could be reduced further by dietary and other changes.

Cancers tend to be the second leading cause of death and, although the aetiology of most cancers is unknown, many are related to smoking, diet and exposure to carcinogens in the occupational environment. The close relationship between smoking and lung cancer is well documented. Smoking is also a major factor in respiratory diseases such as chronic bronchitis and emphysema, although environmental problems such as air pollution have also been linked to rates of respiratory illness.

Various diseases and/or health problems are associated with alcohol consumption, including cirrhosis, suicide and motor-vehicle and other accidents. It has been estimated that 2% of all deaths are directly attributable to alcohol, with 10% of deaths being alcohol related. Deaths from cirrhosis have increased over the past four decades (Shah 1990) and alcoholism is also one of the main reasons for admission to mental hospitals.

The same principle applies to the other diseases listed above. Once the many risk factors associated with a disease are known, attempts can be made to reduce or eliminate one or more to bring about a corresponding reduction in the social and economic burden of illness.

Primary, secondary and tertiary prevention

Traditional approaches to prevention are based on interventions at three levels: primary, secondary and tertiary prevention (Box 17.3).

BOX 17.3

PRIMARY, SECONDARY AND TERTIARY PREVENTION

Primary prevention: seeks to prevent the onset of disease, e.g. immunization to confer immunity on an individual and changes in behaviours such as smoking.

Secondary prevention: consists of the early detection and treatment of disease or states likely to lead to disease, e.g. screening by a clinician for diseases such as human immunodeficiency virus (HIV) infection, tuberculosis or cervical cancer, or screening for major risk factors such as high blood pressure and cholesterol levels.

Tertiary prevention: seeks to minimize the disability and handicap from a disease state that cannot be cured or leaves the individual with some loss of function.

Screening

Screening can be defined as the active early diagnosis of disease or risk factors for disease as a prelude to intervention designed to prevent onset or progression. It can take one of many forms. Mass screening, such as programmes for breast and cervical cancer, involves large numbers of people who are offered the service and participate on a voluntary basis. Some screening procedures are routine, such as the screening of the newborn for various congenital abnormalities. Screening also occurs as part of the normal course of medical care, where a patient presenting with one condition or complaint is screened for another. In some instances screening may be selective and directed towards high-risk groups. Multiphasic screening involves tests for numerous diseases and/or risk factors at one time.

Limitations of screening

Screening has a certain logic; it can reduce morbidity and save lives by identifying and treating individuals at the earliest possible stage in the disease process. Nevertheless, a number of criticisms have been directed at 'screening programmes'. A major criticism is that, with a few exceptions, they may be of little benefit. Many studies of the outcomes of multiphasic screening, or screening for coronary heart disease, have shown disappointing results, with no differences in the morbidity and mortality experience of screened and non-screened control groups (Stoate 1989).

We are also beginning to recognize that screening has psychological and other costs which must be weighed against any benefits obtained (Marteau 1989). A number of studies of people who have participated in screening programmes have shown that screening can have negative psychological and behavioural outcomes. Revealing previously undiagnosed hypertension resulted in more absenteeism from work, lower self-esteem and disruptions in marital relationships (Haynes et al. 1978; Mossey 1981). Bloom and Monterossa (1981) undertook a study of people who were initially diagnosed as hypertensive but subsequently given a clean bill of health following further testing. They found that such people reported more depression and a lower state of general health than a control group – evidence of the lasting effect of this initial labelling. Even a negative result may have untoward consequences. The 'certificate-of-health effect' noted by Tijmstra and Bieleman (1987) may reinforce unhealthy life-styles and foster the impression that the individual is not vulnerable to this disease.

STRATEGIES FOR IMPROVING HEALTH

Medical approach

For most of this century the **medical approach** has dominated thinking about health and approaches to health care. The essential features of this approach are its focus on disease, a bio-mechanical orientation concerned with repairing disease-induced damage to the body and a narrow conception of the causes of disease and the determinants of health. These causes and determinants are usually framed in microbiological or physiological terms, so that when this approach considers prevention it focuses on risk factors such as high cholesterol levels or high blood pressure and the early detection of disease. From this perspective, pharmacological methods of risk factor reduction are preferred and health is equated with the provision of health services.

Behavioural approach

During the mid-1970s, a number of governments published policy documents which gave official recognition to the emerging debate about the most effective strategy for maintaining and improving health. The Lalonde Report was released by the Canadian Government in 1974 and is now considered a turning point and landmark in the development of a new approach to public health (Lalonde 1974). This report was based on the health field concept, which emphasized the significance of four elements in health: human biology, the environment, life-style and health-care organization. As has already been noted, since the Second World War major efforts to improve health have focused on the formal health-care system and on treating illness already manifest. Yet the pattern of diseases affecting modern populations clearly indicates that the potential for further improvements in health lies with the other three elements.

In 1976 the British Government issued a similar document, *Prevention and Health: Everybody's Business* (DHSS 1976), in which the prevention of the major health problems affecting the British population emerged as a key strategy in improving health. This document identified the causes of these health problems and outlined a response. The diseases of modern populations are 'related less to man's outside environment than to his own personal behaviour; what might be termed our lifestyle' (DHSS 1976). Consequently, 'much of the responsibility for ensuring his own good health lies with the individual' (DHSS 1976). The responsibility of governments and health professionals is limited to ensuring that the public have access to such knowledge as is available about the importance of personal habits to health and, at the very least, no obstacles are placed in the way of those who decide to act on that knowledge' (DHSS 1976).

The implication of this particular view of health is that prevention can be achieved simply by the provision of information to the population about the risks to health posed by aspects of our life-style, like smoking, drinking and an inadequate diet. Although at one point in the document it is acknowledged that the government's role is a broader one, involving fiscal and legal controls on the manufacture and sale of health-damaging commodities, the solution to the problem is largely reduced to one of health education.

Naidoo (1986) has criticized the philosophy of individualism underlying the approach described in *Prevention and Health*. This sees health as a matter of individual responsibility and free choice. It assumes that many of the behaviours damaging to health are freely chosen and can be avoided once the individual is informed of their negative effects. Within the framework of a philosophy which values free choice, education, rather than coercion by legal or fiscal means, is the preferred approach to the prevention of disease. This overlooks the fact that there are social and cultural factors which shape our behaviour and set limits on our capacity to change. For example, diets are influenced by advertising, the decisions taken by food manufacturers and distributors and the price and availability of healthy foods in the neighbourhoods in which we live (Townsend 1990). Consequently, nutrition education may have little effect on the diet of families living in poverty whose choices regarding the purchasing of food are limited by a lack of money (see Chapter 8).

A second problem with this behavioural approach is its ready translation into 'victim blaming' and the attribution of guilt (Allison 1982). This is explicit in the UK document on prevention which ascribed many of Britain's health problem to 'over-indulgence and unwise behaviour' and in statements by Government Ministers which indicate that they see the problem solely as one of 'ignorance' (Townsend 1990).

Socioenvironmental approach

Critics of the behavioural approach do not claim that life-styles and personal responsibility play no part in maintaining or improving health. The claim is that it fails to acknowledge the extent to which health is linked to social, economic and environmental conditions which lie outside the control of the individual (see Chapter 2). The individual is relatively powerless to act against a health-damaging environment produced by a society which frequently values profit and economic expansion above health.

McKinlay (1974) addresses the significance of the social and political environment in his analysis of the political economy of health. According to McKinlay, the efforts of the health-care system can be called 'downstream activities', devoted as they are to the rescue of the sick. However, this type of activity cannot influence the level of health of a population when various interest groups and large-scale profit-oriented corporations are operating 'up-stream', constantly adding to the pool of those in need of rescue. Problems such as lung cancer, heart disease, obesity, alcohol abuse and road-traffic accidents can be linked to organizations such as the food and tobacco industries, who spend billions of dollars promoting unhealthy life-styles. The battle between these 'manufacturers of illness' and health educators is an unequal one. The tobacco industry, for example, commands massive resources and has access to sophisticated techniques of persuasion in maintaining and promoting smoking as a desirable activity. McKinlay believes they are effective because they tie at-risk behaviours such as smoking to dominant cultural themes and images. Because free choice does not operate in these situations, McKinlay advocates legislation to curb the activities of the manufacturers of illness.

McKinlay's approach to improving the health of the population is usually referred to as a 'socioenvironmental' approach. This seeks to improve health by means of strategies to modify the social, political and economic environment in which we live. Such changes only come about as the result of action by governments and communities. From this perspective, part of the task of health educators is to teach individuals and communities to recognize health-damaging aspects of home, workplace and community and to foster community action to deal with them.

A more recent document issued by the UK Government, *The Health of the Nation* (Department of Health 1991), accepted these ideas in calling for greater efforts with respect to prevention and health promotion. Although emphasis continued to be placed on the need for people to change their behaviour, the document recognized that improving health required a balance between individual action and government action. The role of government in promoting health is a broad one. First, it must ensure that individuals have the information necessary to make healthy choices. Second, it must ensure that people live in physical and social circumstances where the exercise of free choice is possible. Third, it must act on behalf of individuals and families, using regulation and legislation to control threats to health. Finally, it recognized that in between individuals and governments were a range of organizations whose actions also had a bearing on the nation's health.

DEFINING HEALTH PROMOTION

Health promotion is often called the 'new public health', a reference to the public-health movement of the nineteenth century which, through sanitary reform, brought about a significant decline in deaths from infectious disease. It has been defined as 'the process of enabling people to increase control over and to improve their health' (World Health Organization 1984). Consequently, health promotion draws on behavioural and socioenvironmental perspectives and consists of a comprehensive set of strategies which go beyond health education and life-style change:

> *Health promotion policy combines diverse but complementary approaches including legislation, fiscal measures, taxation and organizational change. It is coordinated action which leads to health, income and social policies that foster greater equity. Joint action contributes to safer goods and services, healthier public services and cleaner, more enjoyable environments* (WHO 1984).

The joint action referred to above involves governments, health and other social and economic sectors, voluntary organizations, local authorities, industry and the media. It entails the creation of physical environments conducive to health and social and political environments within which people can take action to improve their own health and support each other in managing personal and community health problems.

From this perspective, responsibility for health does not lie with the individual. Individuals can do much to maintain or improve their own health, but only if they are presented with meaningful opportunities for doing so. It is through the collaborative efforts of all sectors of society that such opportunities can be realized and maximized.

HEALTH PROMOTION PRINCIPLES AND CONCEPTS

One of the clearest statements of health-promotion principles is to be found in a discussion document released by the European Office of the World Health Organization (WHO) in 1984 (World Health Organization 1984). It identified five important issues in relation to the development of policies and programmes in health promotion. These are summarized in Box 17.4.

BOX 17.4

HEALTH PROMOTION PRINCIPLES

- Health promotion involves the population as a whole in the context of their everyday lives, rather than focusing on people who are sick or at risk for specific diseases;

- Health promotion is directed towards action on the determinants or causes of health;

- Health promotion combines diverse methods or approaches;

- Health promotion aims at effective and concrete public participation;

- Although health promotion is not a medical service, health professionals have an important role in terms of health education and advocacy.

Reproduced with permission from WHO (1984).

Later documents, produced by the WHO and national governments, described additional concepts and principles central to health-promotion efforts.

Create supportive environments

The inextricable links between the environment and health have already been outlined. Creating supportive environments goes somewhat beyond this; it means ensuring that the physical and social environments in which we live maximize the possibility of leading healthy lives. In short, these are environments which 'make healthy choices the easy choices'. A good example is offered by legislation which has banned smoking in the workplace and other public areas. This makes it much easier for non-smokers to escape the effects of second-hand smoke and also acts to support those who aim to reduce or give up smoking altogether. Since smoking is now accepted as a risk factor for periodontal disease, such actions help promote oral as well as general health.

Build healthy public policy

Mention has already been made of the fact that decisions taken by organizations at all levels can promote or damage our health. Building healthy public policies means working to ensure that all organizations must take account of the potential health effects of the policies they develop and implement. This is particularly important with respect to central government, who control and create policy for diverse sectors such as transportation, agriculture, energy and income, all of which can have important health ramifications. A good example is given by decisions taken by the Government of Ontario when faced with the task of reducing public sector spending. Two options were presented: eliminate 40 000 public sector jobs or implement an across-the-board 5% salary cut for all employees. The latter was chosen on the grounds that its negative health impact was likely to be less than the creation of unemployment for substantial numbers of people.

Strengthen community action

Health promotion involves public participation and works through the actions of communities in identifying priorities, planning strategies and implementing them to enhance health. An important task for health promotion is to increase the ability of communities to recognize and change those aspects of their physical and social environment which are hazardous to health or encourage behaviours likely to damage health. Water fluoridation was implemented in many communities only because dental health professionals were able to work with and obtain the support and involvement of the public in persuading local politicians to implement the measure.

Develop personal skills

Individuals as well as communities can undertake actions to improve their health. However, information and education are necessary to enable them to make choices which promote health and enhance their ability to cope with the stresses and strains of daily life. Such education can be provided in a wide range of settings such as schools and places of work.

Reorient health services

Health services have traditionally been more concerned with curing disease than promoting health. Consequently, the formal health care system needs to expand its activities beyond the provision of clinical services to address the health needs of individuals and communities.

Finally, there are three concepts central to oral health promotion, touched upon in the general description of the approach and its principles, which require further elaboration.

Equity and inequality

Equity and inequality are linked to social justice and human rights. Equity refers to differences in opportunities to be healthy and inequality to actual and measurable differences in health status. Both terms imply that these differences are unfair and unjust and that society has a moral obligation to minimize them as far as possible.

Empowerment

Empowerment is the most important idea within health promotion. It is often a difficult idea for health professionals to grasp since most have been trained in a model in which the health care provider is an expert and the patient is a recipient of this expertise. It may also be difficult for health professionals to accept, since it requires the transfer of responsibility for and control over health from professionals to people. Nevertheless, the empowerment of others is one of the most important functions of health professionals with respect to health promotion. It has been defined as 'the capacity to define, analyze and act upon the problems in one's life and living conditions' (Labonte 1993). It involves the provision of health education, teaching people the skills they need in order to use health information effectively and increasing their confidence that they have a choice and can exercise control over the options available to them. Since powerlessness is a major risk factor for disease and ill-health (Wallerstein 1992) (see Chapter 2), an empowered community is a healthy community.

Advocacy

A second important role for health professionals is that of advocacy for health. This involves educating politicians, community leaders and other influential individuals, such as representatives of the media, in order to influence the decisions that have a bearing on the health of the population. In this role, health professionals need to be both technical experts, providing the scientific basis for decision-making, and political activists in mobilizing support for policies which improve health.

These concepts clearly indicate that the new public health requires a fundamental shift in the distribution of power and resources in society. This highlights the essentially social and political nature of health and takes us a long way from the notion of individual responsibility which underlies traditional approaches to disease prevention.

HEALTH PROMOTION IN ACTION

The health-promotion approach is readily illustrated using motor-vehicle accidents as an example. These are a leading cause of death in young people and, as a result, account for the largest proportion of potential-years-of-life lost.

Motor-vehicle accidents, like any other health problem, can usefully be analysed using the health field concept. The main causes of such accidents are the attitudes of, and risk-taking by drivers, the design of cars and roads, and the availability of trauma services, with the first being by far the most important (Shah 1990). Consequently, life-styles, environment and health-care organization are aspects of the problem needing attention, with human biology being of little or no significance. Motor-vehicle accidents, which fall into the life-style category, can be further differentiated into those that are the result of carelessness, speeding, failure to use seat belts and impaired driving.

Actions to reduce such accidents have largely concentrated on legislation designed to modify these life-style factors. Many countries have adopted legislation to control speeding, enforce the wearing of seat belts and deal with the impaired driver. Young drivers, who are responsible for a high proportion of motor-vehicle accidents, are being singled out for attention. Less effort has been directed towards increasing the safety of cars or changing driver attitudes through controls on advertising, which currently promote counterproductive images of cars and driving. Consumer groups have a role to play in addressing both these issues.

CRITICISMS OF THE HEALTH PROMOTION APPROACH

Health promotion is not without its critics. Some have noted that attempts to implement the health-promotion approach at the national level have not gone much beyond attempts to change individual life-styles by health education or legislation. Attempts to control the 'manufacturers of illness', or to deal effectively with health-related issues such as poverty, housing and the environment, have been much less evident.

A more fundamental critique has been offered by those who are concerned about 'healthism', that is, making health the central cultural value governing individual action and social relationships (see Chapter 12). Becker (1986), for example, cautions against the tyranny of health promotion, in which all aspects of our lives become prescribed in the name of health. This should alert us to the fact that health promotion does not entirely escape the moral dilemmas involved in balancing personal and public responsibility for health.

REFERENCES

Allison, K.   (1982) Health education: self-responsibility versus blaming the victim. *Health Educ.*, **20**, 11–13.
Becker, M.   (1986) The tyranny of health promotion. *Public Health Rev.*, **14**, 15–25.
Bloom, J. & Monterossa, S.   (1981) Hypertension labelling and sense of well-being. *Am. J. Public Health*, **71**, 1228–32.
Department of Health   (1991) *The Health of the Nation*. London: HMSO.
Department of Health and Social Security   (1976) *Prevention and Health: Everybody's Business*. London: HMSO.
Green, L. & Kreuter, M.   (1990) Health promotion as a public health strategy for the 1990s. *Annu. Rev. Public Health*, **11**, 319–34.
Haynes, R., Sackett, D., Taylor, D., Gibson, E. & Johnson, A.   (1978) Changes in absenteeism and psychosocial function due to hypertension screening and therapy among working men. *N. Engl. J. Med.*, **299**, 741–4.
Health and Welfare Canada   (1986) *Achieving Health for All: A Framework for Health Promotion*. Ottawa: Minister of Supply and Services.
Labonte, R.   (1993) Health Promotion and Empowerment. Issues in Health Promotion Series no. 3. Centre for Health Promotion, University of Toronto.
Lalonde, M.   (1974) *A New Perspective on the Health of Canadians*. Ottawa: Minister of Supply and Services, Canada.
Marteau, T.   (1989) Psychological costs of screening. *Br. Med. J.*, **299**, 527.

McKeown, T.   (1979) *The Role of Medicine: Dream, Mirage or Nemesis*? Oxford: Blackwell Scientific Publications.

McKinlay, J.   (1974) A case for refocussing upstream: the political economy of ill-health. In: *Applying Behavioral Science to Cardiovascular Risk*. Proceedings of the American Heart Foundation Conference, Seattle.

Mossey, J.   (1981) Psychosocial consequences of labelling in hypertension. *Clin. Invest. Med.*, **4**, 201–7.

Naidoo, J.   (1986) Limits to individualism. In: *The Politics of Health Education*, ed. S. Rodmell & A. Watt. London: Routledge & Kegan Paul.

Shah, C.   (1990) *Public Health and Preventive Medicine in Canada*. Toronto: University of Toronto Press.

Stoate, H.   (1989) Can health screening damage your health? *J. R. Coll. Gen. Pract.*, **39**, 193–5.

Tijmstra, T. & Bieleman, B.   (1987) The psychological impact of mass screening for cardiovascular risk factors. *Family Pract.*, **4**, 287–90.

Townsend, P.   (1990) Individual or social responsibility for premature death? Current controversies in the British debate about death. *Int. J. Health Serv.*, **20**, 373–92.

Wallerstein, N.   (1992) Powerlessness, empowerment and health: implications for health promotion programs. *Am. J. Health Promotion*, **6**, 197–205.

World Health Organization   (1984) *Health Promotion: A Discussion Document on the Concept and Principles*. Copenhagen: Regional Office for Europe.

World Health Organization   (1986) *Ottawa Charter for Health Promotion*. Ottawa: Health and Welfare Canada, Canadian Public Health Association.

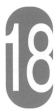

Measuring Health Outcomes

RAY M. FITZPATRICK

In the course of the twentieth century, health problems in the industrialized societies have steadily shifted from the infectious diseases to chronic and degenerative diseases. Health services are now expected to have an impact on a diverse range of health problems that variously involve what we may term the 'five Ds': death, disease, disability, discomfort and dissatisfaction. The health services that have emerged to respond to such demands are of unprecedented size, diversity and complexity. Perhaps the greatest challenge now facing health services is to assess their impact on health problems. Especially now that public funds are an essential component of financial support for health care, governments of all political persuasions have begun to require evidence of the effectiveness of health services. At the same time, the health professions are also beginning to look more closely at the impact that their treatments and interventions may have. The common focus of such concerns is on assessing the outcomes of health care, i.e. the impact on patients and populations of health services.

This chapter examines some of the different ways of conceptualizing and measuring health outcomes and some of the lessons to be gained from such evidence. There is a discussion of the evaluation of health services. It is customary to distinguish between three different components of health-care evaluation.

1. The *structure* of health care, which involves focusing on such matters as the numbers, distribution and qualifications of doctors, nurses and other health professionals.
2. The *processes* of health care, which are concerned with the therapeutic, diagnostic and other activities performed by health professionals for patients.

3. The *outcomes* of health care are the most important focus in evaluation and consider the ultimate results achieved for patients by health services.

MORTALITY

The first measure of outcome is important for a number of reasons. Most obviously it is a central concern of clinicians and society to prevent deaths. From the perspective of measurement it is relatively simple to define compared with most other dimensions of health status. Moreover, particularly in industrialized societies, national recording systems have virtually complete information about deaths, something that cannot be said for most other measures of outcome.

Mortality rates can be used for a number of purposes. Thus they indicate inequalities in health status between different parts of England and Wales. The highest standardized mortality ratios (SMRs) consistently occur in the northern Regional Health Authorities and the lowest in the south and west. The use of SMRs to examine inequalities between social and ethnic groups has been discussed in Chapter 8. Mortality rates can also be used to examine improvements over time. In England and Wales, life expectancy – a summary measure of the mortality rates prevailing at any time – has increased for females from 42 years in 1841 to 78 years in 1990. Most of this improvement has occurred because of reductions in infant mortality; life expectancy at later ages has not improved so markedly. A woman of 65 in 1841 could expect to live another 12 years. This figure had only increased to 18 years in 1990. Nevertheless, mortality rates can be used to show significant progress in some areas in the recent past. Thus, among young men, there has been a dramatic 44% reduction in lung cancer in the period 1975–87, a change almost entirely due to reductions in smoking and the tar content of cigarettes (Doll 1990). Over the same period, mortality rates due to some other cancers, such as Hodgkin's disease, leukaemia and cancer of the testis, have declined markedly due to medical interventions such as radiotherapy and chemotherapy. This is persuasive evidence that counterbalances the more pessimistic analyses of progress against cancer.

Infant mortality tends to be used as a particularly sensitive measure of the overall health of a country. Variations between countries in infant mortality are considered to be a reflection of social and economic conditions generally as well as the quality of maternity and neonatal care.

Avoidable mortality

One important approach to mortality statistics is to focus on deaths from certain conditions considered amenable to health-service intervention. Maternal and infant mortality may be used as indicators of the quality of obstetric and infant care. This approach has been extended to other causes of death where variations in death rates may indicate limitations of health-care provision, particularly if deaths below particular ages are the focus of attention. For example, cervical cancer is regarded as in principle avoidable by a combination of screening and early treatment by surgery or radiotherapy. Similarly, preventive immunization or drug therapy for established cases is highly effective against tuberculosis, so that most mortality is in principle avoidable. Hypertensive disease can be detected by screening and ought to be amenable to dietary and smoking advice together with drug management (Box 18.1). A study in Finland showed that over the period 1969–81 death rates for causes amenable to medical intervention declined by two-thirds for individuals aged 64 years or less (Poikolainen and Eskola 1986).

Hospital deaths

Deaths may nevertheless be an important alarm signal in health care and, as information systems become more effective and public concern over issues of quality increases, it can be expected that increasing attention will be given to hospital mortality data. A great deal of controversy followed the publication in the USA of the death rates for different hospitals of public sector (Medicare) patients. For example, mortality in a 30-day period following admission for pneumonia varied from 0 to 60% between different hospitals. It was argued that such evidence pointed to serious potential deficiencies in the quality of care of certain hospitals about which the public had a right to know. On the other hand, technical objections may be raised regarding the quality of mortality data and incautious interpretations regarding their significance. In particular, account needs to be taken of the variation in the severity and complexity of illness of patients admitted to different hospitals. A study of patients admitted to NHS intensive care units found substantial and significant differences in death rates between units, with the worst mortality rate more than two and a half times higher than the most favourable (Rowan et al. 1993). However, when the study took account of severity of illness in the patients, variations in mortality were explained away for the majority of units, although 15% of units still had significantly higher death rates. Of course, for many other kinds of hospital admissions, such as end-stage cancer, death may be the inevitable and accepted outcome and other criteria, such as the dignity of care, would be the most appropriate measure of quality (Kahn et al. 1988). Again, as with avoidable mortality, there is a practical problem that death for particular hospital units are mercifully too infrequent an event to rely on for purposes of assessing outcomes and quality of care.

BOX 18.1

AVOIDABLE DEATHS AND THE NHS

1. Avoidable death rates vary in different areas of Britain

   - Rates are influenced by social and environmental factors, e.g. deaths due to hypertensive/cardiovascular disease

   - Figures for health authorities, when controlled for social and environmental factors, show variation (Charlton et al. 1983)

   - This variation is greater than could have occurred by chance

2. Are they due to the quality of health services?

   - The positions of health authorities on 'league tables' of avoidable deaths has remained stable (Charlton et al. 1986).

   - Information on mortality is used as an indicator of quality of medical care, but have the social factors been properly allowed for in the analysis?

HEALTH STATUS AND QUALITY OF LIFE

For many health problems treated by health services, not only is death an uncommon and inappropriate measure of outcome but also, more importantly, the primary purpose of treatment is to improve patient's functioning and well-being. Consider, for example, drug treatment for rheumatoid arthritis, epilepsy or migraine, hospice care of the terminally ill, or surgery for ulcerative colitis. In all such instances we are concerned with the broad, pervasive effects that health problems have on the patient in terms of pain, disability, anxiety, depression, social isolation, embarrassment, or difficulties in carrying on daily life. From the patient's perspective, health care is largely judged in terms of impact on these broader aspects of personal well-being. Patients themselves advocate that more research be conducted into the impact of treatments on these aspects of their lives (Goodare and Smith, 1995). In recent years outcome measures have emerged in an attempt to capture such aspects of patients' experiences. Frequently termed quality-of-life measures, they may often also be referred to as health-status instruments.

An early attempt to assess quality of life in patients systematically was the Karnofsky Performance Index (Karnofsky and Burchenal 1949) (Table 18.1). The scale was designed particularly for use in the field of cancer and involves the clinician making a simple rating of the patient. It is still one of the more frequently used 'quality-of-life' scales. The scale is very useful in drawing attention to those factors that matter to patients. It also helps health professionals predict which patients on a ward may require more attention and need more time and resources. Some of its disadvantages are considered here.

1. Is quality of life unidimensional? Fallowfield (1990) points out the fallacy behind the use of a unidimensional scale. Such a scale requires the assumption that a bed-bound person must have a quite poor score even if, for example, he or she is well adjusted to illness, receives full social support and sees life as fulfilling. Conversely, someone ambulant but otherwise depressed, isolated, with low self-esteem and anxious about health status would, nevertheless, receive a favourable score. In other words, instruments such as the Karnofsky Performance Index do not allow for the multidimensional nature of quality of life.

TABLE 18.1 *The Karnofsky Performance Index.*

Description	Score (%)
Normal, no complaints	100
Able to carry on normal activities; minor signs or symptoms of disease	90
Normal activity with effort	80
Cares for self. Unable to carry on normal activity or to do active work	70
Require occasional assistance but able to care for most of his needs	60
Requires considerable assistance and frequent medical care	50
Disabled; requires special care and assistance	40
Severely disabled; hospitalization indicated although death not imminent	30
Very sick. Hospitalization necessary. Active supportive treatment necessary	20
Moribund	10
Dead	0

Reproduced with permission of Souvenir Press from Fallowfield (1990).

2. Is the scale reliable? It is not surprising, in view of the complex nature of quality of life, that the index is deficient in a basic requirement for such instruments in that it is not reliable; different raters disagree in applying the scale to patients.

3. Is the scale valid? As serious a deficiency is that clinicians disagree with patients' self ratings on the scale. Indeed it has more generally been found to be the case across a wide range of health care settings that health professionals make significantly different judgements of their patients' quality of life than patients themselves (Sprangers and Aaronson 1992). Such problems have underlined the need for instruments that patients may, whenever possible, complete themselves.

Health-status instruments

Systematic reviews have shown that a large proportion of published clinical trials purporting to assess the impact of therapies on patients' quality of life rely on inaccurate evidence, such as the doctor's opinion, or inappropriate laboratory measures (Schumacher et al. 1991). Where patients' perceptions of their health or quality of life are obtained in clinical trials, often the questionnaires are unvalidated or simplistic and leave the patient little scope for expressing their feelings (Gill and Feinstein 1994).

A number of instruments (variously termed 'health-status', or 'quality-of-life', instruments) have therefore emerged, designed to be used as questionnaires for self completion. An instrument quite widely used in the UK is the Nottingham Health Profile (NHP) (Hunt and McEwen 1980). The NHP contains 38 simple statements (such as 'I sleep badly at night' or 'I am in pain when I walk') to which the respondent gives 'yes' or 'no' answers. The items fall into one of six scales addressing different aspects of subjective health: physical mobility, pain, sleep, energy, social isolation and emotional reactions. Each item has a weighted score obtained from panels of judges who have rated the relative severity of different statements. Subjects completing the questionnaire thus get a score for each of the six scales determined by the proportion of items to which they give positive answers. The designers of the instrument have made considerable effort to establish that the instrument is reliable (i.e. produces consistent responses if completed on different occasions not too far apart), and is able to distinguish individuals with different types and severity of health problem. The NHP has now been used to examine the impact on individuals' subjective health of a number of different health-care interventions, ranging from heart transplants, intensive care and elective surgery, through trials for anti-inflammatory drugs and hospital management of diabetes and rheumatoid arthritis.

There are a large number of health-status or quality-of-life measures now available. Although different in style, content and general approach to measuring patients' problems, they generally tend to focus on those aspects of patients' daily lives that are most affected by ill-health (Fitzpatrick et al. 1992) (Table 18.2).

Instruments such as the NHP are ambitious in that they are intended to assess the impact on the patient's well-being and quality of life of a wide range of different health problems. Often it is necessary to assess the patient's perspective with an instrument more specifically designed to be sensitive to one particular disease. One very typical and quite successful instrument of this kind is the Arthritis Impact Measurement Scale (AIMS) which, by means of simple questions,

TABLE 18.2 *Dimensions of quality of life usually assessed in health status instruments.*

Physical function, for example, mobility, ability to look after self

Emotional well-being, for example, depression, anxiety, self esteem

Social function, for example, close attachments, social support, social integration

Roles, for example, paid work, housework, child care

Pain, for example, severity, frequency

Other symptoms, for example, nausea, stiffness, fatigue

Reproduced with permission from Fitzpatrick et al. (1992).

assesses the impact of rheumatic disease on patient well-being in areas such as mobility, dexterity, household activities, pain and depression. The instrument has been shown to be sensitive to improvements in patients within just 4 weeks of treatment with non-steroidal anti-inflammatory drugs (Anderson et al. 1989). In a chronic disease, such as rheumatoid arthritis, where improvements to the patient's condition may be quite subtle and undramatic, such instruments have a vital role to play in improving our understanding of outcomes, especially in view of evidence in rheumatology that they may be no less reliable and accurate than conventional laboratory and radiological measures and often provide the clinician with more meaningful information on the impact of treatment (Deyo 1988). Box 18.2 shows an example of how a questionnaire to assess patients' quality of life has been constructed in one particular field of medicine.

Some observers argue that questionnaires such as those just described are still limited because they ask a standard set of fixed questions of everyone and do not leave much room for individuals' personal concerns or problems to be expressed if they happen not to be included as a questionnaire item (O'Boyle et al. 1992). For this reason several instruments have recently been developed in which respondents identify their own most important areas of life (family, religion, leisure activities or whatever) rather than respond to questionnaire items determined by the investigator (Ruta and Garratt 1994). They can then rate how well they are doing in these personally nominated areas of life and also on subsequent occasions judge any changes for better or worse in these domains. Such approaches attempt to address the concern that quality of life is an essentially individualized and personal judgement.

Adverse consequences of health care

Many medical treatments have harmful side-effects. This may be the case in, for example, cancer therapies which are designed to prolong life but which may have a variety of adverse effects at the same time. Cytotoxic chemotherapies may produce nausea, vomiting, hair loss and tiredness, as well as mood effects such as depression. In some cases the costs to the patient from treatments may outweigh benefits to be gained in terms of longevity. Quality-of-life measures allow us to give some quantitative expression to such adverse effects. Thus Croog et al. (1986) used a

---

BOX 18.2

CONSTRUCTING A QUALITY OF LIFE INSTRUMENT

- Objective. Parkinson's disease (PD) is a chronic degenerative disease mainly affecting individuals at older ages. There is no cure and treatment is designed to arrest the progression of symptoms and improve the quality of life. However, there is no specific measure of quality of life in (PD).

- Step one. Identify the problems
  Interview individuals with the problem. Allow them to say in their own words how PD affects them. Content analysis of interviews (tape recorded) draws out a rich variety of themes.

- Step two. Draw up questions
  Draw up a long list (65) of questions based on step one. Ask individuals with PD in the community to complete the questionnaire. Ask for their comments on items. Analyse results to find redundant or difficult items. Statistical analysis found that 39 questionnaire items could be used to assess nine important areas of life: mobility, activities of daily living, emotional well-being, stigma, social support, cognitions, communication, bodily discomfort.

- Step three. Test the questionnaire
  Again ask individuals with PD in the community to complete the (39 item) questionnaire. Ask some to repeat the task. Examine the results for internal consistency and test–retest reliability. Patients in neurological clinics also complete the questionnaire to check that patterns of answers agree with other evidence of neurological problems for purposes of validity.

- Result. A questionnaire that patients find easy to complete, that emphasizes issues that matter to them and that can be used to assess the course of illness and impact of interventions.

Reproduced with permission by Oxford University Press from Peto et al. (1995), Jenkinson et al. (1995).

---

battery of quality-of-life measures to assess the impact of three alternative drugs for controlling hypertension. They measured general well-being, physical symptoms, sexual function, work performance, emotional state, cognitive function (e.g. memory), social participation and life satisfaction. Although achieving similar levels of blood pressure control, one drug stood out from the other two as having less harmful effects on quality of life. They found that some of the harmful side-effects of drugs produced broadly equivalent effects on quality of life to those found by individuals who have just lost their jobs. Another study showed harmful effects on quality of life of transdermal glyceral trinitrate compared with placebo treatment for angina (Fletcher et al. 1988). Possibly because of increased headaches, the active treatment group were less able to maintain social contacts with friends and family. Broadly based measures of quality of life make it possible to detect and assess harmful effects that might occur in any of a wide range of aspects of patients' lives.

Attaching values to health

All health-care systems have to make choices between different health-care interventions; resources are not available to fund and provide all of the treatments that, in principle, are available. This requires extremely difficult choices to be made between interventions for very different health problems, e.g. between coronary bypass surgery, renal transplants, lipid screening and day hospitals for psychiatric patients. One of the many problems complicating such choices is that there is no single numerical scale in terms of which to measure the diverse states of health and illness treated by different health-care programmes. Utility measurement is an approach which can be used to produce numerical values on a scale between 0 and 1 for all possible health states by assessing their relative value to individuals. In principle, it then becomes possible to assess in a standard way the improvements to health that may result from otherwise widely differing medical interventions.

A number of techniques have been developed to elicit how desirable individuals regard one health state compared with another. One such technique is the so-called standard gamble technique (Torrance 1986). At the heart of this approach, a subject is asked to choose between a particular state of ill health on the one hand and a gamble on the other hand. The gamble involves a hypothetical treatment which can cure the individual of the state of ill health, but with a particular probability of death from the treatment. For states of ill health perceived by the subject to be very undesirable one would expect the individual to prefer the gamble even with quite high probabilities of death. This probability is experimentally varied to reveal how ready the individual is to take the gamble rather than choose (hypothetically) to carry on living in the particular state of ill health being investigated. Data can be gathered from a sample of experimental subjects in such a way as to produce numerical values for a range of health states.

An alternative method (magnitude estimation) is to ask subjects to state how much worse they

TABLE 18.3 *Valuation matrix of different health states.[a]*

Disability rating	Distress rating			
	No distress	Mild	Moderate	Severe
No disability	1.000	0.995	0.990	0.967
Slight social disability	0.990	0.986	0.973	0.932
Severe social disability and/ or slight physical impairment	0.980	0.972	0.956	0.912
Physical ability severely limited (e.g. light housework only)	0.964	0.956	0.942	0.870
Unable to take paid employment or education, largely housebound	0.946	0.935	0.900	0.700
Confined to chair or wheelchair	0.875	0.845	0.680	0.000
Confined to bed	0.677	0.564	0.000	−1.486
Unconscious	−1.078	NA	NA	NA

Reproduced with permission by Oxford University Press from Drummond (1989).
[a] *Healthy = 1.0, dead = 0.0. NA, not applicable.*

regard each of a number of ill-health states relative to one standard health state. One research group (Rosser and Kind 1978) asked subjects to rate the relative undesirability of 29 different states of illness produced by a matrix formed from combinations of two dimensions, varying degrees of distress and disability. The resulting relative values or 'utilities' of different health states are shown in Table 3. It is worth noting that some health states were rated as worse than 'dead' by judges. The research group found that values attached to different health states were reliable in the sense that individuals' responses were consistent over time.

QUALITY-ADJUSTED LIFE-YEARS

Some health economists have argued that the values attached to different states of health and ill-ness by methods such as those outlined above can be combined with survival data on years lived as a result of medical treatments to produce a generic output measure, the 'quality-adjusted life-year' (QALY) (Williams 1985). This standard, unitary means of expressing the benefits of medical treatments permits comparisons across treatments. Typically, information on QALYs has been combined with information about the costs of different treatment programmes (cost–utility analysis) and comparisons between programmes expressed in terms of costs per QALY gained, as in Table 18.4. It is argued that health authorities, faced with a scarcity of resources to meet all health problems, need to maximize their use of resources. The methodology of QALYs identifies treatments that maximize the use of resources by obtaining the greatest gain in terms of health for a unit of resource. Table 18.4 indicates that general practitioners giving advice to stop smoking is a dramatically more effective use of resources than, say, hospital haemodialysis. Such information appears to provide a more explicit and more rational basis for making decisions about the allocation of resources. However, the approach outlined above has generated intense debate (Box 18.3).

TABLE 18.4 *'League table' of costs and QALYs for selected health-care interventions (1983–84 prices).*

Intervention	Present value of extra cost per QALY gained (£)
GP[a] advice to stop smoking	170
Pacemaker implantation for heart block	700
Hip replacement	750
CABG for severe angina LMD	1040
GP control of total serum cholesterol	1700
CABG for severe angina with 2VD	2280
Kidney transplantation (cadaver)	3000
Breast cancer screening	3500
Heart transplantation	5000
CABG for mild angina 2VD	12600
Hospital haemodialysis	14000

Reproduced with permission by Oxford University Press from Drummond (1989).
[a] *CABG, coronary artery bypass graft; LMD, left main disease; 2VD, two vessel disease; GP, general practitioner.*

BOX 18.3

DEBATE ABOUT QALYS

Arguments against

- There are no agreed methods – at least six methods have been developed (Froberg and Kane 1989).

- People's values differ and health means different things to different people.

- Doctors' rate states of ill health as less desirable than do patients (Rosser and Kind 1978).

- Even if the principle of 'league tables' is accepted the methods of assessing costs and outcomes varies, therefore the results are problematic (Mason et al. 1993).

- Can moral judgements be made scientific?

- QALYs condone cutting health-care resources.

- QALYs have unfair consequences, systematically disadvantaging some social groups, e.g. the elderly and terminally ill.

Arguments in favour

- The current system of resource allocation is worse.

- QALYs make decisions more open and accountable.

PATIENT SATISFACTION

The patient's perspective

One source of evidence about the outcomes of health care that has, until recently, been all too frequently neglected is the patient's view. This neglect was partly due to the widespread assumption that the patient is insufficiently well informed to comment on his or her health care. Undoubtedly there is also a tendency in many large bureaucratic organizations such as the National Health Service (NHS) to pursue internally generated routines and objectives without seeking external evidence of their reception by users. It should be clear that a primary objective of any health-care system is to provide services in a manner that is acceptable to the patient. The Griffiths NHS Management Inquiry was highly critical of the NHS's failure to act on this principle by systematically obtaining consumer feedback about the quality of services (DHSS 1983). Since that report, most health authorities have made much more effort to conduct such surveys.

There is also ample evidence from social scientific research to indicate how important the issue of patient satisfaction is. Patients who are dissatisfied with their health care are more likely not to follow the medical advice or regimen that they receive. In a sample of patients attending a neurological clinic for chronic headache, those who when interviewed after their consultations were more dissatisfied with the consultation were significantly less likely to take the medication that had been prescribed for them (Fitzpatrick and Hopkins 1981). Similar results have been obtained between satisfaction and compliance in hypertension and paediatric clinics, and in general practice. Dissatisfied patients may be less likely to reattend for further care (Orton et al. 1991) or may change their doctor (Rubin et al. 1993). Satisfaction may also be an indication of how successful a treatment has been (Fitzpatrick et al. 1987).

A common distinction made in relation to health care is that between the technical and interpersonal aspects of care. Technical aspects of care refer to the technical competence with which treatment is provided. Interpersonal aspects focus on how doctors, nurses and other health professionals treat the patient – in other words, the degree of personal care and concern shown. Patient satisfaction is a particularly important indicator of interpersonal aspects of care. Thus, in a study of mothers attending a paediatric clinic with their children, the medical consultations were tape-recorded and analysed and mothers independently interviewed by researchers after the consultation to assess satisfaction (Korsch et al. 1968). Satisfaction was higher when the doctor displayed a friendly manner to the mother. Satisfaction was also positively related to directly questioning mothers early in the consultation as to the main worries and concerns that had prompted the consultation. In a similarly designed study of general medical clinics in which analyses of tape-recorded consultations could be related to subsequent patient satisfaction, those patients who were given encouragement by the doctor to explain their medical problem in their own terms were significantly more satisfied than patients who reported their symptoms in response to more structured doctor-focused questioning (Stiles et al. 1979).

One of the more important of interpersonal skills in health care is giving information. Failures in this area are one of the most important sources of patient dissatisfaction. It can also be shown experimentally that efforts to improve the communication of information are appreciated by patients. Ley (1982) reported a study in which medical inpatients were allocated to one of three different patterns of communication. A 'placebo' group experienced the normal and routine pattern of communication from doctors. A 'control' group received in addition one visit from a junior doctor who discussed general matters not specifically related to the patient's admission. In the 'experimental' group the junior doctor, in the one visit to the patient, made a point of giving an explanation to the patient of the treatments and procedures he or she was receiving. All three groups subsequently completed questionnaires and the 'experimental' group produced significantly higher satisfaction scores.

There are two distinct ways in which we can go about obtaining individuals' views in a survey on a subject like health care (Box 18.4). The choice will depend on circumstances. A general problem with all methods is that patients of different backgrounds tend to differ in readiness to express critical comments about health services. Younger patients, those with poorer health status and individuals with higher levels of education are more likely to express dissatisfaction.

Surveys in the NHS

In order to aid its deliberations, the Royal Commission on the NHS commissioned a survey of a sample of patients who had recently experienced either inpatient or outpatient treatment. The results of the national survey carried out by the Office of Population Censuses and Surveys are

---

BOX 18.4

OBTAINING VIEWS IN A SURVEY

There are two basic strategies to finding the views of patients. Either respondents are given a questionnaire to complete themselves or personal interviews are conducted to ask the questions.

Advantages of the two approaches

Self-completed questionnaire	*Interview*
Questions easy to standardise and process	More appropriate for sensitive or complex material
No interviewer bias	Easier to clarify ambiguous items
Low cost of data gathering	Rapport results in completion of questionnaire
Less need for trained staff	Scope to follow-up non-respondents

Reproduced with permission from Fitzpatrick (1991).

---

likely to be very similar to those that are obtained in local surveys of a particular hospital or district (OPCS 1978).

Table 18.5 shows that much of the dissatisfaction could be traced to problems of having to wait for outpatient appointments or hospital admission and to the length of time waiting to see a doctor. Other complaints focused on amenities such as food and washing facilities in wards and the waiting room in outpatient clinics. A particularly large number in both patient groups were dissatisfied with information. A more recent survey of over 5000 patients attending 36 NHS hospitals found problems of communication still as the main source of dissatisfaction, with 16% of patients receiving no explanation about their condition from the doctor and 60% receiving no advice about activities to do or not do after discharge (Bruster et al. 1994).

It might be noted that absent from either study are any views from patients about the value in terms of outcomes of medical care. Indeed a systematic review of a wide range of studies of

TABLE 18.5 Dissatisfaction with regard to aspects of the NHS.

Outpatients	%	Inpatients	%
Information about progress	37	Woken too early	43
Time waiting for hospital transport	28	Information about progress	31
Waiting for first appointment	21	Food	21
Length of time at hospital	19	Waiting for admission	20
Adequacy of waiting room	18	Washing and bathing facilities	19
Length of wait to see doctor	16	Toilet facilities	15

Reproduced with permission of the Controller of HMSO and the Office for National Statistics OPCS (1978).

patient satisfaction found that only 8% of studies included outcomes as a subject on which to elicit patients' views (Wensing et al. 1994). Investigators appear to avoid this subject, either because of limited faith in patients' competence to judge the benefits of treatment, or because this subject is perceived as a purely clinical matter to be assessed solely by professional criteria. As a result we know far less than we should about patients' perceptions of the value of medical care.

OUTCOMES AND THE EVALUATION OF SERVICES

Evaluation and the medical profession

One of the features that may distinguish a profession from other kinds of occupations is that it retains a very high level of control in assessing the value and quality of the product it provides to the public (see Chapter 15). The medical profession has historically exercised this control by means of a number of methods such as monitoring the content and standards of the training provided for new or established members of the profession, or by penalizing individual doctors who fail to uphold required professional standards. In Britain the General Medical Council was established after lengthy negotiations between the state and the newly emerging medical profession in the middle of the nineteenth century as one of the main institutions to ensure satisfactory performance by doctors. However, health care has now become so complex and costly that traditional methods of upholding professional standards are no longer sufficient. Moreover, society has profoundly changed since the nineteenth century. The state is now intimately involved in health care through funding medical services with public money. It seeks evidence that such funds are well spent. In the USA, in addition to the Federal Government's concern about public health-care spending, industry has become concerned about the value of medical services because so much is paid for from employers' insurance contributions. In other words, powerful forces such as government and business are seeking clearer evidence of the value of health care. In addition, the consumer has also become more knowledgeable, more demanding and more sceptical in dealing with health professionals.

The medical profession has not only faced external pressures to evaluate its activities. From within, epidemiologists such as Cochrane (1972) have argued that insufficient attention has been given to the scientific appraisal of the impact on health of medical interventions. The response of the medical profession to such pressures has been to take more seriously its responsibility to examine and monitor the quality and value of its services, in particular by practising medical audit. Medical audit has been defined as 'looking at what we are doing with the aim of making improvements in patient care and use of resources' (Difford 1990). It is conventional to distinguish between audit of process, in which the focus is the evaluation of medical activities (normally against agreed standards), and audit of outcome in which the question concerns the impact of activities upon illness. The latter is, as this chapter establishes, more difficult, so that most audit has been concerned with examining process, by methods such as reviewing samples of case notes, analysing hospital statistical data or comparing local use of procedures such as X-rays against published expert advice (McKee et al. 1989).

However, audit is still not widely practised. This has been interpreted by some as evidence of complacency or indeed defensiveness on the part of a profession anxious not to expose its limitations (Wilding 1982). The White Paper *Working for Patients* insists that all doctors in the NHS should take part in audit, and urges that hospital units only be allowed to train junior doctors if adequate audit is in operation (Secretaries of State for Health, Wales, Northern Ireland and Scotland 1989). It does not, however, specify what constitutes adequate audit and leaves much of the detail to professional peer control. Thus it may be that other sections of the White Paper will provide greater incentives to impose explicit audit of outcomes. District Health Authorities, as part of their contract to purchase health care from hospitals, will be obliged to ensure the quality of the care provided for the local population. With these statutory obligations it will be very hard for both authorities and hospitals to avoid examining the impact of treatments on outcomes such as mortality, quality of life and patient satisfaction.

Evaluation and the future of health care

There are at least three different views that can be taken of the impact that measurement of outcomes may have on health care. For many observers the evaluation of outcomes will be a fundamental turning point in the history of medicine, allowing for explicit, rational, scientific answers to all the problems arising from current uncertainties as to the value of medical treatments. As is examined in Chapter 19, outcomes research must address the enormous variations in the rates at which many medical and surgical treatments are performed, even among populations with similar levels of medical need. The hope is that all parties – the doctor, the patient and the purchaser – will have access to clearer information as to the likely results of investigations and treatments, and will, therefore, be able to make more informed decisions about health care. A second position about future developments in this area is to adopt a more cautious stance and to argue that at present the advocates of outcomes measurement are expressing something of an article of faith. Despite enormous advances in computers and information systems, we are a very long way from the kinds of integrated systems that can monitor the longer-term impact of medical interventions in populations, and the kinds of practical and valid measures of outcome that can be used on a large scale are only just now beginning to be developed and examined. To understand the outcomes of most procedures, long-term studies integrating hospital and community data, to an extent that is not yet feasible outside of very special research contexts, will be required.

There is also a third, longer-term view of these developments. Analysts of both British and American health care (Ham 1981) have suggested that two distinct interest groups have tried to shape the future of health care. One group – the 'professional monopolizers' – have sought to defend the traditional privileges and practices of the medical profession, particularly the clinical autonomy of the doctor. A second group – 'the corporate rationalizers' – emphasize the many irrationalities and inefficiencies that bedevil health-care systems when traditional professional autonomy is left unchecked by planning and evaluation. According to such analyses there has for a very long time been a stalemate in health policy between these two conflicting philosophies, and the present debate over outcomes is unlikely to result in decisive shifts. According to this view, for the foreseeable future health services will defy precise measurement of their value because of the inherent uncertainties and complexities of medical practice. Whatever the future direction of medical care, the assessment of outcomes will remain a central concern of health services.

REFERENCES

Anderson, J., Firschein, H. & Meenan, R. (1989) Sensitivity of a health status measure to short term clinical changes in arthritis. *Arthritis Rheum.*, **32**, 844–50.

Bruster, S., Jarman, B., Bosanquet N. et al. (1994) National survey of hospital patients. *Br. Med. J.*, **309**, 1542–6.

Charlton, J., Hartley, R., Silver, R. & Holland, W. (1983) Geographical variation in mortality from conditions amenable to medical interventions in England and Wales. *Lancet*, **i**, 691–6.

Charlton, J., Lakhani, A. & Aristidou, M. (1986) How have 'avoidable death' indices for England and Wales changed? 1974–78 compared with 1979–83. *Community Med.*, **8**, 304–14.

Cochrane, A. (1972) *Effectiveness and Efficiency*. London: Nuffield Provincial Hospitals Trust.

Croog, S., Levine, S., Testa, M. et al. (1986) The effects of antihypertensive therapy on the quality of life. *N. Engl. J. Med.*, **314**, 1657–64.

Department of Health and Social Security (1983) *NHS Management Inquiry*. London: HMSO.

Deyo, R. (1988) Measuring the quality of life of patients with rheumatoid arthritis. In: *Quality of Life: Assessment and Applications*, ed. S. Walker & R. Rosser. Lancaster: MTP Press.

Difford, F. (1990) Defining essential data for audit in general practice. *Br. Med. J.*, **300**, 92–4.

Doll, R. (1990) Are we winning the fight against cancer? An epidemiological assessment. *Eur. J. Cancer*, **26**, 500–8.

Drummond, M. (1989) Output measurement for resource allocation decisions in health care. *Oxford Rev. Econ. Pol.*, **5**, 59–74.

Fallowfield, L. (1990) *The Quality of Life: The Missing Measurement in Health Care*. London: Souvenir Press.

Fitzpatrick, R. (1991) Surveys of patient satisfaction: I – Important general considerations. *Br. Med. J.*, **302**, 887–9.

Fitzpatrick, R. & Hopkins, A. (1981) Patients' satisfaction with communication in neurological outpatient clinics. *J. Psychosom. Res.*, **25**, 329–34.

Fitzpatrick, R., Bury, M., Frank, A. & Donnelly, T. (1987) Problems in the assessment of outcome in a back pain clinic. *Int. Disabil. Stud.*, **9**, 161–5.

Fitzpatrick, R., Fletcher, A., Gore, S. et al. (1992) Quality of life measures in health care. I: Applications and issues in assessment. *Br Med J.*, **305**, 1074–7.

Fletcher, A., McLoone, P. & Bulpitt, C. (1988) Quality of life on angina therapy: a randomised controlled trial of transdermal glyceral trinitrate against placebo. *Lancet*, **ii**, 4–9.

Froberg, D. & Kane, R. (1989) Methodology for measuring health-state preferences – III: Population and context effects. *J. Clin. Epidemiol.*, **42**, 585–92.

Gill, T. & Feinstein, A. (1994) A critical appraisal of the quality of quality-of-life measurements. *J. Am. Med. Assoc.*, **272**, 619–26.

Goodare, H. & Smith, R. (1995) The rights of patients in research. *Br. Med. J.*, **310**, 1277–8.

Ham, C. (1981) *Policy Making in the National Health Service*. London: Macmillan.

Hunt, S. & McEwen, J. (1980) The development of a subjective health indicator. *Sociol. Health. Illness*, **2**, 231–46.

Jenkinson, C., Peto, V., Fitzpatrick, R. et al. (1995) Self reported functioning and well-being in patients with Parkinson's disease. *Age Ageing*, **24**, 505–9.

Kahn, K., Brook, R., Draper, D., Keeler, E., Rubenstein, L., Rogers, W. & Kosecoff, J. (1988) Interpreting hospital mortality data: how can we proceed? *J. Am. Med. Assoc.*, **260**, 3625–8.

Karnofsky, D. & Burchenal, J. (1949) The clinical evaluation of chemotherapeutic agents in cancer. In: *Evaluation of Chemotherapeutic Agents*. Symposium at New York Academy of Medicine, New York, ed. C. Macleod, pp. 191–205. New York: Columbia University Press.

Korsch, B., Goszzi, E. & Francis, V. (1968) Gaps in doctor patient communications: 1. Doctor patient interaction and patient satisfaction. *Paediatrics*, **32**, 855–71.

Ley, P. (1982) Satisfaction, compliance and communication. *Br. J. Clin. Psychol.*, **21**, 241–54.

McKee, C., Lauglo, M. & Lessof, L. (1989) Medical audit: a review. *J. R. Soc. Med.*, **82**, 474–8.

Mason, J., Drummond, M. & Torrance, G. (1993) Some guidelines on the use of cost effectiveness league tables. *Br. Med. J.*, **306**, 570–2.

O'Boyle, C., McGee, H., Hickey, A. et al. (1992) Individual quality of life in patients undergoing hip replacement. *Lancet*, **339**, 1088–91.

Office of Population Censuses and Surveys (1978) *Royal Commission on the National Health Service: Patients Attitudes to the Hospital Service*. London: HMSO.

Orton, M., Fitzpatrick, R., Fuller, A. et al. (1991) Factors affecting women's response to an invitation to attend for a second breast cancer screening examination. *Br. J. Gen. Pract.*, **41**, 320–3.

Peto, V., Jenkinson, C., Fitzpatrick, R. & Greenhall, R. (1995) The development and validation of a short measure of functioning and well-being for individuals with Parkinson's disease. *Quality of Life Res.*, **4**, 241–8.

Poikolainen, K. & Eskola, J. (1986) The effect of health services on mortality: decline in death rates from amenable and non-amenable causes in Finland 1969–81. *Lancet*, **i**, 199–202.

Rosser, R. & Kind, P. (1978) A scale of valuations of states of illness: is there a social consensus? *Int. J. Epidemiol.*, **7**, 347–58.

Rowan, K., Kerr, J., Major, E. et al. (1993) Intensive Care Society's APACHE II study in Britain and Ireland – II: Outcome comparisons of intensive care units after adjustment for case mix by the American APACHE II method. *Br. Med. J.*, **307**, 977–81.

Rubin, H., Gandek, B., Rogers, W. et al.   (1993) Patients' ratings of outpatient visits in different practice settings. *J. Am. Med. Assoc.*, **270**, 835–40.

Ruta, D. & Garratt, A.   (1994) Health status to quality of life measurement. In: *Measuring Health and Medical Outcomes*. ed C. Jenkinson. London: UCL Press.

Schumacher, M., Olschewski, M. & Schulgen G.   (1991) Assessment of quality of life in clinical trials. *Stat. Med.*, **10**, 1915–30.

Secretaries of State for Health, Wales, Northern Ireland and Scotland   (1989) *Working for Patients*. Cmd 555. London: HMSO.

Sprangers, M. & Aaronson, N.   (1992) The role of health care providers and significant others in evaluating the quality of life of patients with chronic disease: a review. *J. Clin. Epidemiol.*, **45**, 743–60.

Stiles, W., Putnam, S., Wolf, M. & James, S.   (1979) Interaction exchange structure and patient satisfaction with medical interviews. *Med. Care*, **17**, 667–79.

Torrance, G.   (1986) Measurement of health state utilities for economic appraisal: a review. *J. Health Econ.*, **5**, 1–30.

Wensing, M., Grol, R. & Smits, A.   (1994) Quality judgements by patients on general practice care: a literature analysis. *Soc. Sci. Med.*, **38**, 45–53.

Wilding, P.   (1982) *Professional Power and Social Welfare*. London: Routledge & Kegan Paul.

Williams, A.   (1985) Economics of coronary bypass grafting. *Br. Med. J.*, **291**, 326–9.

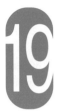

Organizing and Funding Health Care

RAY M. FITZPATRICK

In the twentieth century health care has developed from a collection of small-scale and low-cost services to a complex, labour-intensive and diverse industry. In modern industrialized societies a large and generally growing proportion of resources is now devoted to health care. As the size and scope of this industry have expanded, so too have individuals' rights and expectations with regard to health. Governments have thus become increasingly committed to making health services available to their citizens. The very scale of modern health care has prompted governments of all political persuasions to raise fundamental questions. How effective are health services? How efficient are they in delivering health care? Ultimately, the common theme of such questions concerns the value of modern health care. The answers are often sought by looking for lessons from alternative systems of health care. The most striking feature of modern health care is the diversity of funding and organization in different countries. This chapter describes the different types of health-care systems that have emerged in industrialized societies and the ways they shape the practice of medicine, and then examines the strengths and weaknesses of different systems.

TYPES OF HEALTH-CARE SYSTEMS

A basic requirement for any product or service such as health care is that some method is needed to permit consumers to obtain the product from the producer. The simplest method to understand is the market, wherein the consumer directly purchases the product from the producer at a price agreed between the two parties at the time of the transaction. This is the basic principle behind many transactions in modern industrial societies, and indeed, until quite recently, was the dominant means of providing and obtaining health services. However, health services have tended to evolve away from basic market transactions in two respects. First, potential consumers of health services have increasingly preferred to take out insurance to cover possible costs of health care, rather than face unpredictable and often expensive costs incurred at the time of illness. Second, an additional party has mediated between the producer and consumer of health care to provide resources necessary for the provision of health care. This 'third party', very often the government, but also employers, trade unions, sickness funds, insurance societies and charities, has tended to become increasingly influential in the way services are provided. The more that third parties provide funds directly to the producers (hospitals, doctors and the pharmaceutical industry) to allow them to provide care to those entitled to services, either because of citizenship or an adequate record of insurance contributions, the further the system has evolved away from market mechanisms.

All health-care systems can be understood in terms of the different ways in which transactions occur between these three key parties. In particular, systems differ in the extent to which market versus third-party mechanisms, particularly public provision, dominate transactions and, more specifically, in the ways that individuals obtain insurance against health-care costs. A simple typology distinguishes four major alternative systems of health care that may be found in western industrialized societies (Field, 1973) (Box 19.1).

The socialized systems of health care have probably experienced the most dramatic changes in recent years. In theory these systems provided comprehensive care to all citizens without user charges. Services were centrally planned to maximize efficient and fair use of resources. It

---

BOX 19.1

ALTERNATIVE SYSTEMS OF HEALTH CARE

1　The pluralistic health system

- A wide variety of coexisting schemes (insurance, fee-for-service) provide funds

- Health care facilities owned by wide variety of institutions (private, state, federal)

2　The health insurance system

- Resources gathered by third party as compulsory insurance from individuals and employers

3　The health service system

- Most facilities owned by the state

- Doctors independent but receive most of their income from the state

4　The socialized health system

- All facilities owned by the state

- Most health-care personnel salaried state employees

became increasingly clear, however, that behind this ideal model of health care, there were major deficiencies as the health care system of countries such as Russia received only 2% of Gross National Product, resulting in major shortages of basic drugs and other facilities (Field 1995). Moreover, unofficial bribing was required for patients to obtain adequate care and major inequalities existed in access to health care between political elites and other groups. As the former socialist societies have moved toward markets and privatization, their health care services have also changed, the preferred model now being based on health insurance contributions from employees and their employers which insurance agencies pay as fees to clinics and hospitals (Curtis et al. 1995).

An even greater diversity of forms of health care may be found in non-western societies. A full classification would need to include the traditional systems of healing that have developed in India and China over many hundreds of years. In both these countries traditional medicine has provided sophisticated diagnostic and therapeutic methods that have developed completely independently of western biomedical science. Countries such as India and China are undergoing rapid social and economic changes that are having dramatic impacts on their health care systems. For example, during its socialist period, China evolved a comprehensive system of primary care to cover its largely rural population. 'Bare-foot doctors' with minimal medical training and facilities provided a simple but comprehensive primary care service referring to secondary medical centres the problems that they could not address. The system was funded collectively by the rural commune. However, in the 1980s agriculture was privatized and the collective form of rural medical care virtually disappeared to be replaced by fee-for-service, with the result that illness creates major financial suffering to poorer families (Liu et al. 1995). Meanwhile the growing urban populations of China increasingly receive health care through insurance plans provided by the employer, with marked differences in coverage between plans. Social and economic growth has thus been accompanied by growing inequalities between regions and social groups in China (Hsiao 1995).

Payment mechanisms

In addition to the wide variety of organizational arrangements that have emerged in different western countries, there are also major differences in the methods of paying doctors which can also exert considerable influence on the nature of medical care. We can distinguish three major types of method, although in most health-care systems a mixture of the methods can co-exist and, often, individual doctors may be paid by more than one method.

Fee-for-service involves the patient paying the doctor a fee for each separate item or element of care for which the doctor wishes to charge. In its simplest and historically earliest form, this involves direct patient payments at the time of use. This is still one of the most important methods of paying for health bills in the USA, involving 28% of all personal health expenditure. Insurance systems have emerged in most western countries that reduce or eliminate the need for direct patient payments. However, very often the medical profession has insisted on retaining fee-for-service as their method of payment, with the fees being reclaimed from federal and provincial government (Canada), from the patient's private insurer (USA), or from sickness funds (Germany).

Capitation reimburses the doctor by paying a fixed, usually annual, sum for each patient under his or her care. It is most naturally a method employed in primary care where the doctor has a continuous list or 'panel' of patients for whom he or she is responsible. Britain and Holland are two of the main examples.

Salary is the last method and involves an employer paying the doctor an annual income in return for his or her services. It is the method for paying hospital doctors in Britain, Sweden and Germany.

Unfortunately, there is no perfect method of paying doctors. Each method is known to have certain potentially harmful effects on the provision of health care. The most serious and most clearly documented problems are those associated with fee-for-service. It encourages doctors to perform those procedures specifically rewarded by fees, which in most systems tend to be technical investigations and more interventionist treatments. To put it bluntly, many fee-for-service systems do not recognize talking to the patient as a distinct item of service! Fee-for-service requires more mechanisms than other methods of payment to control potentially wasteful treatments or investigations. Another problem that tends to occur in countries where doctors are paid by fee-for-service is that doctors tend to be poorly distributed geographically, as economic incentives encourage concentrations in more affluent areas. Capitation provides more financial incentives that encourage doctors into underdoctored areas. Among its main limitations are that it does not provide financial rewards for good quality care (as income is unrelated to quality or amount of activity) and may encourage doctors to refer on difficult medical problems. Salaried payment is also not without problems. In principle it requires the doctor to be more concerned about pleasing his or her superiors or employers, who determine rewards and promotions, and less concerned with pleasing the patient. Generally the medical profession has been quite conservative, preferring to keep to the particular system of payment historically established in each country. However, an overall trend can be detected for more doctors to be paid on a salaried basis, typically as employees of an organization.

Health expenditure in different countries

Western countries vary not only in how they organize and fund health services, but also, most dramatically, in the amount of funds devoted to health care. Comparisons of levels of expenditure are not easy because of problems of what is included and excluded in the category of health care in different countries, and also because of unstable exchange rates for countries' currencies. Nevertheless, the most recent figures produced on a systematic standardized basis show differences in levels of expenditure between countries that have remained fairly stable over time (Table 19.1). It is clear that there are considerable differences between countries that might all be regarded as similarly advanced industrial societies, whether expressed as absolute amounts of expenditure or as proportions of the gross domestic product (GDP), used as the most reliable measure of countries' overall wealth. Table 19.1 shows that, for example, the USA spent more than 2.5 times as much per capita as the UK. It is also clear that some countries at very similar levels of wealth in terms of GDP (for example Denmark and Canada) may spend quite different amounts of their wealth on health care.

A number of different explanations have been offered to account for the differences between

TABLE 19.1 *The per capita expenditure on health, the percentage of wealth (GDP) spent on health and the various mortality rates for selected countries for the period 1991–1992.*

Country	Per capita expenditure on health (US $)	Health expenditure as proportion of GDP (%)	GDP[a] per capita (US $)	Life expectancy at birth (years) Male	Female	Infant mortality (% live births)
USA	3094	13.6	21 558	72.0	78.9	8.9
Canada	1949	10.3	18 159	73.8	80.4	6.8
Germany	1775	8.7	19 351	72.9	79.3	6.7
France	1745	9.4	17 959	73.0	81.1	7.3
Holland	1449	7.7	16 898	74.1	80.2	6.5
Sweden	1317	7.9	16 927	74.9	80.5	6.1
Denmark	1163	6.5	18 293	72.2	77.7	7.3
UK	1151	7.1	15 738	73.2	78.8	8.9

Reproduced with permission from Schieber et al. (1994), except GDP per capita from OECD (1995).
[a] *GDP estimates differ slightly from those used to calculate proportions in column two.*

countries in their levels of expenditure. One factor that may play a role is the level of health professionals' earnings, especially those of doctors, which are undoubtedly high in countries such as the USA. A very different explanation would point to the important role of the general practitioner in systems like the NHS in acting as a filter or gate keeper limiting access to more expensive hospital facilities. Another factor that clearly distinguishes systems like the USA and Britain is that the former is an open system in which no actor – the doctor, the patient, the hospital, the insurance company or the government – has the full capacity and incentives to control the volume of medical activities and the costs that ensue. Typically in the USA, doctors or hospitals bill patients' insurance companies who ultimately recover their costs from patients' employers, who hope in turn to pass on these costs to the general public in prices to the consumer. The health-care system in the USA has historically been a highly inflationary one because of this capacity of actors to pass on their costs, and this process stands in direct contrast to the UK where a closed financial system operates in that the total amount of finance available to the NHS is set and controlled centrally by the Treasury and, to a large extent, cannot be expanded further.

However, the most general explanation offered to explain differences in countries' levels of health-care expenditure is that the greater a country's wealth, the greater will be not only the amount but also the proportion of the wealth devoted to health care. Support for this view comes from analyses of data (such as in Table 19.1) for a number of different countries which produce highly significant correlations between countries' GDP and the proportion of GDP allocated to health care (Maxwell 1981). Such analyses may also be used to predict the level of health care that might be expected for a particular country, given its GDP. It has been suggested that, for example, the USA consistently spends more than expected and the UK less than might be expected from its GDP. However, others have argued that such analyses are inappropriate and use misleading exchange rates to calculate standardized expenditures (Parkin et al. 1989).

VARIATIONS IN MEDICAL CARE

It is not surprising, in view of the above differences in funding, to discover that the extent of medical intervention also varies between countries. Thus the rate of surgery in the USA and Canada is at least twice that in the UK, once differences in population size and structure have been taken into consideration. A recent study of hysterectomy (McPherson 1990) showed the age-standardized rate per 100 000 women as 700 in the USA, 600 in Canada, 450 in Australia, 250 in the UK and 110 in Norway. Similar international variations could be shown for tonsillectomy, cholecystecomy and prostatectomy. These international differences are not confined to surgery. Aaron and Schwartz (1984) showed a wide range of differences between the USA and the UK. In the USA, twice as many X-ray examinations were carried out per person; there was six times greater computer tomographic scanning capacity; three times more kidney dialysis treatment was provided; and between five and ten times more hospital intensive-care beds were available.

Variations within countries

Much of the international variation in rates of medical treatments may be accounted for in terms of general differences in economic prosperity of different countries. There is also a tendency for fee-for-service systems of paying the doctor to be associated with higher use of technical procedures such as investigations, and greater resort to active treatments, such as surgery, because such forms of care tend to be more financially rewarding (Abel-Smith 1976). However, it has become increasingly apparent that there are variations in surgical and medical procedures within countries that are as great as those between countries. It is less easy to explain such variation in terms of gross economic incentives. Thus a sixfold variation in tonsillectomy rates and a fourfold variation in hysterectomy rates have been found for different areas within New England (Wennberg and Gittelsohn 1982). Two New England cities which were socially and demographically similar, Boston and New Haven, were examined in more detail. Although Boston had 2.3 times higher rates for carotid endarterectomy, the rates for cholecystectomy and hysterectomy were two-thirds, and for coronary bypass surgery only half, of those in New Haven (Wennberg et al. 1987). Similar variations have been found in different regions of the NHS. For example, rates for hysterectomy per 100 000 women have been found to vary between 181 in Mersey and 287 in North-East Thames, whereas rates for tonsillectomy varied from 144 in Trent to 251 in North-East Thames (McPherson et al. 1981).

Explanations for medical variations

Studies showing variation in the performance of treatments between areas within a country raise fundamental issues. It is extremely unlikely that variation in morbidity in the populations served could explain very much, if any, of the wide variations found in such studies. Moreover, it is unlikely that differences in consumer demand could explain large amounts of the differences in treatment rates prevailing in populations of similar social composition. One factor that is clearly implicated is supply. It can be no coincidence that the twofold differences in surgical rates in the USA compared with the UK is mirrored by there being twice the number of surgeons per capita in the USA. However, where studies have attempted systematically to examine the effects of supply (e.g. McPherson et al. 1981) it has only been possible to explain a small amount of the variation in rates of treatment this way. It is clear that, for many procedures, the main problem is inherent uncertainty about the appropriate indications for treatment and the precise value of treatment in terms of outcomes. It is known that clinicians can vary enormously in the diagnostic and history-taking procedures used in making decisions about elective surgery (Bloor 1976). However, to produce large and consistent differences in rates between areas, such individual differences in clinical opinion and approach must also be influenced by local or regional preferences or customs, otherwise the effects on variations in treatment rates produced by individual differences in clinical style would be cancelled out. Therefore, at the heart of any explanation of variations in treatment rates is professional uncertainty, lack of agreement about the indications for intervention and the value of intervention. Local and international variation is known to be greater for procedures such as tonsillectomy, prostatectomy and hysterectomy where professional uncertainty is greater than for procedures such as cholecystectomy, where some degree of consensus has emerged (Wennberg et al. 1982).

CRITERIA FOR EVALUATING HEALTH SYSTEMS

Health-care expenditure and health status

The main reason why so much uncertainty surrounds many medical and surgical procedures is that they have not been properly evaluated. It is very difficult to distinguish specific effects of a medical therapy from other possible causes of change in the course of illness, such as placebo effects and spontaneous changes in the underlying disorder. For this reason it is often argued that only a randomized controlled trial (RCT), where patients are randomly allocated between the treatment group and a control group and differences in subsequent health status compared between the two groups, is adequate to distinguish real treatment effects. Very few medical interventions have been evaluated by means of such demanding methods (Cochrane 1971). Some would argue that, especially when RCTs might pose ethical problems because of the need to withhold treatment, medical treatments can still be reasonably evaluated by less exact methods such as, for example, longitudinal observational studies in which the impact of therapies on groups of patients are recorded and compared with untreated comparison groups. However, such studies are still all too rare (McPherson 1990).

Greater uncertainty surrounds the relationship between overall levels of health-care expenditure and benefits in terms of health status. In Table 19.1 the expenditure figures for health care in a range of western countries are compared with a number of the most recently available health-status measures. Life expectancy is a global measure that summarizes the mortality rates prevailing at all ages. It is apparent from Table 19.1 that the USA, despite spending much more on health care than other countries, does not enjoy more favourable life expectancy than countries such as Denmark and the UK, with quite low per capita health-care expenditure. The infant mortality rate is a quite widely used indicator not only of infant health status but also of whole populations. Again it is clear that the USA does not enjoy infant mortality rates commensurate with its high health-care expenditure.

Other analyses of the relationship between countries' levels of health-care expenditure and mortality rates have similarly failed to find evidence of the negative correlation that might reasonably be expected (Cochrane et al. 1978; Maxwell 1981). Indeed, the one variable that tends to predict mortality rates from such comparisons of national data is the gross national product (GNP), i.e. the overall level of wealth of the country (Cochrane et al. 1978). This would, of course, be consistent with the arguments of McKeown that social and economic factors have historically exerted far greater influence upon health than have medical measures (see Chapter 1). In view of the evidence that mortality rates are largely influenced by social, economic and environmental factors rather than medical care, it might well be argued that mortality rates are not appropriate measures of health status with which to compare countries' health-care systems. Rather, it might be argued, the main impact of health services is intended to be upon morbidity. In particular, the objectives of health services are to reduce the impact of illness in terms of pain, discomfort, disability and other aspects of health status. However, as indicated in Chapter 18, instruments for measuring these outcomes of health services have only recently been developed and there are numerous logistic and methodological problems that would make the comparative assessment of different health-care systems extremely difficult. At present, therefore, the only available data with which to evaluate the effectiveness, in terms of impact upon health, of different health-care systems is mortality.

Efficiency

There are a number of different ways in which one might evaluate the quality of different health services In Box 19.2 the widely cited criteria of Maxwell (1984) are listed. From what has been said above it should be clear that there are basic difficulties in examining the effectiveness of health-care systems, particularly problems of measuring outcomes. The scope for using the other five criteria are examined briefly below.

Efficiency is a term which is frequently applied to health care but seldom used with much

---

BOX 19.2

CRITERIA TO ASSESS THE QUALITY OF HEALTH SERVICES

Effectiveness

Efficiency

Accessibility

Equity

Social acceptability

Relevance to needs

Reproduced with permission from Maxwell (1984).

clarity. The efficiency of an engine is the relationship between the actual and the theoretically possible amount of energy used to achieve a desired output. The closer the machine gets to the lowest level of energy use considered possible, the greater its efficiency. In human systems one normally compares the costs of two or more alternative ways of achieving the same output or result, with the less costly alternative being regarded as more efficient. The scope for increasing efficiency in health services is potentially enormous. For example, in a wide range of problems, outpatient or day-case care can be substituted for longer inpatient management; or the nurse or general practitioner may replace more costly hospital care. Efficiency is examined by health economists using techniques such as cost–benefit analysis, in which all the costs of two or more alternative therapies or ways of organizing care are compared. This requires taking into account the costs of alternative treatments, such as any additional burden imposed on the family or other carers, as well as formal health-care costs.

The British government sought to achieve numerous 'efficiency savings' from the NHS during the 1980s. However, in practice, this has often meant reducing levels of spending available, which should not be confused with real improvements in efficiency because saving money can often be associated with deteriorating efficiency. Efforts have been made to measure efficiency more directly, but the exercise has proved particularly difficult. One solution has been the development of 'performance indicators' (such as average length of hospital stay, throughput of patients per annum, and turnover interval between cases occupying a bed) that can be measured for different units, hospitals and districts. However, such measures can be quite misleading. A unit may appear to be performing more efficiently if patients' mean length of hospital stay is lower than other units. However, a full cost–benefit analysis might show that this short length of hospital stay involved transferring higher costs to the community by premature discharge, together with unresolved complications of treatment that actually led to many patients being readmitted. It is also possible that varying lengths of stay in different units are due to different levels of severity of disease in the patients admitted.

It is even more difficult to compare health-care systems in terms of efficiency. In general, the length of stay in hospitals in the USA is considerably shorter than in Britain. Economic pressures have been the main factor driving down lengths of stay in the USA. Unfortunately, lengths of stay tend to be a matter of local practice and tradition and optimum length of stay has rarely been subjected to the kind of scientific examination adopted by Deyo et al. (1986), who were able to show from a randomized controlled trial that shorter lengths of bed rest were as effective in the management of back pain as longer stays.

Another aspect of efficiency would include consideration of 'bureaucracy' or administration costs of health care since such costs do not apparently make a direct contribution to patient care. The NHS fares particularly well compared with most other systems. For example, it has been estimated that the USA spends as much as 22% of its health expenditure on administration costs, compared with about 6% required by the NHS (Himmelstein and Woolhandler 1986). High administration costs arise from a combination of fee-for-service and the need to itemize and bill every procedure. It is of note that, as the NHS begins to experiment with 'internal markets', both health authorities and hospitals will require a great deal more information of this kind and administration costs will rise sharply.

Accessibility

This criterion is concerned with how readily available health services are. The health-care system with the most visible problem is the more market oriented one of the USA, in which some 15–20% of the population may have inadequate health-care insurance. No other western health-care system permits this degree of financial inaccessibility. Given that for those who are insured in the USA out-of-pocket expenses at the time of seeking care are higher than in European systems, it is remarkable that consultation rates are no different between systems. A different kind of problem of access is the necessity to wait for admission for treatment. This would appear to be very much more of a problem for the publicly funded and provided services of Britain and Sweden and is one major reason why in both these countries proposals have been implemented to increase the incentives for hospitals to reduce waiting times by a more competitive structure of revenue.

Equity

Equity with regard to health involves addressing some very complex issues, especially when trying to compare the performance of different health-care systems. Thus a distinction can be made between equality of access (the extent to which different social groups have access to health services) and equality of health status (the extent to which different social groups enjoy similar levels of health). As other chapters in this book have shown, social differences in health status can be caused by a wide range of social, economic and environmental factors and the scope for intervention by health services, no matter how broadly defined, may be modest. Some would therefore argue that it is more reasonable to confine attention to comparing the efforts of different health-care systems to achieve equality of access, although even with this more modest criterion there may be substantial social and cultural factors influencing use of health services. Other problems complicating quantitative comparisons of inequalities are that the social groupings (such as classes) are not consistent between countries and that social and cultural factors can influence individuals' perceptions of their health status (see Chapter 3).

With regard to social differences in health status, it is clear that all European and North American societies continue to experience differences in mortality between social groups, and the view that social democratic welfare states or socialist societies have eradicated such differences is misguided (Illsley 1990). Thus a comparative study of Denmark, Finland, Norway, Sweden, Hungary and England and Wales showed that in all countries mortality among men with the highest level of education was 40–60% lower than men of the lowest educational level (Lahelma and Valkonen 1990). In general, some of the lowest inequalities in health status appear to be found in Sweden, a country which has probably the strongest and most active commitment to welfare policies. Nevertheless, even in Sweden there are occupational and regional inequalities in mortality arising from work hazards, dietary- and alcohol-related diseases and other unexplained environmental factors (Diderichsen 1990).

All health-care systems have taken some steps to reduce or eradicate differences of access by income. At one extreme, in the USA a substantial proportion of the population do not have full access to health care because of inadequate insurance. Such individuals have to resort to a 'second-class' system of publicly funded health care which has experienced particularly tight financial restrictions in the last 10 years. At the other extreme, financial barriers to access are largely removed from most European systems, and further steps have tended to be taken centrally to reduce regional inequalities of access. Particularly successful was the impact on the NHS of the Resource Allocation Working Party (RAWP), which resulted in England and Wales having the least regional inequalities in the geographical distribution of doctors when compared to France, Germany and Holland (Townsend and Davidson 1982).

Social acceptability

In those health-care systems where an attempt has been made to assess consumers' views about their health care, the majority of respondents have expressed positive satisfaction. Indeed, a standardized survey of consumers in a cross-national survey that included citizens of Canada, the USA, England, Finland and Yugoslavia found that only 5% of respondents expressed dissatisfaction with their doctor's care, and rates of dissatisfaction did not appear to differ significantly from country to country (Kohn and White 1976). The most common complaint across systems focused on the length of time spent waiting to see the doctor. However, a more recent comparative study of patient satisfaction with primary care has found higher levels of satisfaction in cities in the UK and Greece compared with Belgrade and Moscow (Calnan et al. 1994). Generally such studies suggest that dissatisfaction with information provided by health professionals is also a universal problem. Some health-care systems generate unique complaints. It is unlikely that any other health-care system than the NHS would continue to wake patients up so early that 43% of patients complain about this aspect of being in hospital. Conversely, American consumers focus more critically than the consumers of other health-care systems on the high costs they face from medical care. Americans also differ fundamentally from citizens of other countries in that, although they are generally satisfied with their own care, they view the health-care system as a whole as unsatisfactory and in need of fundamental change (Blendon and Donelan 1990).

Relevance to health needs

Relevance is the last important criterion emphasized in Maxwell's list for evaluating health services. At the extreme it is possible to conceive of a health-care system that takes little or no account of the health needs of the population it served. Thus it has often been a key problem in third world countries that the health-care system has developed largely to conform to the standards of western high-technology medicine and, although relevant to the needs of urban social and political elites, it has failed to address the often more basic health needs of the rural majority populations. Such stark failures of relevance are less easy to identify in western health-care systems and involve major initial difficulties in defining the health needs of populations.

Nevertheless, one very promising line of research has begun to open up the more focused and manageable issue of appropriateness. To what extent are the treatments provided in a health-care system appropriate to the patients who receive them? The methodology for addressing this question is complex and may take different forms, but one approach essentially involves asking representative samples of relevant clinicians to rate the appropriate indications for a particular medical or surgical intervention (for example, which test results, past medical history and other patient characteristics would be appropriate indications for someone to undergo coronary artery bypass graft (CABG)). These agreed indications are then used to analyse the characteristics of samples of patients who have actually undergone the particular procedure. This methodology has been largely used in the USA and has produced quite startling results. Retrospective analyses of case records showed that for patients who received carotid endarterectomy, about one-third were rated as appropriate, one-third equivocal and one-third inappropriate. Similarly, one-quarter of coronary angiographies and one-quarter of endoscopies were rated as equivocal or inappropriate (Brook 1990). These studies give support to the view that a substantial proportion of the treatment provided in the USA may be of questionable value in terms of outcomes and may occur as much out of a more general optimistic bias and faith in technology in US culture or, more cynically, because of strong financial rewards built into fee-for-service medicine.

This methodology has now been applied cross-nationally. Two panels of physicians and surgeons, one from the USA and one from the UK, were asked to rate a large number of indications in the form of elements of case histories, in terms of appropriateness for coronary angiography and also for CABG (Brook et al. 1988). The US panel of doctors rated a much larger number of case-history indications as being appropriate for either procedure. The two panels' agreed sets of indications were then applied to real case histories. First, they were applied to two samples of US patients who had undergone coronary angiography. The US panel's ratings resulted in 17% and 27% being rated as inappropriate, whereas the UK panel's ratings identified 42% and 60% as inappropriate. The ratings of indications were then applied to another sample, US patients who had undergone CABG. By the US criteria 13% and by the UK criteria 35% of operations were inappropriate. There are, therefore, quite powerful differences of views about the scope for benefit from medical treatment in medicine, despite the fact that medical science and medical training are very similar in the two countries.

MARKETS VERSUS REGULATION IN HEALTH CARE

In many respects the many complex difficulties faced by health-care systems can be subsumed into two broad types of problem. First, health-care systems need to obtain adequate funds to pay for the health-care needs of the populations they serve and mechanisms are required to ensure that such funds do not outstrip the capacity of the funder to pay. Second, mechanisms are required to improve the effectiveness and efficiency of health services, particularly in the light of evidence of ineffectiveness and inefficiency of the kind briefly reviewed in this chapter. No health-care system appears to have addressed either problem satisfactorily and there is a constant and increasingly international search for solutions to both problems. Again in order to simplify the discussion, it is possible to detect two alternative strategies that have been pursued by governments, sickness funds, health providers and other agencies concerned with the provision of health care in attempts to address the twin problems just identified. One strategy has focused on competition. It has sought to intensify the scope of market forces in the field of health care. The hope has been that competition between providers of health care would force them to reduce their costs as well as maximize their efficiency and effectiveness in accordance with the logic of market competition in other spheres of commerce. The second and contrasting strategy has been to introduce regulation into the operations of the health-care system. Faced with evidence of inefficiencies such as wide and unaccountable variations in clinical practice and use of resources, this solution has attempted to use methods of centralized planning and managerial control of health budgets. The competitive strategy is best characterized by the US system and the regulation/planning strategy is more typical of European systems.

The competitive strategy was pursued in the USA throughout the 1980s. Government finance for planning of health services was withdrawn and instead support was given to encourage competition, especially to promote the development of Health Maintenance Organizations (HMOs). HMOs were established in which a group of health providers offered a complete package of health-care services to consumers at an annually agreed price. It was hoped that HMOs would compete with each other in terms of the attractiveness of the package of services offered and their price. Finally, competition was encouraged by increasing the proportion of health bills paid out of pocket by the patient in the hope that this would increase consumer sensitivity to costs. To date there has been little evidence that pro-competitive strategies have succeeded in the main objective of driving down the highly inflationary costs of US health care.

The planning and regulatory strategies of European health services are too diverse to encompass in a brief chapter. To varying degrees in each country regulation has included efforts to set overall limits to expenditure on health care, particularly in the hospital sector, by setting doctors' fees, regulating the introduction of high-technology medicine. This strategy has been largely successful in containing costs, but analysts are less happy with the evidence of continued inefficiencies and unexplained variations in most European systems, and countries such as Sweden and Britain continue to be concerned with the unresponsiveness of their health-care systems to the consumer and the persistence of waiting lists as unresolved problems.

Partly because of their perceived lack of consumer responsiveness but more particularly in order to control costs, many European systems have in the 1990s been subjected to major changes intended to induce greater market competitiveness. In the very different systems of Britain, Holland and Sweden, the distinction between purchasers and providers of care was sharpened and providers (particularly hospitals) were given greater incentives to compete for patients on whose behalf the health authorities in Britain and Sweden and the sickness funds in Holland purchased care (Ham and Brommels 1994). However, the benefits of competition predicted by neoclassical economic theory have not produced greater efficiency and effectiveness in the field of health care whether in Europe or in the United States (Glaser 1993). Some of the problems exacerbated by greater competition such as the perceived oversupply of hospitals in large cities have needed traditional European mechanisms of planning and regulation to address them (Ham and Brommels 1994)

Convergence of health-care systems?

Some observers (Enthoven 1990; Ham et al. 1990) have argued that pure strategies of either market competition or central planning and regulation have failed to address the key problems of health services and have suggested that there is now evidence in many health-care systems of a convergence towards a mixed approach combining elements of both strategies. Again it is impossible to encompass all the varieties of strategy emerging in each country, but some commonly occurring themes can be detected. One theme is that of 'peer review', in which particularly clinical decisions that may result in large use of resources such as admission to hospital and decisions about surgery are subject to external review by colleagues. This has gone much further in the USA where peer review is current and intended directly to influence use of resources, whereas in Europe it has, to date, largely been retrospective and used more for educational purposes as in medical audit.

The second theme is the development of information systems to monitor and measure the activities and outcomes of health care. The intention is to use increasingly sophisticated information technology to inform all the parties to health care – the doctor, the patient and the purchaser in particular – about the efficiency and effectiveness of health-care activities (Ellwood 1988).

A third common theme emerging in health-care systems to varying degrees is the desire to separate out the purchaser of health care (such as the health authority or sick fund) from the provider (such as hospitals) and to increase the degree of choice that the purchaser has between different providers. In systems such as those in Britain, Holland and Sweden the intention is to induce competition within a publicly funded system. The hope is that a system which incorporates all three elements (peer review, increased attention to audit of outcomes and scope for funders to choose between providers who compete in terms of quality and price) will produce a solution to the many dilemmas of modern medical care.

The need to ration

One of the most controversial problems facing health-care systems of all types is the need to decide mechanisms of allocating limited health care resources in relation to competing demands. 'Rationing' is an emotive short-hand term used in this context and suggests a process of explicit and deliberate decisions about resource allocation. In reality, many health-care systems have implicitly rationed without formally deciding to do so, because, for example, low income individuals are not able to purchase health care or because delays or queues discourage numbers of patients from obtaining care.

However, as medical technology continues to develop and new treatments and health-care costs escalate, governments across Europe and North America have had to devise more morally explicit principles whereby health care resources are allocated. There are a number of alternative principles that could be used (Box 19.3). Unfortunately these principles may conflict with each other (Harrison and Hunter 1994). For example, patients for whose health problems current treatments are ineffective would be denied health care if the criterion of effectiveness were strictly applied, whereas they would receive services under principles of need or equity. All of the principles are difficult to operationalize. There are, for example, no agreed ways of defining or determining need. Any health care system is therefore likely to have to make trade-offs or compromises between principles rather than rigorously adhere to one.

Health authorities are also increasingly consulting the public about how health services should be prioritized by means of postal surveys or public meetings. However, the results of such consultation exercises have only served to complicate decisions, partly because public responses are substantially influenced by the wording with which questions are posed and partly because the public makes choices on different principles from those considered important by doctors or managers. The

---

BOX 19.3

ALTERNATIVE PRINCIPLES FOR ALLOCATING HEALTH CARE
RESOURCES BETWEEN CONFLICTING DEMANDS

Effectiveness
Resources are allocated to those treatments that have the greatest effect on outcomes in terms of health.

Cost effectiveness
Resources are allocated according to the principle of effectiveness, but also take account of costs in relation to effectiveness (i.e. favouring treatment with the best cost–benefit ratio).

Need
Resources are allocated to those patients or patient groups with the greatest need.

Equity
Resources are allocated on a principle of a basis of fairness or equity between individuals and patient groups.

Chance or 'fair goes'
Resources are allocated by some form of random process so that everyone has a similar chance of care, or 'first come first served' principles.

Reproduced with permission by the Institute for Public Policy Research from Harrison and Hunter (1995).

---

public appears more impressed by the acute and high technology services and to value less preventive interventions such as health education or services for mental illness (Brown 1995).

There are therefore no simple solutions to the problem of providing health services that meet every desirable objective for health. This chapter has illustrated the diversity of forms that advanced health-care systems have adopted in the search for optimal solutions.

REFERENCES

Aaron, H. & Schwartz, W.   (1984) *The Painful Prescription.* Washington, DC: The Brookings Institution.
Abel-Smith, B.   (1976) *Value for Money in Health Services.* London: Heinemann.
Blendon, R. & Donelan, K.   (1990) The public and the emerging debate over national health insurance. *N. Engl. J. Med.,* **323**, 208–12.
Bloor, M.   (1976) Bishop Berkeley and the adenotonsillectomy enigma. *Sociology,* **10**, 44–61.
Brook, R.   (1990) Relationship between appropriateness and outcome. In: *Measuring The Outcomes of Medical Care,* ed. A. Hopkins & D. Costain. London: Royal College of Physicians.
Brook, R., Park, R., Winslow, C. et al.   (1988) Diagnosis and treatment of coronary disease: comparison of doctors' attitudes in the USA and the UK. *Lancet,* **i**, 750–3.
Brown, S.   (1995) Assessing public opinion on investment in health services. *Int. J. Health Sci.,* **6**, 15–24.
Calnan, M., Katsouyiannopoulos, V. & Ocharov, V.   (1994) Major determinants of consumer satisfaction with primary care in different systems. *Family Pract.,* **11**, 468–78.
Cochrane, A.   (1971) *Effectiveness and Efficiency.* London: Nuffield Provincial Hospitals Trust.
Cochrane, A., St Leger, A. & Moore, F.   (1978) Health service input and mortality output in developed countries. *J. Epidemiol. Community Health,* **32**, 200–5.
Curtis, S., Petukhova, N. & Taket, A.   (1995) Health care reforms in Russia: the example of St Petersburg. *Soc. Sci. Med.,* **40**, 755–66.
Deyo, R., Diehl, A. & Rosenthal, M.   (1986) How many days of bed-rest for acute low back pain? A randomised clinical trial. *N. Engl. J. Med.,* **315**, 1064–70.

Diderichsen, F. (1990) Health and social inequalities in Sweden. *Soc. Sci. Med.*, **31**, 359–67.

Ellwood, P.   (1988) Outcomes management: a technology of patient experience. *N. Engl. J. Med.*, **318**, 1549–56.

Enthoven, A.   (1990) What can Europeans learn from Americans? In: *Health Care Systems in Transition*. Paris: OECD.

Field, M.   (1973) The concept of the 'Health System' at the macrosociological level. *Soc. Sci. Med.*, **7**, 763–85.

Field, M.   (1995) The health crisis in the former Soviet Union: a report from the 'post-war' zone. *Soc. Sci. Med.*, **41**, 1469–78.

Glaser, W.   (1993) The competition vogue and its outcomes. *Lancet*, **341**, 805–12.

Ham, C. & Brommels, M.   (1994) Health care reform in the Netherlands, Sweden, and the United Kingdom. *Health Affairs*, **13**, 106–19.

Ham, C., Robinson, R. & Benzeval, M.   (1990) *Health Check: Health Care Reforms in an International Context*. London: Kings Fund Institute.

Harrison, S. & Hunter, D.   (1994) *Rationing Health Care*. London: Institute for Public Policy Research.

Himmelstein, D. & Woolhandler, S.   (1986) Cost without benefit: administrative waste in US health care. *N. Engl. J. Med.*, **314**, 441–5.

Hsiao, W.   (1995) The Chinese health care system: lessons for other nations. *Soc. Sci. Med.*, **41**, 1047–56.

Illsley, R.   (1990) Comparative review of sources, methodology and knowledge. *Soc. Sci. Med.*, **31**, 229–36.

Kohn, P. & White, K.   (1976) *An International Study*. Oxford: Oxford University Press.

Lahelma, E. & Valkonen, T.   (1990) Health and social inequalities in Finland and elsewhere. *Soc. Sci. Med.*, **31**, 257–66.

Liu, Y., Hsiao, W., Li, Q. et al.   (1995) Transformation of China's rural health care system. *Soc. Sci. Med.*, **41**, 1085–94.

Maxwell, R.   (1981) *Health and Wealth*. Lexington, MA: Lexington Books.

Maxwell, R.   (1984) Quality assessment in health. *Br. Med. J.*, **288**, 1470–2.

McPherson, K.   (1990) International differences in medical care practices. In: *Health Care Systems in Transition*. Paris: OECD.

McPherson, K., Strong, P., Epstein, A. & Jones, L.   (1981) Regional variations in the use of common surgical procedures. *Soc. Sci. Med.*, **15A**, 273–88.

Organization for Economic Co-operation and Development   (1995) *Monitoring the World Economy 1820–1992*. Paris:OECD

Parkin, D., McGuire, A. & Yule, B.   (1989) What do international comparisons of health care expenditures really show? *Community Med.*, **11**, 116–23.

Schieber, G., Poullier, J. & Greenwald, L.   (1994) Health system performance in OECD countries, 1980–1992. *Health Affairs* **13**, 100–12.

Townsend, P. & Davidson, N.   (1982) *Inequalities in Health: The Black Report*. Harmondsworth: Penguin.

Wennberg, J. & Gittelsohn, A.   (1982) Variations in medical care among small areas. *Sci. Am.*, **246**, 120–34.

Wennberg, J., Barnes, B. & Zubkoff, M.   (1982) Professional uncertainty and the problem of supplier-induced demand. *Soc. Sci. Med.*, **16**, 811–24.

Wennberg, J., Freeman, J. & Culp, W.   (1987) Are hospital services rationed in New Haven or over-utilised in Boston? *Lancet*, **i**, 118.

Note: Most references are to United Kingdom, except where otherwise stated